HUMAN ENDOCRINOLOGY
AN INTERACTIVE TEXT

MELVIN J. FREGLY
Department of Physiology
University of Florida College of Medicine

WILLIAM G. LUTTGE
Department of Neuroscience
University of Florida College of Medicine

ELSEVIER BIOMEDICAL
New York • Amsterdam • Oxford

Elsevier Science Publishing Co., Inc.
52 Vanderbilt Avenue, New York, New York 10017

Sole distributors outside the United States and Canada:

Elsevier Science Publishers B.V.
P.O. Box 211, 1000 AE Amsterdam, The Netherlands

Library of Congress Cataloging in Publication Data

Fregly, Melvin J.
    Human endocrinology.

    Bibliography: p.
    Includes index.
    1. Endocrinology. I. Luttge, William G. II. Title.
    [DNLM: 1. Endocrine glands—Physiology. WK 102 F858h]
QP187.F675   612'.4   82-2526
ISBN 0-444-00662-1   AACR2

Manufactured in the United States of America

CONTENTS

PREFACE

This book is designed for preprofessional and graduate students in the health sciences. It provides up-to-date coverage of most of the major endocrine systems, including the molecular and physiologic effects of hormones as well as the clinical significance and applications for that information.

The text is written in a Socratic fashion with numerous questions designed to stimulate the student's interaction with the material. Learning objectives are provided with each section of the ten chapters, and students are tested on their attainment of those objectives at the end of each section. Questions are also asked in the text itself to highlight important points. Answers to these "text questions" are provided in Appendix 1. The student should be forwarned that some of these questions have no clear-cut answers. They are provided to provoke thought and speculation about particular aspects of the subject being considered. In other cases, these questions are correlative and attempt to stimulate the student to think about general principles and similar situations, which are covered in other chapters. Finally, students can assess their overall mastery of the subject with the comprehensive questions provided in Appendix 2. The answers to these questions, and in some cases explanations for those answers, are provided in Appendix 3.

Selected references are provided at the end of each chapter for students interested in obtaining additional information. Our selection is biased in favor of review articles and books rather than primary sources in order to be able to cover a wide range of information while still keeping the magnitude of the list of references within reasonable limits. Additional references are provided at the end of the book and are arranged by chapter; they represent the source of many of the figures and tables.

Each chapter is written in a similar format. Anatomy, histology, and embryology are covered briefly in the initial section. Subsequent sections are concerned with the characteristics of the hormone: its chemistry, production, secretion, and transport, its mechanisms of action at target tissues, its metabolism, the factors controlling its secretion, and the physiologic consequences of its actions. Additional sections describe ways this basic information is used clinically in tests of the functional integrity of each endocrine gland. It is our belief that this standardized approach will be helpful in developing an understanding of each hormone as well as in developing an appreciation for the similarities between the various hormone systems.

The sequence in which the chapters are arranged is one we have found to be successful in our own teaching experience. We admit, however, that other sequences may be just as successful. The chapters are complete within themselves so that a course in endocrinology could begin with any of them.

Our emphasis has been on the endocrinology of the human. For many of the endocrine glands, the differences between man and either laboratory or domestic mammals will be relatively minor but for others, particularly the endocrinology of reproduction, there will be major differences. Those interested in comparative endocrinology will find this book useful as a reference for comparison with other species.

Endocrinology is a rapidly progressing field of research that is often difficult for the preprofessional student to understand in the limited time available in today's often highly intensive and condensed curricula. Our objective in writing this book is to provide a consistent framework on which to build the information available for each endocrine gland. We hope that by guiding each student in this way, by asking pertinent questions in the text, and by providing learning objectives and examinations, we will facilitate the process of learning. This text has been used in our classes during the past five years and we are grateful to our students for their helpful comments.

Some teachers of endocrinology may find that a new or nearly new hormone has been omitted from the text. We have relied on our experience and judgment as teachers and on the extent of reliable information to guide us regarding the relative importance of newer hormones to the student studying endocrinology for the first time. Because of the rapid growth of endocrinological research, we are certain that subsequent editions of this text will contain many hormones not mentioned in this one.

To those who object to the "educationally oriented" aspects of this text, we can only state our belief that we have tried to write a book that is thorough, up-to-date, easily readable, and fun to use. Our objective is that each student's experience with endocrinology will be remembered as a pleasant one. We hope that the devices we have used will facilitate learning. In addition, we hope that by challenging the student to think about the spectacular recent advances in endocrinological research and the numerous areas where information is still incomplete, that some of them will choose to devote their postgraduate years to research in basic and/or clinical endocrinology.

Gainesville, Florida   Melvin J. Fregly
June 19, 1981   William G. Luttge

1

ORGANIZATION AND CONTROL OF ENDOCRINE SYSTEMS

SECTION 1-1: GENERAL CHARACTERISTICS OF ENDOCRINE GLANDS AND HORMONES

OBJECTIVES:

The student should be able to:
1. Recite the classical definition of an endocrine system.
2. Discuss the limitations of this definition.
3. Discuss some general characteristics of hormones.

A. A BRIEF HISTORY OF HORMONES

As knowledge and experience in the use of the microscope advanced, it became clear that there were glandular tissues that contained no ducts for the release of their secretions. These became known as the "ductless glands." Even after it was recognized that they secreted directly into blood, their specific physiologic functions were unclear for many years.

The concept that substances were produced that could somehow permeate the body and affect both health and personality probably existed before written history. It was formalized in a Greek medical school known as the Hippocratic school, which advocated a system of medicine based on four humors. They were recognized as blood, phlegm, yellow bile, and black bile. The content of these substances in the body was purported to influence not only health but personality as well. For example, a person said to have a predominance of blood humor was termed "sanguine" and usually was a ruddy-faced, pleasant individual. A predominance of phlegm was supposed to result in a "phlegmatic" individual with a personality characterized by dullness and apathy. Individuals who were said to have a predominance of either yellow or black bile were called choleric or melancholic, respectively. The choleric individuals were said to be quick tempered and irascible, while the melancholic were, of course, sad.

Since these notions could never be verified experimentally, they fell into disrepute. It remained for the famous French physiologist Claude Bernard to demonstrate "internal secretion." He was the first to show that the liver releases glucose into blood, by which it is transported to all cells of the body. Although glucose is a nutrient, not a hormone, this basic observation reintroduced into physiology the recognition that substances produced by specific organs can be released into blood, which transports them throughout the body.

It was not until the midnineteenth and early twentieth centuries that investigators first recognized that certain glands without secretory ducts could have a secretory function. The idea was expressed first probably by Berthold in 1849 when he demonstrated that transplantation of one testis from a rooster into the abdominal cavity of another castrated young rooster maintained the growth of the comb and wattles and the typical behavioral characteristics of an intact rooster. Berthold predicted that something produced by the testes was responsible for the growth of the cock's comb. Since all nerves had been severed as a result of the transplantation, this substance must have been carried by the blood from the testes to the comb and wattles. We know now that this substance is the androgen testosterone. Berthold's findings were lost sight of apparently, and more than half a century passed before it became accepted generally that endocrine glands produce substances that are discharged into blood and carried to specific tissues and cells where they exert an effect. The term "hormone" (from Greek for "to arouse to activity") was first suggested by W. B. Hardy of Cambridge University, and was first used textually in 1905 by the English physiologist Ernest Starling, to describe the gastrointestinal hormones secretin and gastrin, which Hardy and his colleague L. E. Bayliss had discovered.

B. DEFINITION OF A HORMONE

To have a firm grasp of the physiology of any hormone, one must understand the factors affecting its production, secretion, and metabolism, as well as the factors affecting its transport in blood and the number and sensitivity of its receptors in target tissues. One, and occasionally several, of these factors can be altered by disease processes, by drugs, and even by the hormones themselves.

In introducing this subject to students, it seems of obvious importance to define an endocrine system and a hormone. Classically, the endocrine system is often thought of as a group of glandular organs that do not possess ducts for the release of their secretions. The secretory products are released into extracellular spaces and from there into blood, which transports them throughout the body. Classically, secretion has been considered to be independent of the nervous system. These secretory products are the substances that are usually called hormones. Thus, hormones were said to be produced by an organ at a particular site in the body and transported by blood to another different site (target cells), where they exerted a regulatory function. It was believed originally that hormones could only stimulate or increase activity at the target cells at which they act, but it is now known that hormones also can inhibit the activity of these cells. For this reason, hormones must be considered to "regulate" function at target cells.

Even with this qualification, one finds quickly that the classical definition of a hormone is not satisfactory. For example, there are certain cellular products that are either secreted or released into extracellular spaces, are carried by blood, and exert a regulatory effect at a target site. Yet we do not usually consider them to be hormones. One such substance is carbon dioxide. It is released as a result of cellular metabolism, is transported by blood, and exerts effects on the respiratory center in the medullary portion of the brain, which is responsible for controlling respiratory activity. In spite of this, carbon dioxide is not classified as a hormone. It has been suggested that substances like carbon dioxide, which are produced by all cells of the body as a result of cellular metabolism, not by a specific group of cells, be called "parahormones."

The classic definition of a hormone included the property that secretion did not depend on stimulation of the secretory organ by the nervous system. This definition appears to be too restrictive, since the secretion of norepinephrine, epinephrine, oxytocin, vasopressin, and other hormones is influenced by neural stimulation. These substances have been called "neurohormones."

More recent studies have also shown strong neural influences on hormones secreted by the hypothalamus. These hormones are secreted into the hypothalmohypophyseal portal vessels, where they are transported to the anterior pituitary gland. Here they regulate the secretion of such tropic hormones as thyroid stimulating hormone (TSH), adrenocorticotropic hormone (ACTH), and luteinizing hormone (LH). These hypothalamic hormones are referred to as "hypothalamic hypophysiotropic hormones" (HHHs). We see in later chapters that the secretion of these hormones is influenced by hormones from the target organs.

Figure 1-1 summarizes the characteristics of secretion of the different hormones discussed above. This figure does not include the mechanism by which another important hormone, angiotensin II, is produced: this hormone is different from all the others because it is formed from the union of an enzyme and a substrate in the blood itself. The enzyme, renin, is secreted into blood by the kidneys, while the substrate, renin substrate, is secreted into blood by the liver. This means that angiotensin II is not secreted by a specific organ. Thus angiotensin II fails to conform to the classic definition of a hormone.

In further contrast to the general scheme presented in Figure 1-1, some hormones can be secreted and act locally without the necessity of being carried throughout the body by blood. This could be said to be the primary characteristic of norepinephrine, a neurohormone.

It should be obvious at this point that it is difficult to define a hormone. However a

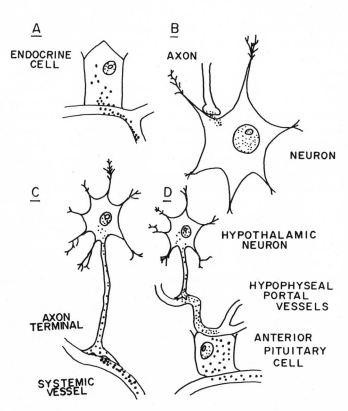

FIGURE 1-1: Summary of the different characteristics of secretion by endocrine glands: A) endocrine cell secreting its hormone into blood; B) axon secreting from its nerve ending a neurohormone that affects the activity of an adjacent neuron; C) nerve cell secreting a hormone that passes down its axon to a storage site at the nerve ending (this is characteristic of neurohypophyseal hormones, and stimulation of the nerve results in release of the stored hormone into blood); D) hypothalamic neuron that secretes a hypophysiotropic hormone into capillaries that transport the hormone via hypophyseal portal vessels to the anterior pituitary gland, where specific cells are stimulated to secrete particular tropic hormones.

general definition can be provided as follows: 1) a hormone is a substance secreted by living cells into the environment outside them (extracellular fluid, synaptic cleft, etc.), where 2) it is transported to its target site, 3) the hormone interacts with its target site by way of a specific receptor, 4) to regulate a cellular reaction, not to initiate it. 5) Hormones are not used as sources of energy.

C. GENERAL CHARACTERISTICS OF HORMONES

Even though a hormone is difficult to define precisely, hormones do have certain general characteristics that can be discussed.

1. The time required for a hormone to manifest an effect is slow compared to that of the nervous system. In fact, this latency of response often makes it difficult to perform experiments with hormones in the student laboratory unless the animals are prepared days or weeks in advance. Whereas stimulation of the nervous system induces responses in milliseconds or seconds, hormones usually require hours or even days to induce a response. However, it must be recognized that there is considerable variability among the hormones with regard to the latent period for a response. For example, milk ejection in response to administration of the hormone oxytocin requires only a few seconds in lactating animals. This contrasts with the latent period for a metabolic response to thyroxine, which can take as long as 3 days. The more usual latent period for a response to a hormone is probably hours.

The latency of response suggests that hormones either produce or undergo chemical alterations in blood or at the target organ before they can exert their effect. Although we have a large number of hormones in chemically pure form, the latency for response may mean that what is administered and what the receptors of the target organ recognize as the hormone may differ. We also learn in a later section of this chapter that certain hormones must interact with their receptors on target cells to activate transport mechanisms, enzymes, and so on. This probably also accounts for a part of their latency for response.

2. A second characteristic of hormones is that they promote homeostasis; that is, they play a role in the maintenance of a relatively stable internal environment. This is accomplished by negative feedback processes, which are discussed later in this chapter. A constant internal environment is essential for health and well-being: death may occur if concentrations of either calcium or potassium in blood are changed drastically, or if the concentration of glucose in blood, or the total volume of fluids in the body, is reduced greatly. These physiologic variables, and others, are controlled by hormones.

3. A third characteristic of hormones is that they seem to control the rates of certain critical (or rate-limiting) cellular reactions and processes. They do not usually initiate either processes or reactions not existing already. They generally accelerate the rate of existing reactions. For example, the hormone thyroxine, produced by the thyroid gland, increases cellular metabolism and the rate of oxygen utilization, but the use of oxygen does not drop to zero in the complete absence of thyroxine. Of course, there are exceptions that must be pointed out. An obvious one relates to the cessation of ovarian follicular growth and maturation when follicle stimulating hormone is absent.

4. A fourth characteristic of hormones is that they produce their effects when present in the blood in very low concentrations. Experimentalists are often misled with respect to the amount of hormone required to elicit a physiologic response because the mode of administration of a hormone is very important. Hormones taken by mouth may be inactivated partially or totally by the gastrointestinal tract, particularly if they are protein or polypeptide substances. Other hormones, such as steroids, may not be inactivated in the gastrointestinal tract but may be inactivated by the liver following absorption into blood. Similar results can occur with both intramuscular and intraperi-

toneal injections. This generally means that to effect complete replacement, larger amounts of a hormone must be given exogenously than are actually secreted by an organ.

5. The fact that hormones can act when present in minute concentrations in blood indicates that they have great specificity with respect to the tissues or cells on which they exert their effects. This specificity is most likely related to the specificity of the cellular receptors that mediate their intracellular effects. Thus, TSH from the anterior pituitary gland stimulates thyroid tissue to secrete thyroid hormones but does not exert a stimulatory activity on either adrenal glands or gonads.

6. Under normal conditions, hormonal equilibrium exists in the body; that is, the rates of secretion and metabolism (or inactivation) of a hormone must come into equilibrium. Perturbations in the rate of secretion of a hormone may occur temporarily as a result of many factors (e.g., excitement, stress). A rise in the concentration of certain hormones in blood may be followed by both an inhibition of the secretory activity of the endocrine gland producing the hormone (negative feedback) and an increase in the rate of inactivation of the hormone. As mentioned above, the liver is one of the organs responsible for much of the inactivation of hormones. It continuously extracts hormones from the blood and metabolizes them for excretion or reutilization. Any situation altering hepatic function seriously can potentially affect its rate of metabolism of hormones. In humans, for example, passive congestion of the liver, which often accompanies congestive heart failure, reduces the rate of metabolism of steroid hormones. This contributes to a vicious cycle that allows the hormone aldosterone, which is responsible for retention of sodium by renal tubules, to remain in the circulation for a longer period of time (i.e., an increased half-life). The result of this is that more sodium and water are retained by the kidneys and the congestive failure worsens.

One may wonder why the body contains an endocrine system that secretes a hormone and then proceeds to inactivate a fair proportion of what is secreted before it can be used. Maintaining hormonal equilibrium is somewhat analogous to maintaining the temperature of a room. This could be accomplished by heating only, but the temperature variation would be rather large. We could prevent excessive variation in temperature if a cooling unit were pitted against the heating unit and were programmed to turn on when room temperature surpassed the desired temperature by a certain amount. At the same temperature differential, the heating unit would turn off. The reverse situation would be programmed to take place when room temperature decreased by a certain amount below the desired room temperature. Within certain limits, the body appears to secrete and inactivate hormones in blood in an analogous way. This accomplishes the task of preventing large variations in the concentration of these hormones in blood much better than secretion alone could have done it. Thus, it appears that the body has sacrificed economy for control.

SECTION 1-1: POST-TEST QUESTIONS

1. The classic definition of an endocrine system includes the following.
   a.
   b.
   c.
2. Why does this definition now appear to be too restrictive?
   a.
   b.
   c.

3. What is a reasonable working definition of a hormone?

4. List six general characteristics of hormones.
   a.
   b.
   c.
   d.
   e.
   f.

SECTION 1-1: POST-TEST ANSWERS

1. a. The organ secreting the hormone does not contain a duct.
   b. Secretion is not affected by the nervous system.
   c. The hormone is transported by blood to a distant site, where it regulates function at target cells.
2. a. The nervous system is now known to play a significant role in the secretion of a number of hormones.
   b. At least one hormone, angiotensin II, is not secreted by a particular organ but is formed as a result of the union of an enzyme (renin) with a substrate (renin substrate) in blood.
   c. Hormones do not need to be transported by blood to a distant site to regulate function. Neurohormones are secreted and act locally to produce their effects.
3. A hormone is a substance secreted by living cells into the environment outside them, where it is transported to its target site. The hormone interacts with its target site by way of receptors specific to it, to regulate and not initiate a cellular reaction. Hormones are not used as sources of energy.
4. a. A long latency for response.
   b. They promote homeostasis.
   c. They control rates of certain critical cellular reactions or processes.
   d. They produce their effects when present in the blood in very low concentrations.
   e. They have great specificity in their action.
   f. Under normal circumstances, the rates of secretion and metabolism are in equilibrium.

SECTION 1-2: CHEMICAL STRUCTURE, SYNTHESIS, AND SECRETION OF HORMONES

OBJECTIVES:

The student should be able to:
   1. State the two classes into which hormones can be divided according to their chemical structures.
   2. Discuss in a general way the steps involved in the synthesis of a protein-type hormone within an endocrine cell.
   3. Discuss how secretion may occur in endocrine cells secreting protein-type hormones.
   4. Discuss the synthesis and secretion of steroid hormones.

A. CHEMICAL STRUCTURE OF HORMONES

Based on their chemical structure, mammalian hormones may be grouped into two major types: proteins, peptides, and amino acid derivatives, and steroids and steroidlike chemicals.

Many of the protein-type hormones are synthesized as prohormones, which must be altered after synthesis (i.e., they undergo posttranslational modifications) by the secretory cell to produce the biologically active hormone. Thus, proinsulin is the prohormone of insulin and consists of a single helical chain of amino acids with the two ends of the molecule connected by two disulfide bonds. Just before secretion, the central segment, or C-peptide, is removed by a specific peptidase in the pancreatic cell to form the characteristic double chain of insulin (see Chapter 9). A number of other hormones is also formed from prohormone precursors, including parathyroid hormone, glucagon, ACTH, oxytocin, and vasopressin. In circumstances of abnormal secretion by an endocrine organ producing a protein-type hormone, excessive quantities of the prohormone may be produced and appear in the circulation in higher than normal amounts (e.g., pancreatic or parathyroid adenoma). In certain assay systems (e.g., radioimmunoassay) the prohormone may not be distinguished from the hormone, although the biological activity of the prohormone may be significantly less than that of the hormone.

The biologically active portion of a protein-type hormone may be much smaller than the actual molecule. The presence of additional amino acid residues may be used to extend the duration of action of the hormone, since the ultimate fate of polypeptide hormones is inactivation by hydrolysis. The inactive portion of the molecule may also serve to solubilize the hormone in serum as well as to add additional recognition signals for the hormonal receptors on cell surfaces. The smaller peptide hormones do not have the benefit of a large inactive portion of their molecule to prolong activity. These molecules are often modified at each end by the pharmaceutical industry to decrease the rate of their hydrolysis by peptidases in the serum and liver.

The second group of hormones is the steroid group. These are hydrophobic, lipid-soluble substances consisting of three cyclohexyl and one cyclopentyl carbon ring combined into a single structure (see Figure 5-2). Hormones such as cortisol, testosterone, estradiol, and aldosterone are steroids. These hormones are synthesized from cholesterol by similar biosynthetic pathways, discussed in greater detail below. Vitamin D is a modified steroid (one of the cyclohexyl rings is split during the activation of the vitamin; see Chapter 10), which also shares a similar mechanism for cellular activation with the gonadal and adrenal steroids.

B. SYNTHESIS AND SECRETION OF HORMONES

When considered in the broadest sense, endocrine tissues may be said to store their hormones intracellularly. One can recognize two main forms of storage: membrane-bound secretory granules in cells of endocrine glands that secrete protein-type hormones, and storage of a precursor (cholesterol) in cells of endocrine glands secreting steroid hormones. The thyroid gland appears to be the single exception, since it stores its hormone extracellularly in the lumen of its follicles.

A large number of the endocrine glands that secrete protein-type hormones store their secretory products in subcellular granules. These include cells of the anterior pituitary gland, the islets of Langerhans of the pancreas, the adrenal medulla, the parathyroid glands, the parafollicular cells of the thyroid gland, and the axon terminals of the neurosecretory cells of the hypothalamic-neurohypophyseal system. Because all these organs contain subcellular secretory granules, it is likely that the mechanisms of synthesis and secretion are similar.

It has been established by both electron microscopic and biochemical analyses that the granules of a secretory cell contain the hormone. Centrifugation and subcellular fractionation techniques have isolated secretory granules from other subcellular elements. Chemical analysis has proved the presence of the hormone in the granules, at least in the case of the adrenal medulla and its granules containing epinephrine and norepinephrine. Electron microscopic analysis of the granules has revealed that they are enclosed in a membrane. We will see that this membrane is important ultimately in the release of the contents of the granules from the cell.

The mechanism of storage of hormones in granules is important physiologically because a) it allows the concentration of the hormone in the granule to reach very high levels and thus provides a large storage capacity, b) the hormone is protected from metabolism, and c) the granules of a given tissue are approximately the same volume. This means that similar amounts of hormone are released (quantum amounts) when the contents of each granule are extruded from the cell. This is of particular importance for the nervous system, which may regulate the strength of contraction of skeletal muscle by changing the number of granules containing acetylcholine, the neurotransmitter substance, that are released per unit time at the nerve ending. d) Granules also appear to be important for the movement of the hormone within the secretory cell. This may be seen especially clearly in the neurohypophyseal neurons, which transport granules containing oxytocin and vasopressin from the hypothalamus to the posterior pituitary gland. e) The membrane surrounding the granule fuses with the cellular membrane to provide a mechanism by which the contents of the granule may be extruded from the cell (exocytosis).

Eukaryotic cells (i.e., cells containing distinct nuclei) have elaborately folded intracellular membranes known as endoplasmic reticulum. The endoplasmic reticulum may be divided into various subdivisions, which may be located in specific areas within a secretory cell. For example, in the B-cells of the islets of Langerhans in the pancreas, the rough endoplasmic reticulum is generally at the base of the cell; the Golgi zone is just above the nucleus, and the granules (i.e., zymogen granules containing proinsulin, insulin, C-peptide, and other chemicals) are at the apex. The endoplasmic reticulum divides the cell into two compartments known as the cytoplasmic matrix and the cisternal space. In highly organized cells, many secretory products are made on the rough endoplasmic reticulum by ribosomes that pass them into the cisternal space. From there the products pass to the Golgi zone in the smooth endoplasmic reticulum, where they are concentrated, condensed, often enzymatically altered, and finally "packaged" (i.e., a membrane is enclosed around them to form the granules). A number of different products may be packaged in the final granule. These then migrate toward the apex of the cell, where the contents of the granule are extruded from the cell by the process of exocytosis. The direction of flow of secretory products within a secretory cell appears to be well established (i.e., from rough endoplasmic reticulum to smooth endoplasmic reticulum to Golgi apparatus to secretory granules). The mechanism by which the flow occurs is much less well understood.

Also poorly understood is the mechanism by which the membrane of the granule fuses with the membrane of the cell. It appears at present that fusion can take place only at certain sites on the cell membrane. How the granule recognizes this segment of the membrane is unknown. Furthermore, although the granular membrane appears to become part of the cell membrane during fusion, it is thought that the membrane is taken back into the cell by endocytosis after secretion has occurred. These "empty vesicles" (i.e., coated vesicles) may then be dismantled by lysosomes and recycled to form new membranes (see Figure 2-16). (*Q. 1-1*) *What would you expect to happen to the secretory cell if endocytosis of granule membranes was inhibited?*

Energy is required for the release of secretory products from cells. Secretion can be blocked by means of inhibitors of oxidative phosphorylation and glycolysis. Since these processes are important in the generation of adenosine triphosphate (ATP), it seems likely that ATP is important for secretion. Calcium ions are involved in the process of providing the energy for secretion, but details of the mechanism are speculative at present. Calcium ions are however, required for secretion to occur. The positively charged calcium ions (Ca^{2+}) may play a role in the fusion of granular and cellular membranes or they may be important for a contractile event necessary for the release of the hormone. (*Q. 1-2*) *Can you explain how calcium might be expected to play a role in these two hypothetical mechanisms of action?*

In the case of all steroid hormone-producing glands, synthesis occurs via the same biosynthetic pathways, even though the hormonal end products secreted by each gland are different. This is readily understandable if one recognizes that the synthetic process is directed toward one or another hormonal end product by the absence of a key enzyme in the biosynthetic pathway (see Figure 1-2). For example, the absence of a 21-hydroxylase enzyme in a particular endocrine tissue would be expected to direct synthesis toward production of testosterone and estradiol. (*Q. 1-3*) *In what endocrine tissues would you expect this to occur?* A detailed knowledge of all the intermediate

FIGURE 1-2: An abbreviated biosynthetic pathway for the synthesis of steroid hormones, showing the type of change that occurs in each structure as a result of enzymatic action on it. Notice that three major routes may be taken by precursors of steroid hormones to produce the major steroid hormones aldosterone, cortisol, testosterone, and 17-β-estradiol. The hormone produced by an endocrine gland depends on the absence (or presence) of certain key enzymes.

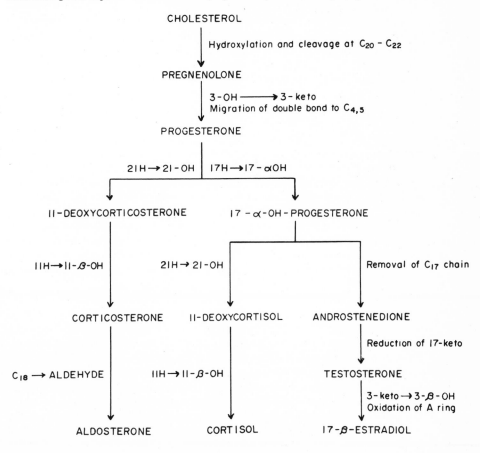

hormones in the biosynthetic pathway for steroids is not important to memorize at this time, but it is important for the health scientist to be able to recognize at least the major steroid hormones and their biosynthetic pathways. Figure 1-2 shows these pathways and contains examples of the enzymatic alterations of the steroid as it moves along the pathway. Note that cholesterol is the ultimate precursor of all steroid hormones. An understanding of this abbreviated biosynthetic pathway is important for an understanding of the physiology, biochemistry, and pathology of the steroid secreting endocrine glands. It is referred to frequently in subsequent chapters.

Since steroid secreting endocrine glands store the precursor, cholesterol, not their products, secretion must first involve an increased production of the hormone via the biosynthetic pathway. The process of releasing the steroid hormone from the secretory cell is relatively simpler than that for protein-type hormones because of the lipid solubility of the steroids and their relatively free permeability of cellular membranes.

SECTION 1-2: POST-TEST QUESTIONS

1. Name the two general types of hormone, based on their chemical structure.
   a.
   b.
2. What are prohormones?

3. How may one explain a high concentration of a peptide hormone in plasma found by radioimmunoassay when a bioassay suggests a normal concentration of the hormone?

4. A number of endocrine glands store their hormones in subcellular granules. Which general type of hormones are these? _____
5. In the B-cells of the islets of Langerhans of the pancreas, synthesis of proinsulin takes place on the a. _____ of the cell. From there the hormone moves into the b. _____ From which it passes to the c. _____. Here the hormone is d. _____ (i.e., it becomes enclosed in a membrane). This then becomes a e. _____ _____ and moves toward the f. ____(what portion?)____ of the cell.
6. How does secretion of a hormone enclosed in a granule occur?

7. Does this type of secretion require the generation and expenditure of metabolic energy? Why?

8. Are calcium ions essential for this type of secretion to occur? _____

9. The common precursor for the synthesis of all steroid hormones is _____ _____.

10. All steroid producing glands also have in common the same a. _____ _____. In spite of this, different hormonal end products can be secreted by different glands because b. _____ _____.

11. Why is the translocation of steroid hormones from blood plasma into cells a simple process compared to that for proteinlike hormones?

12. Is calcium required for secretion of steroid hormones? _____

SECTION 1-2: POST-TEST ANSWERS

1. a. Protein, peptide, or amino acid
   b. Steroid
2. Prohormones are generally proteins that contain in their structure the active hormone. Release of the active hormone depends on cleavage of the prohormone at specific sites by specialized enzymes in the secretory cell, often in the Golgi apparatus.
3. This can be explained by the hypersecretion of a prohormone that cross-reacts immunologically with the active hormone but lacks the biologic activity of the active hormone.
4. Protein-type hormones.
5. a. rough endoplasmic reticulum
   b. cisternal space
   c. Golgi apparatus
   d. "packaged"
   e. secretory granule
   f. apex
6. Secretion occurs by the fusion of the membrane surrounding the secretory granule with a specific site on the cellular membrane. This process is known as exocytosis.
7. Yes. Because secretion can be blocked by means of inhibitors of oxidative phosphorylation and glycolysis, both of which are important for the generation of ATP.
8. Yes
9. cholesterol
10. a. biosynthetic pathway
    b. certain key enzymes are deficient in them
11. Steroid hormones have a high lipid solubility and the cellular membrane is freely permeable to them.
12. No

SECTION 1-3: TRANSPORT OF HORMONES AND THEIR MECHANISMS OF ACTION AT THEIR TARGET SITE

OBJECTIVES:

The student should be able to:
1. Discuss the transport of hormones in blood and its biologic significance.
2. Discuss the predominant mechanism by which certain protein-type hormones stimulate their target cells to activity.

3. Discuss the predominant mechanism by which steroid hormones stimulate their target cells to activity.
4. Describe an experimental technique for measurement of receptor number and affinity.
5. Discuss some examples of hormonal interaction.
6. Describe the principle of radioimmunoassay.

A. TRANSPORT OF HORMONES IN BLOOD

Hormones are transported to their target tissues generally by blood. The transport of certain hormones (e.g., steroids) presents difficulty because their solubility in plasma is low. If this were the only way these hormones could be transported, the maximal amounts available to the cells of target tissues would be limited by the solubility in plasma of the hormones. This potential problem has been bypassed because most of the steroid hormones are transported in blood bound to a plasma protein. These protein-bound hormones are in equilibrium with the free, or unbound, hormones. It should be recognized that it is the free hormone that is important physiologically.

The binding of steroid hormones to low-affinity plasma proteins, such as albumin, permits the release of the hormone to occur at the site of utilization. If the utilization is large, more bound hormone will dissociate to its free form because of the equilibrium that exists between the bound and free forms of the hormone. (Q. 1-4) *What difference does it make if the steroid is bound to a high-affinity plasma protein, such as transcortin or testosterone binding globulin rather than to a low-affinity plasma protein?* The fact that the hormone is bound to protein also provides a mechanism for storage of the hormone. If the protein that binds a particular hormone increases in concentration, the total bound hormone concentration in blood will increase. However, this increase need not be accompanied by a change in the free hormone concentration. For example, the concentration of thyroxine bound to plasma proteins increases during pregnancy or as a result of chronic ingestion of an oral contraceptive agent because the concentration of thyroxine binding protein in blood increases. In spite of this, the concentration of free thyroxine in blood is unchanged and there is no measurable metabolic effect. This may be accomplished by an increase in the rate of dissociation of the bound hormone. (Q. 1-5) *Can you think of any other possible explanations?*

Another advantage gained physiologically by the binding of a hormone to plasma protein is that the hormone is protected both from metabolism and from excretion. Most free hormones can pass through the glomerular membranes of the renal tubules. Therefore, if hormones were not bound, they could easily be excreted into urine. They could also be either metabolized or conjugated with glucuronide or sulfate by the liver. It is interesting in this regard that one steroid hormone, aldosterone, is bound to plasma protein only to the extent of about 20%. It has been shown experimentally that virtually all the free aldosterone is extracted from the blood by the liver in one passage through it.

Since the bound hormone is usually present in blood in great excess relative to the free hormone, any outside influence that alters the binding properties of the protein or competes with the hormone for binding sites on the carrier protein can have physiologic consequences. Thus, aspirin affects the binding of thyroxine to its carrier protein, resulting in larger quantities of free thyroxine in plasma. While this increases initially the availability of free thyroxine for use by the cells of the body, it also increases the rate of metabolism of thyroxine by the liver. The net result for aspirin and other compounds with a similar mechanism of action is a much greater turnover of thyroxine (production and metabolism) with little change in total body metabolic rate.

It is sometimes difficult to recognize that the concentrations of binding proteins as well as hormones in blood are not static. Hormones and binding proteins are being produced and metabolized constantly and their rates of production and metabolism are subjected to change by both internal and external influences. For example, later chapters discuss the phenomenon of normal circadian variations (i.e., variations with the time of day) in the concentrations of certain hormones in blood.

B. PERIPHERAL EFFECTS OF HORMONES

1. *The Role and Classification of Receptors.* All hormones may be present in the extracellular fluid at a given time, yet the response to each hormone occurs only in specific tissues and cells. This specificity of action of hormones appears to reside in two distinct and separable functions of the receptors on, or in, particular cells (i.e., the target cells): a) recognition, in which the receptor binds specifically the hormone; and b) transduction or actuation, in which the hormone-receptor (ligand-receptor) interaction is translated by the cell into a change in its biochemical function. These properties can be grouped into five basic *criteria for defining a receptor*: a) strict structural and steric specificity for the hormone, b) saturability, indicating a finite number of receptors at any time, c) high affinity for the hormone, especially in consideration of the low concentration of the hormone in blood, d) kinetic reversibility, which accords with a decrease in biologic response upon removal of the hormone, and e) tissue specificity, in agreement with the specificity of the biological response.

Receptors have been identified for a long list of ligands. The receptors for water-soluble ligands that cannot readily penetrate the cellular membrane are located usually in the cellular membrane and are thought to be glycoprotein in structure. These are known as fixed receptors (see Figure 1-3). (*Q. 1-6*) *Which type(s) of hormones would you expect to be bound to this type of receptor?* There is a second class of receptors referred to as mobile receptors. They are found in the cytoplasm (and nucleoplasm) of target cells. (*Q. 1-7*) *Which type(s) of hormones would you expect to be bound to this type of receptor?*

2. *Mechanisms of Hormone Action: Protein, Peptide, and Amino Acid Derivative Hormones.* The mechanism by which the fixed receptors mediate a change in the activity of certain secretory cells has been worked out to a considerable extent (see Figure 1-3). When a protein-type hormone such as either TSH or a catecholamine couples with its receptor on the cell membrane of a target cell, the adenylate cyclase system is activated. The information that the receptor has been activated by the hormone is transmitted through the membrane by a transducer, the mechanism and structure of which are not yet understood clearly. The transducing mechanism may involve guanosine triphosphate (GTP) and a nucleotide regulatory component. The transducing mechanism is necessary for activating the membrane-bound enzyme adenylate cyclase, which, in turn, converts MgATP to cyclic adenosine monophosphate (cAMP). The cAMP activates a protein kinase enzyme. The protein kinase enzyme consists of at least two subunits; one is catalytic and the other is regulatory or inhibitory. When the two subunits are complexed together, the enzyme is inactive. Activation occurs when cAMP complexes with the inhibitory subunit and allows the enzyme to become active. The active protein kinase now converts inactive phosphorylase kinase to active phosphorylase kinase by phosphorylation through ATP. The active phosphorylase kinase then converts inactive phosphorylase "b" to active phosphorylase "a" by phosphorylation. In the case of the liver cell, phosphorylase "a" would then stimulate the breakdown of glycogen to glucose.

The majority of protein kinases described to date are activated by cAMP, specifically

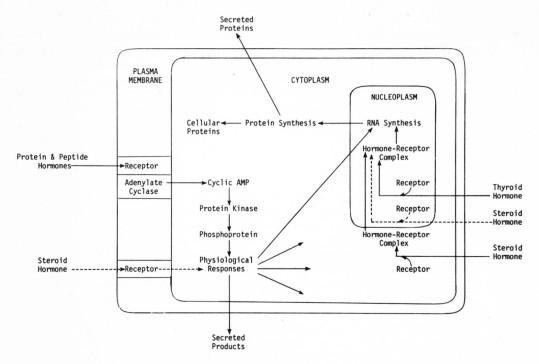

FIGURE 1-3: A simplified schema of the putative mechanisms of action of hormones in eukaryotic cells. Further details and exceptions are noted in the text of this and subsequent chapters. Dashed lines indicate mechanisms which are not as well established as those indicated with solid lines. (*Adapted from*: Martin et al. 1977.)

by the complexing of cAMP with the inhibitory subunit of the kinase enzyme. This frees the catalytic subunit to do its work. Although there are many protein kinases, there is, apparently, a degree of similarity among them. For example, it has been shown that a protein kinase from one type of cell will phosphorylate proteins from other types of cells. This suggests that specificity of response depends on the membrane receptor protein and on the specific intracellular protein available for phosphorylation. The synthesis of these proteins is, of course, dependent on the particular genetic makeup of the target cell. Because of its role in mediating these hormonal effects, cAMP has been called the *second messenger*.

An important characteristic of this system is the amplification of the original stimulus that it provides. For example, when epinephrine acts on hepatic cells to induce the release of glucose, it has been estimated that one molecule of this catecholamine hormone can induce the release of 10^8 molecules of glucose. Hormones acting through the cAMP system may initiate a variety of cellular responses. These include: a) activation of the transport of substances across cellular membranes, b) synthesis of protein in the endoplasmic reticulum, c) nuclear reactions in cells such as DNA and RNA synthesis, differentiation, and microtubular secretion, d) lipolysis (formation of fats from stored triglycerides), and e) glycogenolysis (formation of glucose from stored glycogen). Many other cellular responses are also mediated by the cAMP system.

Although many hormones stimulate the cAMP system to activity, there are also a number of other hormones that inhibit it. These substances produce a cellular response when cAMP is inhibited. One example is insulin. Some investigators have suggested a role for cyclic guanosine monophosphate (cGMP) as the mediator inhibiting the responsiveness of cellular mechanisms to cAMP. It has also been suggested that the response of a cell is the resultant of the relative activities of cAMP and cGMP induced by stimulation of the membrane-bound receptor. Alternate theories, including changes in intracellular calcium ions, have also been proposed. It can be assumed at present that the responses of secretory cells to stimulation by certain hormones can be explained reasonably by mediation of the cAMP system. It must also be remembered, however, that we have no adequate explanation for the cellular responses of certain other hormones that cannot traverse the cellular membrane and are known to inhibit the cAMP system.

3. Mechanisms of Hormone Action: Steroid and Steroid-Derivative Hormones. In the case of steroid hormones (and steroid derivatives such as vitamin D; see Chapter 10), passage through the cellular membrane presents no problem. Once inside the cell, the steroid hormone couples with a cytoplasmic receptor, called a mobile receptor. The receptor-hormone complex undergoes a poorly understood "activation" process that facilitates its interaction with chromatin acceptor sites but does not affect its transport through the nuclear membrane. Within the nucleus, the activated steroid-receptor complex facilitates the transcriptional production of specific messenger RNA (mRNA) species, which code for a number of types of proteins including regulatory and catalytic enzymes, additional steroid receptors, intracellular structural components, and proteins that control membrane transport of amino acids, ions, glucose, and so on. (see Figure 5-11). The particular protein synthetic mechanism initiated by the mRNA depends on both the target cell and the steroid hormone. Effects of specific steroid hormones are covered in detail in later chapters.

It should be noted that although steroid hormones can diffuse through plasma membranes and initiate subsequent genomic responses through interactions with cytoplasmic (and nucleoplasmic) receptors and chromatin acceptors, they can also exert nongenomic responses through interactions with receptors found in the plasma membrane of the target cell (see Figure 1-3). Numerous examples of this alternative (and still poorly understood) mechanism of action of steroid hormones can be found in the central nervous system. Recent experiments with laboratory animals have shown that certain steroid hormones can either increase or decrease the rate of firing (i.e., action potentials) of target cell neurons within milliseconds after exposure to the hormone. In one study it was also shown that the decrease in the rate of firing was accompanied by an increase in the permeability of the neuronal membrane to chloride and potassium ions. This change in ionic fluxes resulted in a hyperpolarization of the neuron similar to that produced by certain "inhibitory" neurotransmitters such as γ-aminobutyric acid (GABA).

The thyroid hormones thyroxine and triiodothyronine have also been purported to exert genomic responses in certain target cells through a direct interaction with nucleoplasmic receptors (i.e., without interacting with cytoplasmic receptors) (see Figures 1-3 and 3-8). The details of this novel, and still controversial, ligand-receptor-acceptor interaction are not well understood. Further discussions on the mechanisms of thyroid hormone actions are provided in Chapter 3.

4. Regulation and Quantification of Receptor Number and Affinity. Although receptors may appear to be fixed entities, it is now clear that they may increase and decrease in response to particular stimuli. One such stimulus for an increase in the number of receptors is a relative deficiency of the hormone that normally couples to it. This is called "up-regulation" of receptors and, in many respects, it is similar to the denervation supersensitivity response observed in striated muscle following the removal of its normal synaptic contacts. In the opposite situation, "down-regulation" occurs. Examples of both these forms of regulation are given in subsequent chapters. In addition to the change in the number of receptors, a change in their binding affinity may also occur. This situation may also translate into a change in the responsiveness or sensitivity of the target cell to the hormonal ligand. It is further possible to have an alteration in the efficiency with which a hormone-receptor complex produces its biologic response (e.g., a desensitization of the target cell following a reduction in the efficiency of coupling of the hormone-receptor complex with a chromatin acceptor or some other biochemical effector). Changes in either the number or affinity of receptors (or in the efficiency of the biologic response elicited by the hormone-receptor complex) may also be induced by hormones (and drugs) other than those that normally couple to it. This type of interaction between different hormones is discussed further below.

Quantification of the number and affinity of receptors for specific ligands can be achieved experimentally through the use of radioreceptor assays. These assays focus attention on a single step in the hormonal response, namely, the formation of the hormone-receptor complex, and they normally require the use of a hormonal ligand that has been made radioactive (e.g., the hormone is labeled with ^3H, ^{14}C, ^{125}I, or some other isotope). In the simplest case of a single ligand and a single class of identical, noninteracting receptor sites, the hormone-receptor binding relationship can be expressed as follows:

$$H + \underset{k_2}{\overset{k_1}{\rightleftharpoons}} H\text{---}R \tag{1}$$

where

$\qquad$ H ≡ hormonal ligand (unbound or free hormonal ligand ≡ F)

$\qquad$ R ≡ receptor

H---R ≡ hormone-receptor complex (bound hormonal ligand ≡ B)

$\qquad$ k_1 ≡ rate constant for binding association

$\qquad$ k_2 ≡ rate constant for binding dissociation

According to the law of mass action, the rates of association and dissociation of the hormone-receptor complex must be equal at equilibrium, thus

$$k_1[F][R_t - B] = k_2[B] \tag{2}$$

where R_t ≡ total concentration (i.e., number) of receptors = R + H---R. Rearranging equation (2) we have

$$\frac{k_1}{k_2} = \frac{[B]}{[F][R_t - B]} \equiv K_a \equiv \frac{1}{K_d} \tag{3}$$

where

$\qquad$ K_a ≡ the association or affinity constant (with units of liters/mole)

$\qquad$ K_d ≡ the dissociation constant (with units of moles/liter)

These constants are used interchangeably by scientists and clinicians. Rearranging equation (3) we can produce the highly popular Scatchard equation

$$\frac{B}{F} = K_a \cdot [R_t - B] = K_a \cdot [R_t] - K_a \cdot [B] \tag{4}$$

which is often used in the graphic determination of K_a and R_t. Thus, plots of B/F on the ordinate versus B on the abscissa yield $-K_a$ from the slope and R_t from the intercept on the abscissa. (*Q. 1-8*) *Does a receptor with a K_d of 10^{-8} mole/liter have a higher or lower affinity for its ligand than a receptor with a K_d of 10^{-10} mole/liter?*

In actual practice the determination of K_a and R_t are more difficult than is indicated in the simplified derivation outlined above. The most common problem relates to the existence of nonspecific binding (e.g., steroid binding to intra- or extracellular albumin). This problem is most often approached by adding a large excess of unlabeled ligand to one set of assay tubes, to saturate the specific (i.e., high-affinity, limited-capacity) binding but leaving the nonspecific (i.e., low-affinity, large-capacity) binding. The contribution of the nonspecific binding to the total binding observed in tubes lacking the large excess of unlabeled ligand is subtracted and the remainder is assumed to represent the specific binding. Other problems with the simplified model outlined earlier relate to the existence of multiple or interacting ligands and nonidentical receptor sites. Details of how these problems are approached in the research and clinical laboratory are beyond the scope of this text.

C. HORMONAL INTERACTIONS

Changes in the concentration of one hormone in blood may influence both the production of another hormone and the response to it. There is a great deal of hormonal interaction that is not apparent in most textbooks of endocrinology, where one endocrine organ is considered generally as if it functioned independently of other endocrine glands.

An example of one type of interaction between two endocrine glands and their secretions is illustrated when the rate of secretion of thyroxine by the thyroid gland increases. One of the physiologic responses is an increase in the rate of cellular metabolism, including the cells of the liver. A consequence of this is an increased rate of metabolism of hormones by the liver. Thus, the steroid hormone cortisol, produced by the adrenal cortex, is metabolized at a faster than normal rate in the presence of excess thyroxine and, to maintain the concentration of this hormone at normal levels in blood, the adrenal cortex must secrete at a faster rate. This means that in hyperthyroidism cortisol is turning over at a faster than normal rate. This is called an indirect hormonal interaction.

An example of a direct interaction is illustrated by the fact that growth hormone, a hormone secreted by the anterior pituitary gland, which is responsible for somatic growth, will not stimulate growth in hypophysectomized rats (i.e., rats whose pituitary gland has been removed) unless thyroxine is present. However, thyroxine alone will not stimulate growth in the hypophysectomized rats. The ultimate mechanism is not clear, but it may relate to changes in receptor number and sensitivity in the hypophysectomized rat. This type of interaction has been termed a permissive action because a particular hormone is essential for a biologic response to occur, although the hormone itself does not normally initiate or regulate the response.

D. USE OF INHIBITORS OF PROTEIN SYNTHESIS TO STUDY THE MECHANISM OF ACTION OF HORMONES

To determine whether a hormone exerts its characteristic effect by stimulating the synthesis of proteins, several important chemical tools are available. Actinomycin D, a substance that blocks the transcription phase of protein synthesis, may be used. Other compounds such as puromycin and cycloheximide block protein synthesis at the translational step. Thus, with proper selection of inhibitors, the site of action of hormones on protein synthesis may be determined. (*Q. 1-9) Could such a study be done in the living animal?* This technique is referred to in subsequent chapters in which the cellular mechanism of action of specific hormones is discussed.

E. ASSAY OF HORMONES

The measurement of the concentration of hormones in blood has always provided a serious problem for the research scientist and clinician. The concentrations of some hormones (or groups of hormones) in blood are relatively simple to measure by chemical means (e.g., the Porter-Silber fluorometric assay for 17-ketosteroids; see Section 5-4). Other hormones, however, offer a more serious analytical challenge. Most of these hormones are present in plasma and/or serum in extremely low concentrations. In some cases these hormones can be measured by bioassay techniques. These assays involve the ability to measure a sensitive biologic response in the whole animal (e.g., blood pressure, body growth) or in tissues (e.g., rate of oxygen consumption, target tissue weight) that is affected by the hormone and relatively specific for it. With proper precautions and extreme care, the bioassay technique is a valuable tool that is still used today. (Q.1-10) *Why might a bioassay be preferential to the chemical assay for the same hormone?*

Over a decade ago, the radioimmunoassay for measurement of the concentrations of hormones in plasma and serum was introduced. This approach is based on the antigenic properties of the hormone itself or of a hormone-protein complex. Proteins and peptides isolated from human beings, whether hormonal or not, may be capable of eliciting the production of high concentrations of antibodies when injected into a laboratory animal (rabbits and sheep are used commonly for this purpose). However steroids are not antigenic normally and therefore must be linked covalently to a protein to stimulate the production of antibodies, which hopefully will recognize some unique property of the steroid rather than simply the protein to which it is attached. Problems of cross-reactivity (i.e., nonspecific binding of the antibody to other hormones or unrelated biochemicals) can be reduced if the hormonal antigens used to produce the antibodies are very pure. Cross-reactivity in the final assay can also be reduced using chemical means to remove the cross-reactant (e.g., a chemically similar hormone) prior to the assay. For example, a radioimmunoassay for a given steroid hormone can often be improved markedly by subjecting the sample to a chromatographic purification step to remove other steroids before the assay. Antibodies with multiple or less-specific binding can also be removed before the assay by allowing these antibodies to bind to hormones with antigenic properties similar to the one under investigation. It is very important to keep in mind that radioimmunoassays measure the immunologic activity, not the biologic activity of a hormone. (Q. 1-11) *Do you recall a situation in which the bioassay and radioimmunoassay for a hormone are known to differ?* (Hint: The example was cited in Section 1.2)

In practice, a measured amount of the antibody and a measured amount of the pure hormone (both radiolabeled and unlabeled) are added to assay tubes. Since only a small amount of antibody is added, and its capacity to bind the hormone is limited, only a fraction of the hormone will be bound. Since the antibody does not differentiate between the labeled and unlabeled hormone (under most conditions), both these ligands are able to compete for the limited number of binding sites on the antibody molecules. As the amount of unlabeled hormone is increased relative to the concentration of labeled hormone, the amount of labeled hormone bound to the antibody will naturally be decreased. Thus it is possible to construct a standard curve comparing the amount of radiolabeled hormone bound to the antibody with the amount of pure unlabeled hormone added to the assay tubes. By replacing the pure hormone with a sample of hormone contained in a serum or plasma sample, the concentration of the hormone (i.e., as determined by its immunologic properties) in the sample can be determined directly.

Radioimmunoassays have opened areas for research that were unassailable by other techniques. With their aid, a great deal of new information has become available. There are at present radioimmunoassays available for virtually all the protein-type hormones, including catecholamines, as well as for a number of steroid hormones.

SECTION 1-3: POST-TEST QUESTIONS

1. Carriers are required for most protein-type hormones in blood. (True/False)
2. Why is the binding of hormones to proteins in blood important?
   a.
   b.
   c.
3. Different hormones use different carrier proteins for transport in blood. (True/False)
4. Why is the cellular response of a particular tissue specific for a particular hormone?

5. The hormone-receptor interrelationship involves two distinct and separable functions. What are they? a. _____, b. _____. How does a competitive inhibitor react with respect to these two functions? c.

6. Name five characteristics of receptors.
   a.
   b.
   c.
   d.
   e.
7. Receptors located on the surface of cellular membranes are called a. _____ _____ receptors. Those located in cytoplasm are called b. _____ receptors.
8. Which type of hormone initiates cellular activity by way of receptors bound to cellular membranes?

9. Steroid hormones may not require proteins for transport across cellular membranes because _____ _____.
10. Cyclic AMP has been called the a. _____ . It is known to activate a b. _____ enzyme, which is responsible for the activation of a number of enzymes, including the c. _____ _____.
11. Although a number of different cells are activated by cAMP, explain the fact that their responses differ.

12. When a steroid hormone interacts with its cytoplasmic receptor in neurons, a cellular response occurs more quickly than when the same hormone interacts with its membrane receptor. (True/False)

13. Both the concentration and the affinity of specific receptors may either increase or decrease depending on physiologic conditions. (True/False) These parameters may be measured by means of a a. _____ assay using a graphic means that relies on the b. _____ equation.

14. What is meant by "the permissive action of a hormone"?

15. What chemical substances could be used to verify the suspicion that a hormone acts on a specific tissue by stimulating the synthesis of another protein-type hormone? a. _____, b. _____. At which step in the synthetic process does each act? c. _____ _____ d. _____ _____.

16. Bioassays are used to estimate the concentration of a hormone in a body fluid by determining its effects in inducing a specific biologic response in the whole animal or in tissues from an animal. (True/False)

17. What are the necessary conditions to develop a radioimmunoassay for a hormone.
    a.
    b.
    c.

SECTION 1-3: POST-TEST ANSWERS

1. False. Carriers are required for steroid-type hormones.
2. a. It solubilizes the hormone.
   b. It protects the hormone from metabolism and excretion.
   c. It serves as a storage depot for the hormone in blood.
3. True. However some plasma proteins can bind, and therefore carry, more than one type of hormone. For example, testosterone binding globulin can carry both androgens and estrogens.
4. Receptors in target cells show high specificity and affinity for the hormone.
5. a. Recognition
   b. Transduction or activation
   c. A competitive inhibitor competes with the hormone for a site on the receptor. However, once on the receptor it cannot act (or is much less efficient in its role) as a transducer or activator of cellular responses.
6. a. They have strict structural and steric specificity for the hormone.
   b. They are saturable (i.e., there are a finite number of receptors at any time).
   c. They have a high affinity for the hormone.
   d. There is kinetic reversibility.
   e. There is a tissue specificity with respect to the receptors.
7. a. fixed
   b. mobile
8. This is commonly considered to be the protein-type hormones. However, steroid hormones are also known to interact with receptors found in plasma membranes of

certain neurons in the brain. This interaction acutely alters the firing rate of these neurons.

9. The cellular membrane is freely permeable to them.
10. a. second messenger
    b. kinase
    c. conversion of inactive phosphorylase kinase to active phosphorylase kinase.
11. The specificity is a function of the cellular receptor for the hormone and the genetic makeup of the cell.
12. False. A change in the firing rate of a neuron may occur within a few milliseconds following the interaction of a steroid with its membrane receptor.
13. True
    a. radioreceptor
    b. Scatchard
14. This relates to the fact that a particular hormone is essential for a biological response to occur, although the hormone itself does not normally initiate or regulate the response.
15. a. Actinomycin D
    b. Puromycin or actidione
    c. Actinomycin D inhibits protein synthesis at its transcription step
    d. Puromycin and cycloheximide inhibit protein synthesis at its translational step
16. True
17. a. A highly purified hormone.
    b. An appropriate animal that can produce high titers of a very specific antibody to the hormone.
    c. A radiolabeled, highly purified hormone.

SECTION 1-4: ENDOCRINE CONTROL MECHANISMS

OBJECTIVES:

The student should be able to:
1. Discuss the concepts of negative and positive feedback mechanisms as they apply to endocrine systems.
2. Describe four types of control mechanisms that influence the secretion of hormones by the body.
3. Discuss by example the variable that is being regulated in each case.
4. Describe the importance of the set-point mechanism in the control of endocrine secretion.
5. State the difference between vertical (hierarchic) and horizontal control systems.

Physiologic control of the rate of secretion of most hormones occurs by way of negative feedback. A negative feedback system can be illustrated simply, but not completely correctly, by the following:

$$A \xrightleftharpoons[\text{- - - -}]{+} B$$

In this situation, an increase in rate of secretion of hormone A increases the rate of secretion of hormone B, which then feeds back (dashed line) on A to decrease its rate of secretion. One can imagine that in this simplified situation, there is a concentration of B that, if exceeded, feeds back on A to reduce its rate of secretion. Conversely, if the concentration of B in blood falls below this level, the rate of secretion of A increases. Negative feedback is used to produce stability in a system.

A positive feedback system is also one in which an increase in the rate of secretion of A increases the rate of secretion of B. However, in contrast to the negative feedback system described above, an increase in rate of secretion of B induces a further increase in the rate of secretion of A. Such positive feedback is inherently unstable, producing ultimately either physiologic breakdown or wildly oscillating rates of secretion of both A and B. This is characteristically what happens when a speaker from a public address system is held too close to its microphone. Positive feedback is found only rarely in biologic systems. One example is discussed in Chapter 7 with respect to the effect of increasing concentrations of estrogen in blood in increasing the rate of secretion of the pituitary tropic hormones, follicle stimulating hormone, and luteinizing hormone.

There is a hierarchic system of complexity used by the body to control the rates of secretion by the various endocrine glands. The simplest type appears to be a system in which the hormone acts on specific cells to promote a change in a regulated variable in the extracellular fluid which, in turn, controls the output of hormone by the gland (see Figure 1-4).

Although this system operates as a closed-loop, negative feedback system, its particular setting can be changed by endocrine, neural, or other influences. As shown in Figure 1-4, such factors may act either on the endocrine gland (C_1) or on the cell (C_2). Examples of factors that may act at the levels of the endocrine gland and cell include changes in acid-base balance, diurnal factors, and changes in cellular receptor number and sensitivity. The regulated variable in this system is generally a constituent of plasma or extracellular fluid (e.g., calcium, glucose). Examples of this type of system include the interrelationship between the rate of secretion of insulin by the pancreas and the concentration of glucose in blood, and the rate of secretion of parathyroid hormone by the parathyroid gland and the concentration of calcium in blood. The major features of this system are the absence of direct control by either the hypothalamus or the anterior pituitary glands and the fact that the regulated variable is a constituent of plasma and extracellular fluid.

The second type of control system is somewhat more complicated and operates to control the rate of secretion of aldosterone by the adrenal cortex (see Figure 1-5). In this case, renin substrate is secreted into the blood by the liver, where it is acted on by the enzyme renin, which is secreted into blood by the kidneys. The result of the action of the enzyme on its substrate is the eventual production of angiotensin II, an octapeptide, which stimulates the production of aldosterone by the adrenal cortex. Aldosterone then exerts its effect on the renal tubules of the kidney to alter electrolyte excretion into urine. The increase in the concentration of sodium, and the decrease in the concentration of potassium, in plasma serve to feed back on the kidney to decrease the production of renin. If the system was stimulated to secrete by an acute fall in blood pressure, the

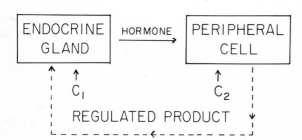

FIGURE 1-4: The type 1 control system in which an endocrine gland produces a hormone that acts on a peripheral cell to influence its secretion of a certain product. This, in turn, feeds back on the endocrine gland to inhibit its production of hormone.

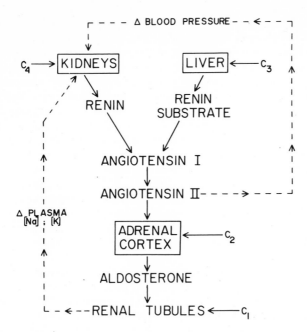

FIGURE 1-5: The feedback mechanism controlling the secretion of angiotensin and aldosterone (see text for discussion). The dashed lines represent feedback mechanisms that are important in the control of secretion of renin.

increase in the rate of secretion of angiotensin II, a potent vasoconstrictor agent, would return blood pressure to normal levels, which would turn off the system.

The regulated variables in this system are the concentrations of sodium and potassium in plasma, as well as blood pressure. Therefore, two independent negative feedback loops seem to be required for regulation; both loops modulate the production of renin by the kidneys, while renin substrate is effectively unmonitored. Certain physiologic factors (e.g., changes in receptor number and sensitivity) can operate independently at C_1 (renal tubules), C_2 (adrenal cortex), C_3 (liver), and C_4 (kidneys) to change their responsiveness. The unusual feature of this system is that the production of angiotensin II results from the union of an enzyme and a substrate in blood. Hence, no specific organ can be said to produce it. An additional feature of this system is that there appears to be no significant control exerted on it by either the hypothalamus or anterior pituitary gland.

The next order of complexity of endocrine control systems is the third type in which the endocrine gland is under control of the hypothalamus, which is located in the brain (see Figure 1-6). Endocrine control is achieved by a hierarchy that consists of the

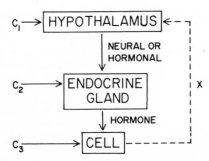

FIGURE 1-6: The feedback mechanism controlling the secretion of such hormones as antidiuretic hormone from the posterior pituitary gland (see text for discussion). The dashed line represents the feedback mechanism to the hypothalamus.

hypothalamus, then the endocrine gland, and then the target cell. The signal originating from the hypothalamus to activate the system may be either neural or hormonal. The release of the hormone is accompanied by a change in a plasma constituent (X in Figure 1-6), which in turn affects hypothalamic activity, as opposed to the hormone from the endocrine gland itself. C_1, C_2, and C_3 represent additional factors that modulate the activity of the hypothalamus, the pituitary gland, and the cell, respectively. This type of system appears to operate in the case of the secretion of antidiuretic hormone (ADH) from the posterior pituitary gland. The prohormone for ADH is produced by neurons in the hypothalamus and is transported within the axons of these neurons to the posterior pituitary gland. The hormone ADH can be released from the posterior pituitary gland by an increase in the osmolality of plasma. The released ADH acts at the level of the cells of the renal tubules to increase their reabsorption of water from urine back into blood. The osmolality of the plasma seems to be the regulated variable in this system and is sensed by osmoreceptors that appear to be located in or near the hypothalamus. We see later (Chapter 8) that the mechanisms controlling the secretion of growth hormone by the anterior pituitary gland may be characterized by this type of feedback mechanism, except that the regulated variable is less clear.

In the fourth type of control system, the activity of the final endocrine effector is controlled by the anterior pituitary gland; however, its activity is, in turn, regulated by the hypothalamus (see Figure 1-7). Endocrine control in this system is achieved by a hierarchy that begins with the hypothalamus, proceeding to the anterior pituitary gland, then the endocrine gland, and finally the cell that is the target for the hormone produced by the endocrine gland. It should be noted that feedback control is exerted primarily at either the level of the anterior pituitary gland, the hypothalamus, or both, and usually by the hormone secreted by the endocrine gland rather than by some product elaborated by the final effector cell. Each step from the hypothalamus to the final endocrine gland and return is mediated hormonally (i.e., H_1, H_2, H_3). C_1, C_2, C_3, and C_4 are factors influencing independently the activities of the hypothalamus, anterior pituitary gland, endocrine gland, and cell, respectively. This scheme takes into account the fact that the activity of the separate components can be altered by signals from outside the closed loop, which can affect the final hormonal output. This is exemplified by such phenomena as diurnal variations in rates of secretion of many hormones even though the essential feedback relations remain intact.

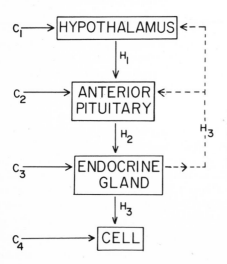

FIGURE 1-7: The fourth type of feedback mechanism controlling the secretion of such hormones as thyroxine from the thyroid gland and cortisol from the adrenal cortex (see text for discussion). The dashed lines represent the feedback mechanisms that are a function of the change in concentration of the hormone (H_3) produced by the endocrine gland.

Hypothalamic control of the secretions of thyroxine and cortisol are examples of the fourth type of system. The control of secretion of the gonadal hormone estradiol is similar but has, in addition, a positive feedback loop, which is discussed in Chapter 7. This serves to initiate the sequential release of hormones from the anterior pituitary gland and ovaries.

An essential element in any feedback control system is the mechanism that controls the "set point" around which the system operates. A device, familiar to all, that operates as a controller of a set point is the room thermostat, which essentially determines when the heating system turns on and off. Mechanisms for controlling the set point in biologic systems are also operative and, like the thermostat, can also be changed. The osmoreceptors that initiate the release of ADH from the posterior pituitary gland represent one type of setpoint device. They are programmed apparently to maintain the osmolarity of the plasma within a set range near 300 milliosmols/liter. Increases in the osmolar concentration of the plasma initiate the release of ADH, whereas decreases in osmolar concentration decrease it. It is worth mentioning that control systems do not really have a set "point," but a set range, within which they operate. If the range is too narrow, the system will turn on and off frequently and "chattering" results. In mechanical devices, this often leads to damage of the controller if the on/off frequency is very high. On the other hand, if the set-point range is too wide and responsiveness of the system is slow, even a negative feedback system will become unstable.

Each hormone, cellular product, or other substance that feeds back on the hypothalamus, anterior pituitary gland, or endocrine gland to influence its rate of secretion presumably affects receptors on or in cells associated with the set-point mechanism in that organ. Certain factors such as stress and disease states may reset the level about which the set point operates and, in this way, influence the level of activity of the control system.

It should be clear from reference to the control systems outlined here that the set point of the system may be influenced by a number of apparently different stimuli. An example of this is the control of the secretion of aldosterone. Here a number of apparently different stimuli (e.g., changes in plasma concentrations of sodium, potassium, catecholamines, and ADH, as well as a change in blood pressure) can influence the rate of secretion of aldosterone. How these diverse stimuli influence and interact with the same cells of the set-point mechanism is not well understood; nor is it entirely clear that there is only one set-point mechanism in this system. However, it does suggest that nature has provided for a certain amount of redundancy in the control of secretion of this important hormone.

This brief discussion of mechanisms for control of the secretion of endocrine glands is meant to provide a general background only. The specific aspects of control mechanisms influencing the secretion of the various endocrine glands are considered in detail in the chapters in which they are discussed. Furthermore, it should be recognized that only hierarchic (vertical) control has been considered here. It is also possible to consider the control of certain endocrine glands to be horizontal (i.e., to have one hormone that initiates secretion of an endocrine gland and another that inhibits secretion). Interaction and coordination between the initiating and inhibiting stimuli would be required. This system is somewhat more complicated than the hierarchic system, but it may be operative physiologically with respect to the control of the concentration of glucose in blood by the hormones, insulin (reduces glucose concentration), and glucagon (increases glucose concentration). The control of the concentration of calcium in blood may also be affected by dual mechanisms (parathyroid hormone increases calcium concentration, whereas calcitonin decreases it). Thus, as more information becomes available, it will become clearer which type of control system is more applicable to the control of secretion by each endocrine gland.

SECTION 1-4: POST-TEST QUESTIONS

1. Biological systems are controlled almost completely by a a. _____ feedback system. This is important because such a control mechanism imparts b. _____ to the system.

2. The simplest of the control systems (type 1) involves the interaction between an endocrine gland and a peripheral cell. This interaction involves a a. _____ from the endocrine gland and a b. _____ from the peripheral cell.

   What is being regulated in this system?
   c.

   What is the feedback limb of this system?
   d.

   This is called a e. _____ system whose functional level can be influenced by factors acting on the f. _____ and g. _____.

3. The second type of control system (type 2) operates to control the rate of secretion of a. _____ by the b. _____.

   Why is this system unusual?
   c.

   What variable(s) is being regulated in this system?
   d.

   What are the feedback limbs of this system?
   e.

   What distinguishing feature do the first and second types of control system have in common?
   f.

4. The third type of control mechanism described here involves control by the a. _____ of the brain. The hierarchic arrangement for control of secretion begins with the b. _____, then proceeds to the c. _____, and finally the d. _____. The signal initiating the system to activity and originating in (b) may be either e. _____ or f. _____.

   What is the regulated variable in this system?
   g.

   At what points can outside factors influence the level of activity of this system?
   h.

What is an example of a hormone whose secretory activity is affected by this type of control mechanism? i. _____. What type of receptor is most likely responsible for initiating an effect on the activity of this system?
j.

5. Describe the hierarchic system used to control the fourth type of endocrine control mechanism discussed in this section.
   a.

   In this system, feedback may be mediated at both the b. _____ and the c. _____.
   What is the regulated variable in this system?
   d.

   What constitutes the feedback limb?
   e.

   Where can stimuli interact with this system to affect its level of activity?
   f.

6. Describe the importance of a set-point mechanism in the control of endocrine secretion.

7. State the difference between vertical and horizontal control systems with respect to control of endocrine secretion.

SECTION 1-4: POST-TEST ANSWERS

1. a. negative
   b. stability
2. a. hormone
   b. product
   c. The concentration of the product in the blood.
   d. The change in concentration of the product in the blood.
   e. closed-loop, negative feedback
   f. endocrine gland
   g. peripheral cell
3. a. aldosterone
   b. adrenal cortex
   c. It involves the union of an enzyme (kidney) and a substrate (liver) in blood to form ultimately a hormone, angiotensin II, which influences the secretion of aldosterone by the adrenal cortex. Thus, no specific organ is responsible for the secretion of angiotensin II.

   d. The concentrations of sodium and potassium in blood as well as blood pressure.
   e. Changes in the concentration of sodium and potassium in blood and changes in blood pressure are known stimuli, among others, that influence the rate of secretion and release of renin from the kidney into blood.
   f. They lack control from either the anterior pituitary gland or the hypothalamus.
4. a. hypothalamus
   b. hypothalamus
   c. endocrine gland
   d. cell
   e. nervous
   f. hormonal
   g. A constituent of plasma.
   f. Inputs into the hypothalamus, the endocrine gland, and the peripheral cell may act independently to influence the level of secretory activity of each.
   i. Antidiuretic hormone
   j. An osmoreceptor located in the region of the hypothalamus.

5. a. Hypothalamus to anterior pituitary to endocrine gland to cell.
   b. hypothalamus
   c. anterior pituitary gland
   d. The concentration in blood of the hormone produced by the endocrine target organ.
   e. The hormone
   f. At the hypothalamus, the anterior pituitary gland, the endocrine gland, and the effector cell.
6. The set-point mechanism in an endocrine control system is responsible for maintaining the regulated variable within certain limits of a desired (set-point) concentration.
7. Vertical control systems are hierarchic, whereas horizontal control systems involve the use of two (or more) hormones to control a regulated variable. The regulation of certain physiologic variables may be explained by way of either vertical or horizontal control systems (e.g., the concentrations of glucose and calcium in blood).

SELECTED REFERENCES

Luttge, W. G., 1982, Molecular mechanisms of steroid hormone actions, in *Hormones And Aggressive Behavior*, B. B. Svare (Ed.), New York: Plenum Press.

Rennels, E. G. and Herbert, D. C., 1979, The anterior pituitary gland—its cells and hormones, *BioScience* 29: 408.

Satir, B., 1975, The final steps in secretion, *Scientific American* 233: 28.

Schally, A. V., 1978, Aspects of hypothalamic regulation of the pituitary gland, *Science* 202: 18.

Trifaro, J. M., 1977, Common mechanisms of hormone secretion, *Annual Review Of Pharmacology And Toxicology* 17: 27.

CHAPTER

2

INTRODUCTION TO NEUROENDOCRINOLOGY: NEUROHYPOPHYSEAL HORMONES

SECTION 2-1: OVERVIEW OF THE ANATOMY AND BLOOD SUPPLY OF THE PITUITARY AND HYPOTHALAMUS

OBJECTIVES:

The student should be able to:
1. Describe the basic anatomy and ontogeny of the major subdivisions of the pituitary.
2. Name the hormones synthesized and/or stored and released from each of the major subdivisions of the pituitary.
3. Describe the basic anatomy, subdivisions and ventricular supply of the hypothalamus.
4. Describe the hypothalamo-pituitary blood supply.

A. PITUITARY ANATOMY, ONTOGENY, AND HORMONES

The pituitary or hypophysis is often referred to as the master endocrine gland since it controls the activity of many of the other endocrine glands in the body. In adult men and women the pituitary is approximately 1 cm in length, 1–1.5 cm in width and 0.5 cm in depth. The pituitary weighs approximately 0.5 g in adult men and slightly more in women. Figure 2-1 illustrates a sagittal view of the pituitary. Note that it rests in a depression in the upper surface of the sphenoid bone in an area called the sella turcica. Note also that the dura mater, a tough fibrous material that encases the entire brain, dips down to line the sella turcica and that a shelf of dura known as the diaphragma sellae extends over most of the top of the gland. Thus, the pituitary is enclosed nearly completely in a protective shell. (*Q. 2-1*) *On the basis of this rather unusual anatomy, in which direction would you predict most tumors of the pituitary to grow and in which tissue(s) would you expect this growth to compress and often damage?*

The pituitary gland may be divided, on the basis of histological criteria, into four major subdivisions (See Figure 2-1). The pars distalis (*adenohypophysis* or anterior pituitary) forms the largest subdivision and is the source of at least six protein and peptide hormones: Thyroid Stimulating Hormone (TSH, see Chapter 3), Adrenocorticotropic Hormone (ACTH, see Chapter 5), Luteinizing Hormone (LH, see Chapters 6 and 7), Follicle Stimulating Hormone (FSH, see Chapters 6 and 7), Prolactin (Prl, see Chapters 6 and 7), and Growth Hormone (GH, see Chapter 8). The pars intermedia or intermediate lobe forms a very small subdivision of the human pituitary and is thought

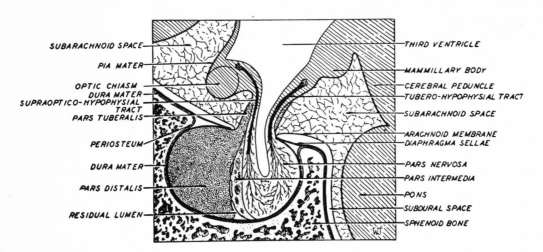

FIGURE 2-1: A diagramatic sagittal section through the human pituitary gland. (*Source:* Turner and Bagnara, 1971.)

to be discernible as a distinct entity only during the fetal period and possibly also during pregnancy. In animals such as the rat, the pars intermedia is believed to be the major source of Melanocyte Stimulating Hormone (MSH), whereas in adult (nonpregnant) humans this hormone is probably synthesized along with ACTH and the endogenous opiod β-endorphin, in the adenohypophysis. MSH, ACTH and β-endorphin are all believed to be posttranslational products of the same large precursor protein (or prohormone) called proopiocorticotropin. The pars tuberalis is a very small subdivision of the pituitary. Since this highly vascularized structure secretes no known hormones, it is conceptually more realistic to consider it as simply part of the continuum between the hypothalamic infundibulum and the last subdivision of the pituitary, the pars nervosa (*neurohypophysis* or posterior pituitary). The neurohypophysis forms the second largest subdivision of the human pituitary and although the peptide hormones, Oxytocin (see Section 2-3 and Chapter 7) and Antidiuretic Hormone (ADH or vasopressin, see Section 2-3), are found in relatively high concentrations in this region of the pituitary, these hormones are in fact synthesized in the brain.

Ontogenetic analyses indicate that the subdivisions of the pituitary are derived embryologically from two different sets of ectodermal tissue. The neurohypophysis is derived from diencephalic neural ectoderm, which also forms a subdivision of the brain known as the hypothalamus (see below). The adenohypophysis and the pars intermedia and tuberalis are derived from ectodermal epithelial cells from the roof of the primitive mouth known as Rathke's pouch. As shown in Figure 2-2, the portion of Rathke's pouch in contact with the diencephalon forms the pars intermedia whereas the remaining portion of the pouch expands to form the pars tuberalis and the adenohypophysis. (*Q. 2-2) On the basis of this differential embryologic origin, which divisions of the pituitary would you predict to receive extensive innervation from the brain?*

B. HYPOTHALAMIC ANATOMY

The hypothalamus is a division of the diencephalon, located in the medial ventral region of the brain directly dorsal to the pituitary (see Figures 2-1, 2-3 and 2-4). The two main types of cells in the hypothalamus, as well as the rest of the nervous system, are the electrically excitable neurons and their supportive cells, the glia. The neurons can

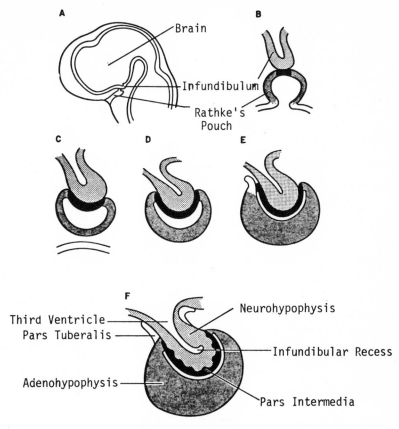

FIGURE 2-2: The ontogenetic development of the pituitary. Note that the neurohypophysis is of neural origin, whereas the adenohypophysis and the pars tuberalis and intermedia are derived from nonneural ectodermal epithelial cells. (*Adapted from:* Villee et al., 1973.)

be separated into groupings known as nuclei on the basis of histological and functional criteria. Examples of the hypothalamic nuclei (with recognized importance in neuroendocrinology) include the arcuate, median eminence, ventromedial, preoptic, paraventricular, supraoptic, and suprachiasmatic nuclei (see Figure 2-4). Some of these nuclei (e.g., arcuate, median eminence, preoptic, and ventromedial) are thought to be involved in the synthesis and/or release of the hypothalamic hypophysiotropic hormones (see Section 2-2). Two of the nuclei (supraoptic and paraventricular) are known to be involved in the synthesis of the neurohypophyseal hormones (see Section 2-3), and at least one of the nuclei (suprachiasmatic) appears to be involved in regulating the diurnal fluctuations of certain adenohypophseal hormones (e.g., ACTH, see Figure 5-4).

C. BLOOD SUPPLY OF THE HYPOTHALAMUS AND PITUITARY GLAND

The principal source of arterial blood for the hypothalamus is derived from the so-called Circle of Willis (see Figure 2-5) which, in turn, derives its input from the basilar and internal carotid arteries and which supplies blood to the rest of the brain through the anterior, middle, and posterior cerebral arteries. The latter set of arteries interconnect to form the "circle" by the anterior and posterior communicating arteries. The

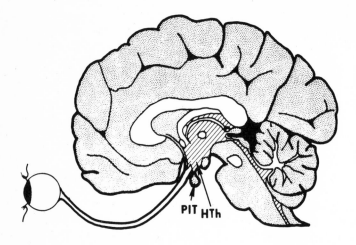

FIGURE 2-3: A diagramatic sagittal section through the human brain. The eye has been included to help in the orientation of the section. The pituitary (PIT) is located just caudal to the termination of the optic tract, while the hypothalamus (HTh) is located just dorsal to the pituitary.

supraoptic-preoptic, lateral and mammillary-posterior areas of the hypothalamus receive their principal arterial input from branches of the anterior, middle, and posterior cerebral arteries, respectively. The median eminence, proximal infundibular stalk, and medial basal hypothalamus are richly vascularized by a capillary network derived from the superior hypophyseal arteries, which are branches of the internal carotid and posterior communicating arteries (see Figures 2-5 and 2-6a). Capillary loops from this external or surface plexus of vessels penetrate into the median eminence where the tuberal-hypophyseal synapses occur. These contacts are probably the major site of release of the hypothalamic hypophysiotropic hormones (HHH) into the vascular supply which eventually reaches the adenohypophysis and hence the target cells for the HHH (see Section 2-2). Additional capillary loops from the internal capillary plexus, a derivative of the external plexus, penetrate deeper into the median eminence where they come into close proximity and often make functional contacts with the ependymal glial cells lining the ventral wall of the third ventricle within the infundibular recess

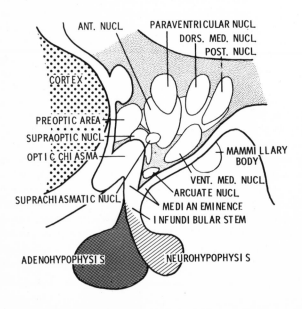

FIGURE 2-4: A diagramatic sagittal section through the human hypothalamus and pituitary. Only the major hypothalamic nuclei have been schematically represented and identified.

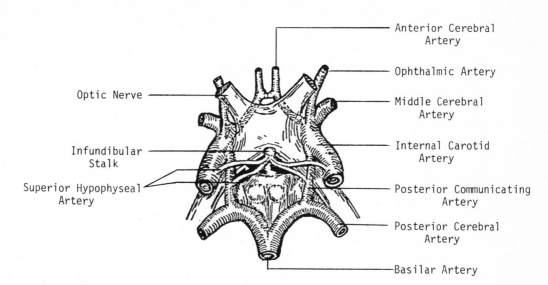

Anterior Cerebral Artery

Ophthalmic Artery

Middle Cerebral Artery

Internal Carotid Artery

Posterior Communicating Artery

Posterior Cerebral Artery

Basilar Artery

Optic Nerve

Infundibular Stalk

Superior Hypophyseal Artery

FIGURE 2-5: A diagrammatic representation of the ventral surface of the hypothalamus (the rest of the brain is not shown). Note the origins and distribution of the arteries in the Circle of Willis and those contributing to the superior hypophyseal arteries.

(see Figures 2-6b, 2-8 and 2-9). These contacts may also be sites of exchange and transport of hypothalamic hypophysiotropic, neurohypophyseal, and/or adenohypophyseal hormones (see Section 2-1D).

The adenohypophysis receives no *direct* arterial supply whereas the neurohypophysis receives direct vascular input from the three hypophyseal arteries: superior, middle, and inferior (see Figure 2-6a). However, the adenohypophysis is interconnected with the neurohypophysis and median eminence by a common capillary bed. Since this dense plexus of vessels between the adeno- and neurohypophysis greatly exceeds the number of vessels that egress directly from the adenohypophysis to the cavernous sinus and hence to the general circulation, much of the blood, rich in hormones, leaving the adenohypophysis does so through the bidirectional capillary vessels, which interconnect the adeno- and neurohypophysis (see Figure 2-6c). (*Q. 2-3*) *If these vessels were veins, could the flow of blood still be bidirectional?* The hypophyseal blood may then drain to either the cavernous sinus through the Y-shaped confluent pituitary veins (see Figure 2-6a) or to the hypothalamus through the infundibular (portal) capillaries, in what could be thought of as a retrograde/dorsal direction from the neurohypophysis (infundibular process) to the infundibular stem and eventually to the infundibulum and median eminence (see Figures 2-6c, 2-6d, and 2-6f). Once in the median eminence, the adeno- and neurohypophyseal hormones may be transported through the external plexus of capillaries to the entire medial basal hypothalamus and even to the third ventricle via the specialized ependymal cells called tanycytes, which line the infundibular recess making functional contacts with the capillary loop of the internal plexus (see Figure 2-6d and Section 2-1D). Since the capillaries lining the surface of the infundibular stalk, infundibulum, and median eminence have fenestrated endothelial cells, the adeno- and neurohypophyseal hormones transported within these vessels can also enter the cerebral spinal fluid (CSF) by diffusing directly into the surrounding subarachnoid space (see Figure 2-6e and Section 2-1D). (*Q. 2-4*) *Are the capillaries in this region of the brain different from those found in other brain regions (Hint: blood-brain-barrier)?*

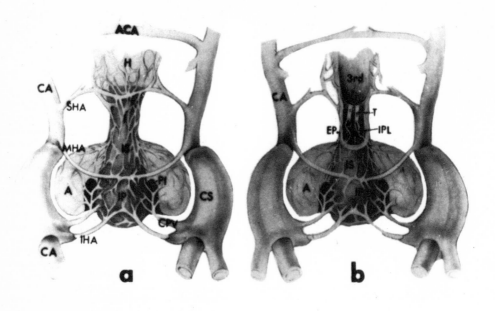

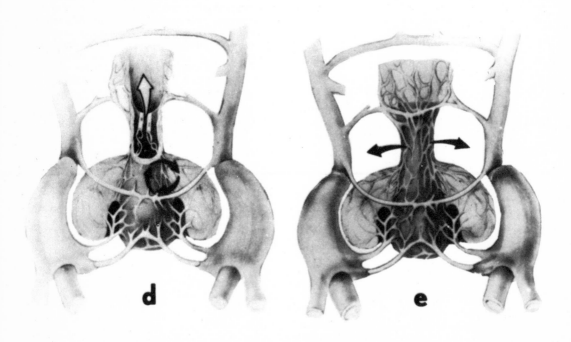

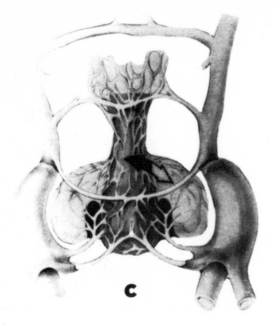

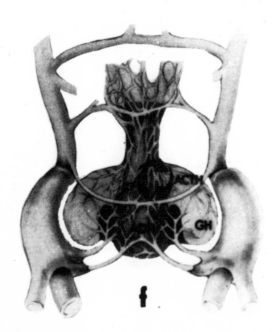

FIGURE 2-6: Posterior view of the vascular relationships in the primate: a) the external surface anatomy is depicted; b) a portion of the median eminence/infundibulum has been removed, c) depicts the bidirectional nature of the dense plexus of capillaries between the adeno- and neurohypophysis, d) illustrates the possibility of a circular blood flow between the adeno- and neurohypophysis, which could supply hormones to the tanycytes which may in turn transport them to the third ventricle; e) illustrates the fact that since the infundiblar (portal) capillary vessels have fenestrated endothelial cells, hormones contained within these capillaries may leak to the surrounding subarachnoid cerebral spinal fluid; f) illustrates the possibility that since the hormones synthesized and/or released within the neuro- and adenohypophysis have a regional distribution pattern, certain hormones may have a greater probability of participating in hypophysial recirculation and/or "retrograde" transport to the hypothalamus. Abbreviations: ACA-anterior communicating artery, H-medial basal hypothalamus, I-median eminence/infundibulum, IS-neurohypophysis/infundibular stem, IP-neurohypophysis/infundibular process, CA-carotid artery, SHA-superior hypophysial artery, MHA-middle hypophysial artery, IHA-inferior hypophysial artery, A-adenohypophysis, PI-pars intermedia, T-tanycytes, EP-external capillary plexus, IPL-internal capillary plexus, RF-hypothalamic hypophyseal hormones, ACTH-adrenocorticotropic hormone, GH-growth hormone, ADH-antidiuretic hormone. (*Source:* Bergland and Page, 1979.)

It should be noted that the Y-shaped confluent pituitary veins are found exclusively in the lower caudal portion of the pituitary and hence provide a direct route of venous drainage for only the caudal adeno- and neurohypophysis. There is no system of direct venous drainage from the infundibulum and median eminence. The extraordinary richness of the capillary bed interconnecting the rostral adeno- and neurohypophysis (i.e., infundibular stalk; see Figure 2-6c), however, facilitates the recirculation and retrograde transport of hormones produced and/or released in this area (e.g., HHH, ACTH, and Prl) as compared to those produced and/or released in the more caudal-lateral portions of the pituitary (e.g., ADH and GH; see Figures 2-6d and 2-6f). This recirculation and/or bidirectional flow of blood forms an efficient pathway for the HHH to get from the brain to their target cells in the adenohypophysis and for the adeno- and

FIGURE 2-7: A diagrammatic sagittal section through the human brain and spinal cord illustrating the circulation (note the arrows) of cerebral spinal fluid (CSF in black) through the ventricular system. The figure also depicts one of the arachnoid villi through which CSF enters venous blood in a dural sinus. Note also the location of the choroid plexuses, which produce approximately ⅔ of the CSF, the third ventricle, and the infundibular recess (not labeled but just dorsal to the infundibular stalk). (*Source:* Rasmussen, 1945.)

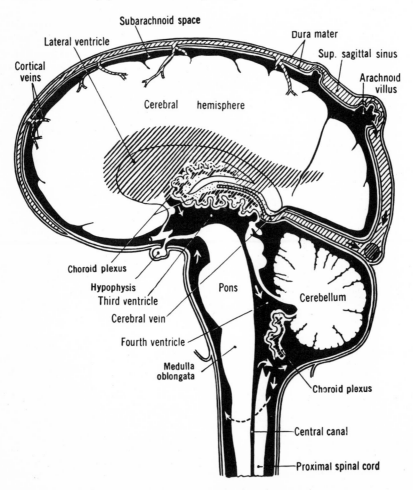

neurohypophyseal hormones to get from the pituitary to their target cells in the brain. This latter route of hormone transport is thought to be important in facilitating the so-called short feedback loop, wherein adenohypophyseal hormones may influence their own secretion through a direct modulation of HHH synthesis and/or secretion (see Section 2-2).

D. HYPOTHALAMIC VENTRICULAR SUPPLY

The neural tube, a major anatomical landmark during the embryological development of the brain, spinal cord, and pituitary (see Figure 2-2), persists throughout adulthood in a modified form known as the ventricular system (see Figure 2-7). The ventricular cavities, encased within the brain, are interconnected through channels known as foramen with the subarachnoid spaces that surround the brain, spinal cord, and infundibular stalk (see Figure 2-6e). This entire system of channels and cavities is filled with a clear fluid, known as cerebral spinal fluid (CSF), which is actively produced by the glial cells (approximately $\frac{1}{3}$ of the total) and the choroid plexuses of the ventricles (approximately $\frac{2}{3}$ of the total). The ventricular system thus provides physical support and protection (i.e., it functions as a shock absorber), as well as a route through which biochemicals (e.g., hormones) can enter and leave the brain, spinal cord, and pituitary (see Figure 2-8). The sites of production and routes of transport for CSF in the human brain are described further in Figure 2-7.

The ventral surface of the third ventricle directly dorsal to the median eminence is known as the infundibular recess (see Figures 2-1 and 2-7). This region of the ventricular system is lined with specialized ependymal cells called tanycytes (see Figures 2-6b and 2-8). These modified glial cells have fingerlike protrusions extending into the third ventricle and long processes which abut with the capillary loops derived from the

FIGURE 2-8: A diagrammatic coronal section through the medial basal hypothalamus illustrating the potential routes of movement of hormone within the infundibular recess of the third ventricle. Note the regional distribution of the ependymal cilia, the bidirectional transport within the processes of the tanycytes, and the intimate contact between the tanycytes and the fenestrated capillaries of the median eminence. (*Adapted from:* Kendall et al., 1972.)

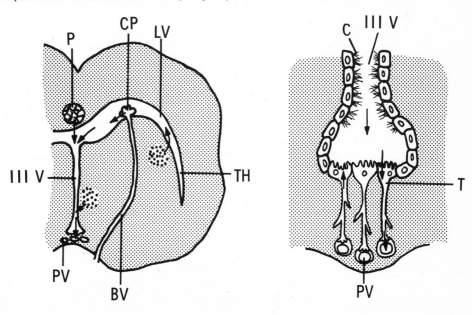

internal plexus of the median eminence. The tanycytes are believed to accumulate and transport HHH from the third ventricle to the capillary plexuses of the median eminence and hence to the adenohypophysis (see Section 2-2). The ependymal cilia found in the upper two-thirds of the third ventricle, but absent from the tanycytes and other ependymal cells lining the infundibular recess, may aid in the transport of the HHH from the ventricle to the infundibular recess. The tanycytes may then accumulate and transport these hormones to the capillary plexuses of the median eminence and hence to the adenohypophysis. The opposite situation may also arise since the tanycytes may serve to accumulate and transport adeno- and neurohypophyseal hormones (derived from the so-called retrograde blood flow from the pituitary to the median eminence) to the third ventricle (see Figures 2-6b and 2-6d).

SECTION 2-1: POST-TEST QUESTIONS

1. Describe the protective shell in which the pituitary is encased.

2. Name the four classic subdivisions of the pituitary in man.
   a.
   b.
   c.
   d.

3. Name the hormones synthesized and/or stored and released from each of these four subdivisions (answer in same sequence as in question 2).
   a.
   b.
   c.
   d.

4. Name the embryological cells of origin for each of these same four subdivisions.
   a.
   b.
   c.
   d.

5. Name the interconnected system of arteries which forms the principal source of the blood for the hypothalamus and adenohypophysis.

6. Name the arteries forming the interconnected system described in question 5.

7. The a. _____, b. _____, and c. _____ _____ areas of the hypothalamus are richly vascularized by branches of the anterior, middle, and posterior d. _____ arteries, respectively.

8. The infundibulum, infundibular stem, and infundibular process (body of the neurohypophysis) are richly vascularized by capillaries derived mainly from the a. _____, b. _____, c. _____, and d. _____ _____ arteries.

9. The adenohypophysis is richly vascularized by capillaries mainly derived from capillaries found in the a. _____ and the b. _____ _____ of the medial basal hypothalamus. The latter capillary plexus receives its vascular input primarily from the c. _____ arteries.

10. Much of the blood in the medial basal hypothalamus appears to flow a. (to/from) _____ the pituitary. However, recent studies have shown that this blood can flow in the opposite direction thus providing an efficient pathway for hormones derived from, but not necessarily synthesized within the b. _____ to gain access to the c. _____ wherein a homeostatic regulation d. _____ _____ hormone synthesis and/or release can occur.

11. The specialized ependymal cells, known as a. _____, found in the b. _____ recess of the c. _____ ventricle, have been shown to accumulate hormones from the d. _____ fluid within the ventricle and transport them to the e. _____ loops derived from the f. _____ _____ plexus of the median eminence. There is growing evidence that g. _____ and _____ hormones may be transported in the h. (same/opposite) direction.

SECTION 2-1: POST-TEST ANSWERS

1. The ventral surface of the pituitary rests in a depression of the sphenoid bone known as the sella turcica. The dorsal surface of the pituitary is partially covered by a shelf of dura known as the diaphragma sellae.

2. a. Adenohypophysis (pars distalis or anterior pituitary)
   b. Neurohypophysis (pars nervosa or posterior pituitary)
   c. Pars intermedia (intermediate lobe)
   d. Pars tuberalis

3. a. TSH, GH, LH, FSH, Prl, ACTH (and MSH and β-endorphin)
   b. Oxytocin and ADH (or vasopressin)
   c. MSH (and ACTH and β-endorphin)
   d. None

4. a. Rathke's pouch (primitive mouth epithelial ectoderm)
   b. Diencephalic neural ectoderm
   c. Rathke's pouch
   d. Rathke's pouch

5. Circle of Willis

6. Posterior, middle, and anterior cerebral arteries and posterior and anterior communicating arteries.

7. a. supraoptic-preoptic
   b. lateral
   c. mammillary-posterior
   d. cerebral

8. a. superior
   b. middle
   c. inferior
   d. hypophyseal

9. a. neurohypophysis (infundibular process)
   b. median eminence (infundibulum or infundibular stalk)
   c. superior hypophyseal

10. a. to
    b. pituitary
    c. hypothalamus
    d. hypothalamic hypophysiotropic

11. a. tanycytes
    b. infundibular
    c. third

      d. cerebral spinal
      e. capillary
      f. internal
      g. adeno- and neurohypophyseal
      h. opposite

SECTION 2-2: OVERVIEW OF THE HYPOTHALAMO-ADENOHYPOPHYSEAL SYSTEM

OBJECTIVES:

The student should be able to:
1. Name the hypothalamic hypophysiotropic hormones and the adenohypophyseal hormones on which they exert their positive and negative regulatory effects.
2. Describe the synthesis, storage, release, and transport of the hypothalamic hypophysiotropic and adenohypophyseal hormones.
3. Describe the various types of feedback mechanisms used to control the homeostasis of the hypothalamo-adenohypophyseal system.

A. HYPOTHALAMIC HYPOPHYSIOTROPIC HORMONES

As described in Section 2-1, there is no direct neural contact between the hypothalamus and the adenohypophysis, yet the hypothalamus can both facilitate and inhibit the synthesis and secretion of the adenohypophyseal hormones. This homeostatic control is mediated through the actions of the Hypothalamic Hypophysiotropic Hormones (HHH, see Figure 2-9): Thyrotropin Releasing Hormone (TRH, see Section 3-8), Corticotropin Releasing Hormone (CRH, see Section 5-7), Luteinizing Hormone and Follicle Stimulating Hormone-Releasing Hormones (LH-RH and FSH-RH, respectively; see Sections 6-4 and 7-5), Prolactin Releasing and Inhibiting Hormones (PRH and PIH, respectively; see Sections 3-8 and 7-5) and Growth Hormone Releasing and Inhibiting Hormones (GH-RH and GH-IH, respectively; see Sections 7-5, 8-2, and 9-4). These hormones are also sometimes referred to as factors (e.g., CRF, PIF, etc.). Since recent evidence suggests that LH-RH and FSH-RH may in fact be the same molecule (see Sections 6-4 and 7-5), it has been proposed that a more appropriate name for this bifunctional hormone is Gonadotropin Releasing Hormone (Gn-RH). Somatostatin (SRIH) is also used by many endocrinologists as the name of choice for GH-IH. Both of these alternative names will be used throughout this text.

Of the HHH whose structures are known, TRH, Gn-RH (LH-RH), and somatostatin are peptides (3, 10, and 14 amino acids in length, respectively), whereas one of the principal candidates for PIH is a catecholamine (dopamine). TRH, Gn-RH, and somatostatin appear to be synthesized by traditional protein synthetic mechanisms. Although it is often speculated that these small peptides are in fact the posttranslational cleavage products of one or more large precursor or prohormone proteins, there is little direct evidence to support this hypothesis at the present time. (Evidence of a somatostatin prohormone being produced in the pancreas has been recently presented, but similar findings have yet to be reported for the brain.) The PIH, dopamine, is synthesized by a well established enzymatic pathway (see Section 4-2). The structures and synthesis of the other HHH have been firmly established, but recent evidence supports the speculation that many of them may be small peptides (e.g., CRH).

Most of the HHH appear to be synthesized in the somas of parvicellular (i.e., small) neurons found in various regions of the hypothalamus (see Figure 2-12). The HHH are then packaged into dense cored vesicles and transported to the axon terminals by an energy-dependent process resulting in a bidirectional flow of axonal neuroplasm. The vesicles are stored within the terminals pending their catabolic destruction (presumably by the actions of lysosomal enzymes) or the receipt of an appropriate depolarization of the axonal plasma membrane, which initiates the release of the vesicles by an exocytotic mechanism (see Sections 1-2 and 2-3). This depolarization-induced exocytotic release has been referred to as stimulus-secretion-coupling to draw the analogy with the process of excitation-contraction-coupling in striated muscle tissue.

Although recent studies have shown that the HHH can act as traditional neurotransmitters when released at interneuronal synaptic contacts, their most important function in neuroendocrine regulation is mediated undoubtedly by their release into either the

FIGURE 2-9: The site of the action of hypothalamic hypophysiotropic hormones (HHH) and the adenohypophyseal hormones whose synthesis and secretion they either facilitate or inhibit. Examples of the actions and/or hormones released by the adenohypophyseal hormones are also shown. (*Adapted from:* Junqueira and Carneiro, 1980.)

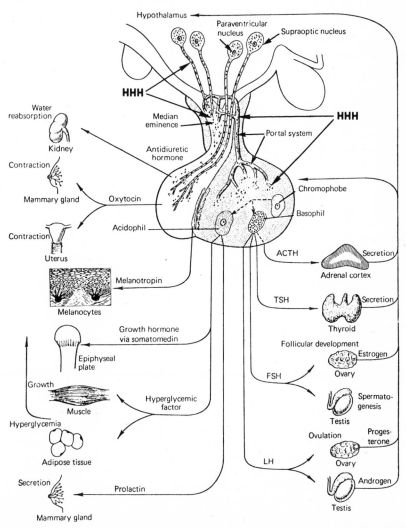

perivascular space in the median eminence or the periventricular space near the third ventricle. In the former site the HHH can diffuse directly into the fenestrated capillary loops of the external plexus, whereas at the latter site the HHH must diffuse through the CSF of the third ventricle to reach the infundibular recess wherein the tanycytes may accumulate these hormones and transport them to the capillary loops of the internal plexus (see Section 2-1). The infundibular (portal) system of capillaries can transport the HHH to the adenohypophysis where these hormones diffuse through the fenestrations in the endothelial cells lining the capillaries and bind to specific receptors on the plasma membranes of their target cells. This binding results in either the stimulation or inhibition of the synthesis and release of the various adenohypophyseal hormones (for details on individual HHH see the appropriate chapters emphasizing each HHH-adeno-hypophyseal hormone system).

B. FEEDBACK LOOP REGULATION

Up to now the hypothalamo-adenohypohyseal system has been described as though it operated without homeostatic controls; however, as discussed in Section 1-4, there are feedback control systems regulating the synthesis and secretion of essentially all of the hormones in the body. Tropic hormones released from the adenohypophysis stimulate a variety of actions in their target tissues in the body, one of which is the synthesis and secretion of still other hormones (see Figure 2-9). These hormones can in turn exert

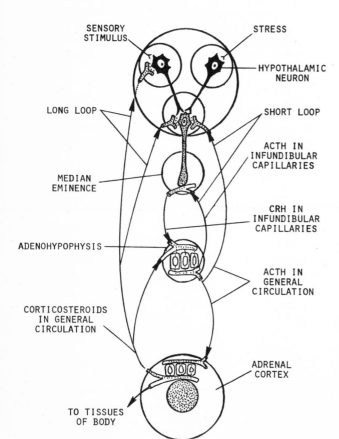

FIGURE 2-10: A diagram illustrating long and short feedback loops using the hypothalamo - adenohypophyseal-adrenal axis as a model (see Section 5-7 for further details). The diagram also depicts the fact that stressful stimuli can directly influence this (and several other) neuroendocrine systems.

many actions in their target tissues in the periphery as well as in the brain where they may influence behavior, neuronal metabolism, and electrical activity and even the synthesis and secretion of the HHH. These hormones may also act at the level of the adenohypophysis to influence the actions of the HHH on their target cells. Thus, in long feedback loops (see Figure 2-10) the hormones produced in these peripheral target organs can travel in the general circulation to reach the brain and/or pituitary and influence the synthesis, release, and/or action of the HHH. (*Q. 2-5*) *Can you describe the various blood vessels through which a hormone must travel (once it reaches the internal carotid and/or basilar artery) in order to influence the cells producing HHH in the ventromedial region of the hypothalamus? (Q. 2-6) What additional and/or different vessels must be traversed in order for this hormone to reach the cells producing the adenohypophyseal hormones?*

In negative feedback loops the hormones produced in the peripheral glands act to inhibit the synthesis, release, and/or action of the HHH (e.g., inhibition of TRH actions in the pituitary by thyroid hormone; see Section 3-8), whereas in positive feedback loops the opposite situation occurs (e.g., stimulation of the synthesis, release, and actions of Gn-RH prior to ovulation by estrogenic hormone; see Section 7-6). In addition and in contrast to these long feedback loops, recent anatomic and physiologic evidence has supported the existence of short feedback loops wherein the adenohypophyseal hormones act in the brain (presumably in the hypothalamus) to directly influence the synthesis and/or secretion of the HHH. (*Q. 2-7*) *Can you describe the most probable vascular route which mediates the effect of this short feedback loop on the adenohypophyseal hormones?* Although the evidence supporting the existence of short feedback loops is increasing (especially for growth hormone and prolactin; e.g., see Section 7-6D), the preeminent importance of the long feedback loops in regulating the day-to-day fluctuations in the secretion of adenohypophyseal hormones appears undeniable.

SECTION 2-2: POST-TEST QUESTIONS

1. Name the seven HHH and the adenohypophyseal hormones whose synthesis and/or secretion they either facilitate or inhibit.
   a.
   b.
   c.
   d.
   e.
   f.
   g.

2. Given that Gn-RH and TRH both stimulate adenylate cyclase activity prior to their selective stimulation of LH (and FSH) and TSH secretion, respectively. Why does Gn-RH fail to stimulate the secretion of TSH?

3. In a. ____(long/short)____ feedback loops the adenohypophyseal hormones directly influence the secretion of HHH, whereas in b. ____(long/short)____ feedback loops their influence on HHH secretion (and/or action) is indirectly mediated through the actions of other c. _____.

4. Of the established HHH, a. _____, b. _____, and c. _____
_____ are peptides of 3 to 14 amino acids in length, while at least one of the
endogenous biochemicals with d. _____ activity is known to be a
e. _____.

5. By what mechanism is each HHH released from its cell of origin? Explain.

6. How do the HHH get from their site of synthesis to their site of action in the
adenohypophysis?

SECTION 2-2: POST-TEST ANSWERS

1. a. Thyrotropin Releasing Hormone (TRH), Thyroid Stimulating Hormone (TSH)
   b. Corticotropin Releasing Hormone (CRH), Adrenocorticotropic Hormone (ACTH)
   c. Gonadotropin Releasing Hormone (Gn-RH), Luteinizing Hormone (LH) and Folli-
      cle Stimulating Hormone (FSH)
   d. Prolactin Releasing Hormone (PRH), Prolactin (Prl)
   e. Prolactin Inhibiting Hormone (PIH), Prolactin (Prl)
   f. Growth Hormone Releasing Hormone (GH-RH), Growth Hormone (GH)
   g. Somatostatin, Growth Hormone (GH)
2. Although it is true that both Gn-RH and TRH appear to stimulate an increase in
   adenylate cyclase activity as a necessary prerequisite to the increased synthesis and
   secretion of LH (and FSH) and TSH, respectively, each of these HHH initiates this
   mechanism by first interacting with an apparently specific receptor on the plasma
   membrane of the gonadotropes (for LH and FSH) or the thyrotropes (for TSH). Thus, it
   is the interaction of the HHH with a receptor at the plasma membranes of a given cell
   type within the adenohypophysis that determines the specificity of the action of the
   HHH.
3. a. short
   b. long
   c. hormones or factors
4. a. TRH
   b. Gn-RH (LH-RH)
   c. somatostatin
   d. PIH (or inhibitory)
   e. catecholamines (dopamine)
5. Exocytosis of the HHH-containing vesicles. The HHH-containing neurons are depolarized by appropriate stimuli, this depolarization travels to the axon terminal
   wherein a so-called stimulus-secretion-coupling process facilitates the fusion of

HHH-containing vesicles with the plasma membrane of the axon terminal. This fusion results in the expulsion of the contents of the vesicles, which in this case includes the HHH. Additional details of this mechanism can be found in Section 1-2.

6. The peptide HHH are synthesized in the neuronal cell bodies, packaged into vesicles, transported to the axon terminal by axoplasmic flow, released from the axon terminal by exocytosis into either the perivascular space near the capillary loops of the external plexus or the periventricular space near the third ventricle. In the former situation the HHH diffuses into the "portal" capillaries, travels to the adenohypophysis, diffuses out of the capillaries and interacts with its target cells. In the latter situation, the HHH must first diffuse through the third ventricle to the infundibular recess wherein it may be taken up by the tanycytes, transported to the capillary loops of the internal plexus and taken up by these capillaries and transported to the adenohypophysis by the same mechanism as described for the former situation.

SECTION 2-3: THE HYPOTHALAMO-NEUROHYPOPHYSEAL SYSTEM

OBJECTIVES:

The student should be able to:

1. Name the locations and describe the basic anatomy of the cells of origin for the neurohypophyseal hormones.
2. Name the neurohypophyseal hormones, and describe their basic chemistry.
3. Describe the synthesis, intraneuronal transport, storage, and release of the neurohypophyseal hormones.
4. Describe the neural control of the synthesis and secretion of the neurohypophyseal hormones.

A. ANATOMY OF THE MAGNOCELLULAR NEURONS

Within the hypothalamus, magnocellular (i.e., large) neurons in the supraoptic and paraventricular nuclei are the major source of production for the neurohypophyseal hormones, oxytocin, and Antidiuretic Hormone (ADH, or vasopressin) (see Figures 2-4, 2-11, and 2-12). Both of these nuclei receive a very dense blood supply from branches of the anterior cerebral arteries. Microscopic examination of the magnocellular neurons reveals that they are specialized for active protein synthesis (see Figure 2-11). For example, during periods of prolonged increases in the synthesis of the neurohypophyseal hormones (e.g., dehydration for ADH and lactation for oxytocin) there is a pronounced increase in the size of the Golgi apparatus and rough endoplasmic reticulum (changes that are thought to reflect the increase in the packaging and synthesis, respectively, of neurohypophyseal hormones) and an increase in the number of large dense-cored vesicles (DCV, approximately 150 nm in diameter) stored in the magnocellular nerve terminals in the neurohypophysis. However, only about 30% of the DCV are found in the axon terminals adjacent to neurohypophyseal capillaries (see Figures 2-11 and 2-13). It is likely that this fraction corresponds to the so-called readily releasable pool of neurohypophyseal hormones (see below). Most of the remaining DCV are found in the axon terminal regions, which are not adjacent to neurohypophyseal capillaries and thus may correspond to a storage pool for the neurohypophyseal hormone. Histological studies with laboratory rodents have revealed that some of the magnocellular neurons send axonal branches to terminate on capillary loops in the median eminence (see Figure 2-12). (*Q. 2-8*) *What does this latter anatomic relationship suggest about the*

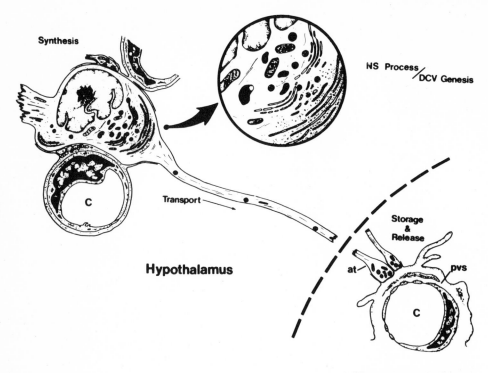

Neurohemal Organ

FIGURE 2-11: A schematic representation of a magnocellular supraoptic or paraventricular neuron. The diagram emphasizes the fact that the neurohypophyseal hormone-carrier protein complex is synthesized by traditional protein synthetic mechanisms. Note the denseness of the rough endoplasmic reticulum shown in the inset. The diagram also emphasizes the close association of the magnocellular cell bodies with blood capillaries (c). The neurohypophyseal hormone-protein complex is packaged into dense cored vesicles (DCV) by the Golgi apparatus (see inset), transported down the unmyelinated axons by an energy-dependent neuroplasmic flow mechanism and stored in the axon terminals (at), pending depolarization-induced exocytotic release into the perivascular space (pvs) within the neurohypophysis. (*Source:* Clattenburg, 1974.)

potential role of neurohypophyseal hormones in the regulation of the secretion of adenohypophyseal hormones?

B. STRUCTURE AND BIOSYNTHESIS OF OXYTOCIN, ADH, AND THE NEUROPHYSINS

Ocytocin and ADH are both octapeptides arranged with a five member ring linked with a disulfide bond and a tail containing three amino acids (see Figure 2-14). With the exception of two amino acids (shown underlined Figure 2-14) these hormones have identical structures. (*Q. 2-9*) *Would you predict the two hormones to have absolutely specific or somewhat overlapping actions?* Experiments with organ cultures have shown that de novo synthesis of these hormones is not possible in either the infundibular stem or the neurohypophysis, whereas synthesis is possible in cultures containing neurons from the SON and PVN. Since the synthesis can be blocked by treatment with either puromycin or cycloheximide, it appears to be mediated by traditional protein synthetic mechanisms. Recent studies have suggested that these peptide hormones (and

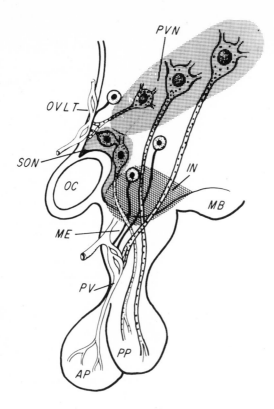

FIGURE 2-12: A sagittal section through the human hypothalamus and pituitary illustrating the magnocellular neurons of the paraventricular (PVN) and supraoptic (SON) nuclei and the parvicellular neurons of the preoptic area (rostral to the PVN), ventromedial (ventral to the PVN) and arcuate nuclei (shown in the shaded infundibular region, IN). Note that the PVN and SON each contain magnocellular neurons which synthesize oxytocin and ADH and that, although most of their axons pass directly through the IN to the neurohypophysis (PP), some deviate from this path to make functional contacts with infundibular (portal) capillary vessels (PV) in the median eminence (ME), thus raising the possibility that the neurohypophyseal hormones may act as HHH. Note also that the parvicellular neurons synthesizing HHH make functional contacts with blood vessels of the organum vaculosum in the lamina terminalis (OVLT) as well as with the PV in the ME. (*Source:* Zimmerman and Antunes, 1976).

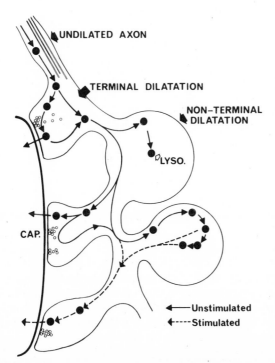

FIGURE 2-13: A schematic representation of a hypothetical path taken by dense-cored vesicles (DCV) within the axons of magnocellular neurons terminating in the neurohypophysis. Note that only about 30% of the DCV are found in the terminal dilations wherein they could be released by exocytosis into the perivascular space surrounding the fenestrated capillaries (CAP) within the neurohypophysis. The remaining DCV are found in either the unmyelinated axons (i.e., still in transit to the neurohypophysis) or in the nonterminal dilations. The DCV within the nonterminal dilations appear to be stored pending either their catabolic destruction by lysosomal enzymes or their diffusion to the terminal dilations where they may be released by exocytosis following the appropriate depolarization of the axon terminal. (*Source:* Cross et al., 1975.)

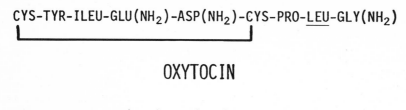

CYS-TYR-ILEU-GLU(NH$_2$)-ASP(NH$_2$)-CYS-PRO-<u>LEU</u>-GLY(NH$_2$)

OXYTOCIN

CYS-TYR-PHE-GLU(NH$_2$)-ASP(NH$_2$)-CYS-PRO-<u>ARG</u>-GLY(NH$_2$)

ANTIDIURETIC HORMONE

FIGURE 2-14: The primary amino acid sequence of the neurohypophyseal hormones, oxytocin and ADH. Note the similarity in the amino acid sequences.

many others, see Section 1-2) may be derived from the posttranslational cleavage of protein prohormones. These proteins are thought to be synthesized on rough endoplasmic reticulum in the magnocellular neurons of the SON and PVN, packaged into large DCV by the Golgi apparatus and then cleaved to form the neurohypophysial hormones and specific "carrier" proteins known as neurophysins (see Figure 2-15). The neurophysins have an approximate molecular weight of 10,000 daltons, and although they appear to be bound to the neurohypophyseal hormones while they are within the DCV, this binding does not persist following their release into the systemic circulation. (Q. *2-10*) *How and why are the neurophysins released from the DCV into the blood supply draining the neurohypophysis?* The circulating neurophysin proteins have no known intrinsic physiologic actions, but a variety of biochemical and immunohistochemical studies have clearly suggested that humans have at least two different neurophysins: Nicotine-Stimulated Neurophysin (NSN) and Estrogen-Stimulated Neurophysin (ESN). The concentration of NSN in blood correlates well with the secretion of ADH, whereas the concentration of ESN correlates with the secretion of oxytocin.

FIGURE 2-15: A diagramatic representation of a neuron in the process of synthesizing oxytocin. Note the proposed synthesis and packaging of a prohormone, which is later cleaved to form oxytocin and estrogen-stimulated neurophysin. (*Adapted from:* Cross et al., 1975.)

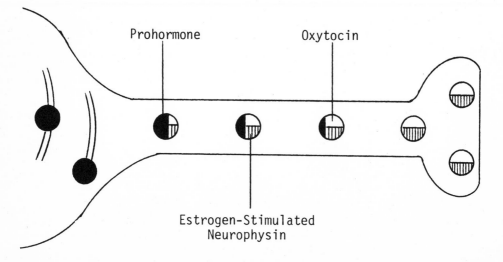

C. INTRACELLULAR TRANSPORT AND STORAGE OF OXYTOCIN, ADH, ESN, AND NSN

Since oxytocin, ADH, ESN, and NSN are synthesized within the cell bodies of magno-cellular neurons found in the SON and PVN regions of the hypothalamus, the DCV containing these biochemicals must be transported to the neurohypophysis where they are stored pending release (see Figures 2-11, 2-13, and 2-15). This energy-dependent transport is analogous to that described earlier for the DCV containing the HHH. It is important to note that the axoplasmic transport of DCV is not unique since mitochondria, enzymes, and other materials are also transported from the neuronal cell body to its axon terminals (and vice versa). Recent experiments have shown that it takes approximately 90 minutes for the synthesis and packaging to occur and an additional 30 minutes to complete the transport of the newly synthesized prohormone-, hormone-, and neurophysin-containing DCV to the neurohypophysis. (Q. 2-11) *Based on this time course, would you predict that the secretion of neurohypophyseal hormones following an abrupt stimulus (e.g., oxytocin can be released within 30 seconds after the onset of suckling stimulation in a lactating woman) is linked to the synthesis of those hormones?* These studies have also suggested that the hormones are segregated into two functional, if not anatomical, pools corresponding to a readily releasable and a storage pool (see Figure 2-13). The mechanism(s) by which the DCV are shuttled from the storage to the readily releasable pool is unknown as is the mechanism(s) by which "aging" DCV are selected for destruction by lysosomal enzymes.

D. EXOCYTOTIC RELEASE OF OXYTOCIN, ADH, ESN, AND NSN

The mechanism of release of neurohypophyseal hormones is analogous to that described earlier for the HHH and can be considered as a model for the release of many other biochemicals stored in the intracellular vesicles (see Figure 2-16). In neurohypophyseal neurons, exocytosis is initiated by the depolarization of the axon terminal. This depolarization is precipitated by the invasion of an action potential traveling down the axon from the neuronal cell body found in the hypothalamus. Although recent

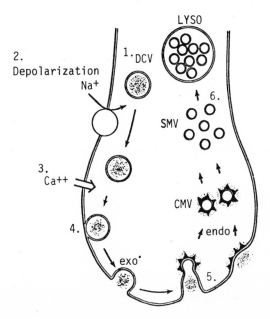

FIGURE 2-16: A schematic representation of the stimulus-secretion-coupled-exocytotic mechanism of release for the neurohypophyseal hormones. The hormones, together with their associated neurophysins are transported to the axon terminal in large dense-cored vesicles (DCV) (Step 1). The actual mechanism of release is initiated by a traveling wave of axonal depolarization (i.e., the action potential) (Step 2), which invades the axon terminal and facilitates the necessary increase in the influx of calcium ions (Step 3), the fusion of the DCV with the plasma membrane (Step 4), the exocytotic (exo) emptying of the vesicular contents, the endocytotic (endo) reuptake of the vesicular membrane forming coated microvesicles (CMV) (Step 5), the conversion of these CMV to smooth microvesicles (SMV) (Step 6), and finally, the destruction of the SMV by the lysosomal (LYSO) enzymes. (*Adapted from:* Douglas, 1974.)

studies have shown that the entry of sodium ions, normally evident during depolarization, is not required for exocytosis, the depolarization-induced influx of calcium ions is an absolute requirement. The DCV fuses with the plasma membrane of the axon terminal and releases its contents (i.e., both the neurohypophyseal hormone and its associated neurophysin) into the perivascular space. Since the plasma membrane of the axon terminal normally does not grow in response to an increase in the secretion of neurohypophyseal hormones, it is apparent that the vesicular membrane does not remain fused with the plasma membrane. The vesicular membrane is in fact taken back into the axon terminal by endocytosis (i.e., the reverse of exocytosis), and in the process forms coated microvesicles which are in turn converted into smooth microvesicles and then destroyed by lysosomal enzymes. As mentioned in Section 2-2, this linkage between depolarization and exocytotic hormone secretion has been termed stimulus-secretion-coupling to point out the similarities between this mechanism and the excitation-contraction-coupling employed by striated muscle. Both mechanisms have an absolute requirement for calcium, and both the striated muscle cells and DCV membranes contain actin-myosin-like proteins. It has been speculated that these proteins may be involved in the actual contraction of the DCV following its fusion with the plasma membrane and thereby facilitate the exocytotic release of the vesicular contents.

E. OVERVIEW OF NEURAL CONTROL AND PERIPHERAL ACTIONS OF OXYTOCIN

The milk let-down reflex is clearly one of the most important examples of the neural control of the release of oxytocin (see Figure 2-17). Stimulation of the areolar region of

FIGURE 2-17: A schema of the milk let-down reflex. Suckling stimulation leads to an increase in the release of oxytocin from the neurohypophysis. Stress can often lead to an inhibition of this process.

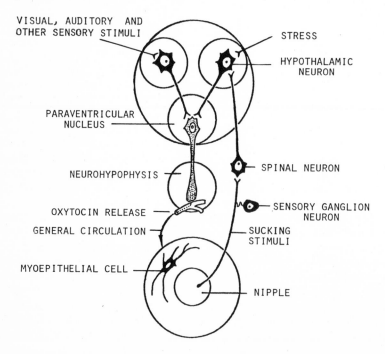

the breast (see Figure 7-2) during suckling activates somesthetic nervous pathways (e.g., lateral spinothalamic pathway) which transmit this signal (through a multisynaptic pathway) to and within the hypothalamus where the discharge frequency (i.e., an index of the degree of neuronal activity) of neurohypophyseal magnocellular neurons in the paraventricular (and supraoptic) nucleus is increased. The increased frequency of depolarization in these neurons activates the stimulus-secretion-coupled-exocytotic secretion of oxytocin from the readily releasable pool of DCV within the neurohypophysis (see Figures 2-13 and 2-16). Prolonged suckling stimulation can eventually initiate an increase in the synthesis of oxytocin. (*Q. 2-12*) *Approximately how long would you guess it to take to transport this newly synthesized hormone to the neurohypophysis?*

Oxytocin induces an increase in the pressure within the gland and the release of milk by stimulating the contraction of the myoepithelial cells, which cover the stromal surface of the epithelium of the alveoli, ducts, and cisterns of the breast (see Section 7-4D and Figures 2-17 and 7-2). The latency from onset of suckling stimulation until the release of milk can be as short as 30 to 60 seconds, but stress can delay or even prevent this response. The mechanism of this inhibition is mediated through an inhibition of the suckling-induced increase in the secretion of oxytocin.

The secretion of oxytocin can be conditioned such that physical stimulation of the nipple is no longer required. For example, it is common, and sometimes inconvenient, that a nursing woman can experience a let-down reflex in response to the sight and/or sound of her own or even someone else's baby. (A similar response can be elicited in dairy cattle by the mere presence of the person who normally performs the milking.) The secretion of oxytocin can also be elicited in response to genital tract stimulation such as that which occurs during either copulation or labor. In women still lactating from a previous pregnancy, it has been reported that milk can be released from the breast in synchrony with labor pains. Oxytocin is thought to aid in the final stages of parturition by stimulating the depolarization of myometrial smooth muscle membranes in the estrogen-primed uterus (see Section 7-40). Even though oxytocin is produced and released in men (e.g., in response to genital tract stimulation), it appears to have no known functions.

F. OVERVIEW OF NEURAL CONTROL AND PERIPHERAL ACTIONS OF ADH (VASOPRESSIN)

The principal stimuli for increasing the secretion of ADH are increases in the osmotic pressure of blood plasma (e.g., due to dehydration or the administration of an oral load of hypertonic saline) and reduction in the total circulating volume of blood (e.g., due to hemorrhage). Conversely, the two principal stimuli for decreasing the secretion of ADH are decreases in the osmotic pressure of blood plasma (e.g., due to excessive drinking of water or other hypotonic fluids) and expansions in the apparent blood volume (e.g., infusion of isotonic saline intravenously). Alcohol and emotional stress can inhibit the secretion of ADH, while nicotine facilitates it (see Figure 2-18). (*Q. 2-13*) *What is the name of the neurophysin that is released in association with ADH?*

The primary physiologic action of ADH is to stimulate an increase in water reabsorption by the kidney, leading to an increase in the concentration of urine and a decrease in the osmotic pressure of blood plasma. Although these antidiuretic actions are well established, ADH can also exhibit potent pressor actions on blood vessels when administered in pharmacologically high doses. Neurophysiological experiments with laboratory animals have shown that there are clear increases in the discharge frequency of magnocellular neurons in the supraoptic nucleus in response to increases in the osmolarity of blood plasma or to an acute decrease in the total volume of blood. Other studies have shown that stimuli arising from changes in osmolarity and blood volume are

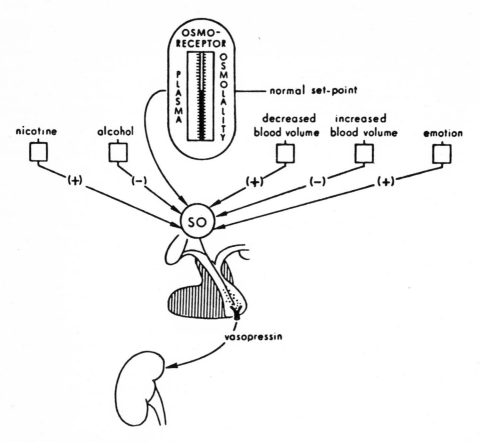

FIGURE 2-18: A review of the various stimuli which either stimulate or inhibit the release of ADH (vasopressin). (*Adapted from:* Ezrin et al., 1979.)

additive with respect to increasing the secretion of ADH; when the stimuli are in opposite directions, neither dominates. (*Q. 2-14*) *Do these data suggest that changes in osmolarity and blood volume increase the secretion of ADH by activating the same or different populations of neurosecretory cells?*

SECTION 2-3: POST-TEST QUESTIONS

1. The a. (size) _____ peptide hormones, ADH and oxytocin are produced in b. (magnocellular/parvicellular/multicellular) neurons in both the c. _____ and d. _____ nuclei of the hypothalamus.

2. Recent studies have suggested that ADH and oxytocin are derived from a protein a. _____ which is later cleaved to yield the peptide hormone and their associated "carrier" proteins called b. _____. This entire complex is packaged into large c. _____ vesicles by the d. _____ apparatus.

3. The neurohypophyseal hormones are transported down the a. (myelinated/unmyelinated) axons via an b. _____-dependent process also utilized for the bidirectional transport of c. _____.

SECTION 2-3: POST-TEST ANSWERS

4. In humans there are two types of neurophysins: a. _____-stimulated and b. _____-stimulated neurophysin. The former is associated normally with the secretion of ADH, while the latter is associated normally with the secretion of oxytocin.

5. The a. _____-_____ coupled b. _____ release mechanism utilized by neurohypophyseal hormones is initiated by the c. _____ _____ of the axon terminal which leads to a necessary d. (increase/decrease) in the e. (influx/efflux) of f. _____ ions. The DCV then g. _____ with the plasma membrane and releases its contents by a process known as h. _____ into the i. _____ space. The vesicular membrane is then taken back into the axon terminal by a process known as j. _____, forming a k. _____ which are then converted into l. _____ _____ prior to their destruction by m. _____ enzymes.

6. Stimulation of the areolar region of the breast during suckling can result in an a. (increase/decrease) in the b. _____ rate of magnocellular neurons in the c. _____ nucleus of the hypothalmus. This response leads to an increase in the secretion of d. _____ which in turn produces an increase in the contraction of the e. _____ cells lining the stromal surface of the epithelium of the alveoli, ducts and cisterns of the breast.

7. What are the two principal stimuli for increasing the secretion of ADH?
   a.
   b.
   What are the two principal stimuli for decreasing the secretion of ADH?
   c.
   d.
   What is the principal physiologic action of ADH?
   e.

SECTION 2-3: POST-TEST ANSWERS

1. a. octa
   b. magnocellular
   c. supraoptic
   d. paraventricular
2. a. prohormones
   b. neurophysins
   c. dense cored
   d. Golgi
3. a. unmyelinated
   b. energy
   c. mitochondria, enzymes and other biochemicals
4. a. nicotine
   b. estrogen
5. a. stimulus-secretion
   b. exocytotic
   c. depolarization
   d. increase
   e. influx
   f. calcium
   g. fuses
   h. exocytosis

      i. perivascular
      j. endocytosis
     k. coated microvesicle
     l. smooth microvesicle
    m. lysosomal

6. a. increase
    b. discharge
    c. paraventricular
    d. oxytocin
    e. myoepithelial

7. a. Increase in the osmotic pressure of blood plasma.
    b. Decreases in the total volume of blood.
    c. Decreases in the osmotic pressure of blood plasma.
    d. Increases in the apparent volume of blood.
    e. Stimulation of an increase in the reabsorption of water from the urine.

SELECTED REFERENCES

Bergland, R. M., and Page, R. B., 1979, Pituitary-brain vascular relations: A new paradigm, *Science* 204: 18.

Bowers, C. Y., Folkers, K., Knudsen, R., Lam, Y.-K., Wan, Y.-P., Humphries, J., and Chang, D., 1979, Hypothalamic peptide hormones; chemistry and physiology, in *Endocrinology*, L. J. DeGroot, G. F. Cahill, Jr., L. Martini, D. H. Nelsen, W. D. Odell, J. T. Potts, Jr., E. Steinberger and A. I. Winegrad (Eds.), New York: Grune & Stratton, Vol. 1, p. 65.

Brownstein, M. J., Russell, J. T., and Gainer, H., 1980, Synthesis, transport, and release of posterior pituitary hormones, *Science* 207: 373.

Martin, J. B., Reichlin, S., and Brown, G. M., 1977, *Clinical Neuroendocrinology*, Philadelphia: F. A. Davis Co.

Motta, M. (Ed.), 1980, *The Endocrine Functions Of The Brain*, New York: Raven Press.

CHAPTER

3

THE THYROID GLAND

SECTION 3-1: ANATOMY AND EMBRYOLOGY OF THE THYROID GLAND

OBJECTIVES:

The student should be able to state:
1. Gross anatomic relationships of the thyroid gland, including vasculature and neural innervation.
2. The components of a follicle.
3. Two developmental abnormalities associated with the gland, specifically the thyroglossal duct.

The thyroid gland lies just anterior to the trachea at the level of the fifth, sixth, and seventh cervical vertebrae. It is a bilobed structure with an isthmus connecting the two divisions (see Figure 3-1). The gland is one of the most highly vascularized areas of the body, receiving a rich supply of blood from the superior and inferior thyroid arteries. Innervation is via sympathetic and parasympathetic fibers arising from the superior cervical ganglion and vagus nerve, respectively (see Figure 4-1).

The basic functional unit of the thyroid is termed the follicle (see Figure 3-2). Each follicle consists of a sphere of epithelial cells (follicular cells) surrounding a colloid core. This colloid material is composed of the glycoprotein thyroglobulin, which acts as a storage depot for thyroxine (T_4) and triiodothyronine (T_3). Generally, the level of secretory activity of the follicular cells can be estimated as a direct function of their height.

A second cell type is also present in the thyroid gland. These are the C-cells or parafollicular cells, which are found in the interstitial spaces between adjacent follicles. These cells synthesize and release calcitonin, a hormone important in calcium metabolism. This subject is discussed in more detail in Chapter 10 in connection with the parathyroid gland.

The thyroid develops initially as a midline evagination from the floor of the embryonic pharynx. The pocket enlarges, grows posteriorly, and then bifurcates. The base of each bifurcation will subsequently give rise to a lobe of the gland. The thyroid and the

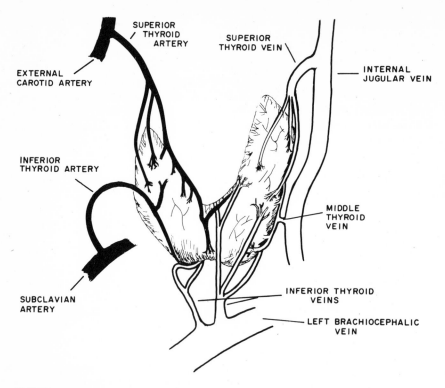

FIGURE 3-1: Gross anatomy and blood supply of the thyroid gland. The arteries are shown only on the left side of the specimen; veins are shown only on the right.

FIGURE 3-2: The histologic appearance of the thyroid gland.

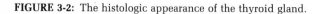

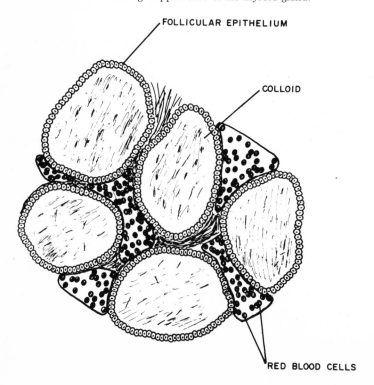

pharynx are connected during early development by a thin tube termed the thyroglossal duct, whose opening in the mouth at the base of the tongue is the foramen cecum. This duct atrophies during the later stages of fetal development. Failure of remnants of thyroid tissue to atrophy results in anomalies such as an ectopic thyroid gland in the musculature of the tongue.

SECTION 3-1: POST-TEST QUESTIONS

1. The thyroid gland lies just anterior to which one of the following structures in the neck:
   a. esophagus
   b. carotid sheath
   c. trachea
   d. thymus
2. Name two different secretory cell types found in the thyroid gland.
   a.
   b.
3. The a. _____ and b. _____ arteries supply the thyroid gland. Capillary networks form from these arteries and supply each c. _____ (i.e., the basic functional units of the thyroid gland).
4. Each follicle possesses a colloid core, which is composed of _____.
5. Follicles containing cuboidal cells are more/less (circle one) active than follicles containing columnar cells.
6. The C-cells are active in synthesis of:
   a. epinephrine
   b. thyroxine
   c. calcitonin
7. The thyroid gland develops initially as a midline evagination from the floor of the _____.
8. The a. _____ and b. _____ are connected during early development by a thin tube called the c. _____, whose opening in the mouth at the base of the tongue is called the d. _____.

SECTION 3-1: POST-TEST ANSWERS

1. c
2. a. C-cells
   b. follicular cells
3. a. superior
   b. inferior thyroid
   c. follicle
4. thyroglobulin
5. less active
6. c
7. pharynx
8. a. thyroid or pharynx
   b. pharynx or thyroid
   c. thyroglossal duct
   d. foramen cecum

SECTION 3-2: HORMONES OF THE THYROID GLAND

OBJECTIVES

The student should be able to:
1. Identify the chemical structures of thyroxine and triiodothyroxine.
2. Describe briefly how iodide is handled by the body.

Thyroxine, triiodothyroxine, and calcitonin are the three major hormones of the thyroid gland. The follicular cells elaborate T_4 and T_3, whereas calcitonin is synthesized by the C-cells. The chemical structures of thyroxine and triiodothyroxine are illustrated in Figure 3-3. Calcitonin is considered in Chapter 10 when the parathyroid gland is discussed.

It is important to note that T_4 and T_3 contain iodide atoms, which are necessary for biologic activity. Since the thyroid gland does not discriminate between nonradioactive and radioactive iodide in the production of thyroid hormones, it has been possible for researchers to learn a great deal about uptake of iodide by the thyroid, its incorporation into thyroid hormones, its storage within the thyroid gland, and its subsequent release into the blood. For example, approximately 1 mg of iodide per week must be ingested to provide sufficient quantities of thyroid hormone to maintain a euthyroid or normal state. Iodide (I^-) contained in food and fluid is absorbed from the gastrointestinal tract into blood and then is rapidly taken up by the richly vascularized thyroid. Iodide is taken into the thyroid from the blood by active transport. It has been shown, for example, that the thyroid gland can transport iodide against an electrochemical gradient and that the concentration of iodide within the thyroid gland is about 25 times that in blood when compared as milligrams of iodide per gram of thyroid tissue versus milligrams of iodide per milliliter of plasma. For this reason the thyroid gland is considered to be an "iodide trap." The rate of uptake of iodide from the blood into the thyroid gland is controlled by the rate of secretion and blood concentration of thyroid stimulating hormone, which is produced by the anterior pituitary gland. The physiologic factors influencing the rate of secretion of TSH and its mechanism of action are discussed in Section 3-8.

FIGURE 3-3: The structures of thyroxine and triiodothyronine.

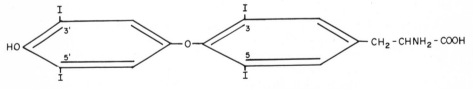

T_4, THYROXINE (3,5,3',5' - TETRAIODOTHYRONINE)

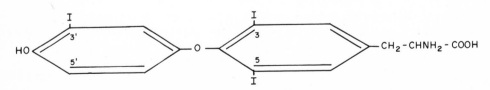

T_3, (3,5,3' - TRIIODOTHYRONINE)

SECTION 3-2: POST-TEST QUESTIONS

1. Which of the following products do the follicular cells synthesize?
   a. thyroxine (T_4)
   b. triiodothyronine (T_3)
   c. calcitonin
   d. corticosteroids
2. The thyroid gland has the ability to take up and concentrate _____ from the blood.
3. To which thyroid hormone does the following structure correspond?

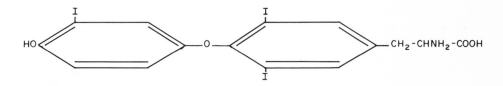

4. The ultimate sources of iodide are _____ and _____.
5. Why is the thyroid gland known as an "iodide trap"?

6. Hypothyroidism may not develop for months after production of thyroid hormones ceases because _____
   _____.

SECTION 3-2: POST-TEST ANSWERS

1. a and b
2. iodide
3. Triiodothyronine
4. food and fluid
5. Because it can transport iodide against an electrochemical gradient and contains 25 times more iodide than plasma.
6. the thyroid gland stores thyroid hormones.

SECTION 3-3: SYNTHESIS AND STORAGE OF THYROID HORMONES

OBJECTIVES:

The student should be able to:
1. State the four general steps in the synthesis of the thyroid hormones.
2. Recall two inhibitors of iodide trapping.
3. State which organ "competes" with the thyroid gland for iodide.
4. Name the enzymes involved in the synthesis of thyroid hormones.
5. State which residues in the thyroglobulin molecule are important for the synthesis of thyroid hormones.
6. State how thyroid hormone is stored.
7. State which hormone, T_3 or T_4, is synthesized in larger amounts by the thyroid gland.

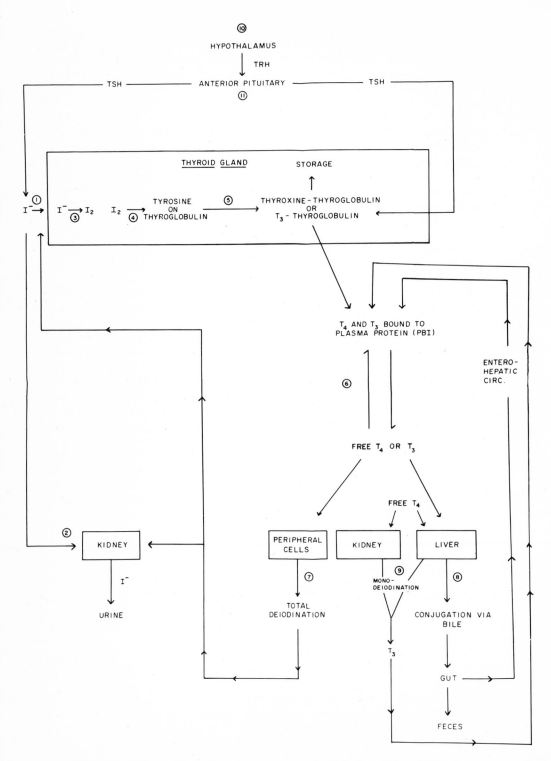

FIGURE 3-4: The iodide cycle and production and metabolism of thyroid hormones.

In Section 3-2, the uptake of iodide by the follicular cells was discussed. As you recall, this is the initial phase of the synthesis of thyroid hormone (step 1, Figure 3-4) and is referred to as "iodide trapping." This mechanism allows the thyroid gland to concentrate I^- to intracellular levels that are 25 or more times greater than that of the serum. There is evidence that the iodide trap is a metabolically driven, active transport system: for example, iodide is transported against an electrochemical gradient, anoxia or cyanide inhibits concentration of iodide by thyroid tissue, and both thiocyanate and perchlorate ions compete with iodide for sites on the transport mechanism.

Competition for iodide also occurs outside the thyroid gland. For example, the kidneys compete with the thyroid gland for iodide ions. About 20% of the cardiac output goes through the kidney, which may be why this organ removes about five times more iodide per unit time than the thyroid gland (step 2, Figure 3-4). Studies using radioactive iodide have shown that the kidney removes 50–70% of the injected dose within 24 hours and excretes it into urine, while 20–30% is taken up by the thyroid gland. The remainder is distributed throughout the body, particularly to the salivary glands and stomach. These organs also have the ability to concentrate or trap iodide ions but cannot make thyroid hormones from the trapped iodide. (*Q. 3-1*) *Can you suggest why?*

Following uptake of iodide by the follicular cells, the ion is oxidized to iodine (I_2) in a reaction catalyzed by a peroxidase enzyme (step 3, Figure 3-4). The same enzyme then iodinates tyrosyl residues contained in the thyroglobulin molecule (step 4, Figure 3-4). Thyroglobulin is a high molecular weight glycoprotein synthesized by the follicular cells of the thyroid gland. Each thyroglobulin molecule contains approximately 115 tyrosyl residues, which act as substrate for the peroxidase enzyme. About 10% of the tyrosyl residues are iodinated to form monoiodotyrosine (MIT) and diiodotyrosine (DIT). By a mechanism as yet incompletely understood, a coupling occurs between iodinated tyrosine residues, perhaps as a result of a conformational change in the thyroglobulin molecule. The coupling results in the formation of T_4 and T_3, but there are 8 to 10 times more molecules of T_4 formed than T_3 (step 5, Figure 3-4).

The most likely site of formation of T_4 and T_3 is the apical border of the follicular cell and the lumen of the follicle. Here electron microscopic photographs show a highly unfolded membrane with many microvilli. When the thyroglobulin molecule is iodinated and T_4 and T_3 are formed in it, the thyroglobulin is transported, perhaps by pinocytosis, across the cell wall into the follicular lumen, where it is stored.

SECTION 3-3: POST-TEST QUESTIONS

1. State the four general steps of thyroid hormone synthesis.
   a.
   b.
   c.
   d.
2. The amino acid contained in thyroglobulin that undergoes iodination to form MIT and DIT is _____.
3. The enzyme that performs the iodination is _____.
4. Name an organ that competes with the thyroid gland for iodide.
5. a. Which organs other than thyroid gland can trap and concentrate iodide?

   b. Why are they unable to synthesize thyroid hormones?

6. Name two compounds that compete with iodide for sites on the transport mechanism.
   a.
   b.
7. Which hormone, T_3 or T_4, is synthesized in larger amounts by the thyroid gland?

8. How are T_4 and T_3 stored in the thyroid gland?
9. Enzymatic iodination of tyrosine can occur only if this amino acid is free in the thyroid gland. (True/False)

SECTION 3-3: POST-TEST ANSWERS

1. a. Uptake of iodide
   b. Oxidation of iodide
   c. Iodination of tyrosine
   d. Coupling of DIT with DIT to form T_4 or MIT with DIT to form T_3
2. tyrosine
3. peroxidase
4. The kidney.
5. a. The salivary glands, the stomach.
   b. These organs do not contain a peroxidase enzyme.
6. a. Thiocyanate
   b. perchlorate
7. T_4
8. Attached to thyroglobulin in the lumen of the follicle.
9. False. Tyrosyl residues contained in the thyroglobulin molecule are the ones iodinated by the peroxidase enzyme of the thyroid gland.

SECTION 3-4: SECRETION OF THYROID HORMONES

OBJECTIVES:

The student should be able to:
1. Describe the process by which T_4 and T_3 are released from thyroglobulin.
2. Name the iodinated products released by the thyroid gland.
3. State whether T_4 or T_3 is released in greater amounts by the thyroid gland.
4. State whether T_4 or T_3 has greater biologic activity.
5. State whether storage of thyroid hormones occurs.

In the stored thyroglobulin of the thyroid gland there are on average about nine molecules of thyroxine for each molecule of triiodothyronine. Enough hormone is accumulated in the colloid to maintain normal serum levels (i.e., a euthyroid state) for approximately 3 months in the absence of the synthesis of T_4 and T_3.

The apical aspect of follicular cells possesses microvilli that penetrate the colloid and aid in both the deposition and the absorption of the glycoprotein, thyroglobulin. When the concentration of thyroid stimulating hormone in blood increases, pinocytotic vesicles containing colloid appear in this area of the follicular cells. These vesicles are acted on by proteolytic enzymes contained within thyroid cells and degradation of thyroglobulin occurs. This yields the products T_4, T_3, MIT, and DIT. The thyroid hormones are

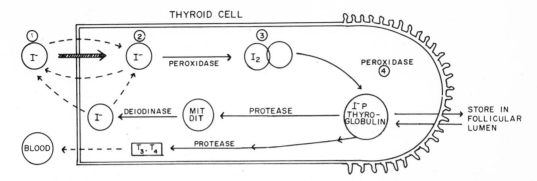

FIGURE 3-5: The production of thyroid hormones in vivo. Iodide ions from plasma are actively transported (dark arrows, step 1) into the thyroid cell (step 2), although some ions diffuse in and others out (dashed lines, step 1), depending on the relative concentrations of each. Iodide ions are oxidized to iodine (step 3), which is used by the peroxidase enzyme to iodinate tyrosine moieties within the thyroglobulin molecule (step 4). Following formation of T_4 and T_3, the thyroglobulin molecule is stored in the follicular lumen. See text for details for release of thyroglobulin from storage.

released into the circulation while MIT and DIT are deiodinated by enzymes within each thyroid cell. The iodide thus released is recycled by the thyroid cell (see Figure 3-5).

It is important to repeat that the only iodinated products released by the thyroid gland into blood are T_4 and T_3. Small amounts of thyroglobulin may leak out of the thyroid glands of normal individuals. Formation of antibodies to thyroglobulin appears to be suppressed under normal circumstances. When suppression does not occur, antibodies to thyroglobulin are formed and a disease known as Hashimoto's thyroiditis may develop.

The normal ratio of T_4 to T_3 released into blood from the thyroid gland is approximately 20:1. About 35% of the circulating T_4 is deiodinated peripherally to T_3. An additional 45% is deiodinated to reverse T_3 (3,5,5'-triiodothyronine) (see Figure 3-6). As a result, the ratio of the circulating level of T_4 to T_3 does not reflect accurately the ratio of these two substances when they were released from the thyroid gland. In man, about

FIGURE 3-6: The pathways for production and metabolism of thyroid hormones in normal man: T_4 and T_3 are secreted by the thyroid gland at rates of 100 and 5 nmole/day. Of the 100 nmole of T_4 produced per day, 35 is converted peripherally to T_3 and 45 to reverse T_3 (rT_3). The remainder is metabolized either by conjugation or oxidative deamination. The thyroid gland secretes negligible amounts (<5 nmole/day) of rT_3.

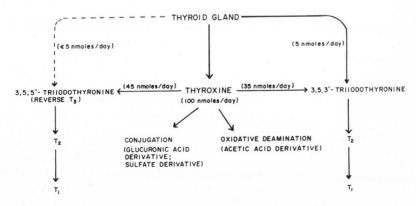

100 nmole of T_4 and about 5 nmole of T_3 are secreted by the thyroid gland daily. Because T_3 has three to five times the biologic activity of T_4, it is difficult to state whether T_3 or T_4 is *"the"* thyroid hormone on the basis of either the daily secretion rate or the biologic activity. We see later, however, that it now appears to be T_3 that is effective at the cellular level.

SECTION 3-4: POST-TEST QUESTIONS

1. What initiates the release of thyroglobulin from storage?

2. What is the first histologic evidence of release of thyroglobulin from storage?

3. a. How are iodinated products released from thyroglobulin? b. Name the products. c. State what happens to them after release from thyroglobulin.

4. What is the normal ratio of T_4 to T_3 released into blood?

5. Which hormone, T_4 or T_3, has greater biologic activity?

SECTION 3-4: POST-TEST ANSWERS

1. TSH
2. Colloid droplets appear in follicular cells.
3. a. By protease enzymes.
   b. MIT, DIT, T_4, T_3.
   c. MIT and DIT are deiodinated by a deiodinase enzyme; T_4 and T_3 are released into blood.
4. 20 : 1.
5. T_3

SECTION 3-5: TRANSPORT OF THYROID HORMONES IN THE BLOOD

OBJECTIVES:

The student should be able to:
1. List three proteins that are important in the transport of the thyroid hormones.
2. State the relative affinity of T_3 and T_4 for these proteins.
3. State why binding of thyroid hormones to plasma proteins is important.

T_4 and T_3 are poorly soluble in saline at physiologic pH (7.4). This property is of no physiologic consequence because these hormones are transported in blood bound to plasma proteins. In fact, the binding of T_4 is so good that 99.97% of the total amount in blood is bound. T_3 is less well bound—only 99.7% of the total amount in blood is bound. Although this difference of ~0.3% may appear unimportant, it constitutes the basis for a clinical test that is used to determine the availability of binding sites for T_4 on plasma proteins.

The three plasma proteins important in the transport of thyroid hormones are thyroxine binding globulin (TBG), prealbumin, and albumin. TBG should not be confused with thyroglobulin in the thyroid gland. Thyroxine binding globulin and albumin carry both T_3 and T_4, whereas prealbumin transports only T_4. In general, T_4 has a higher affinity for plasma proteins than does T_3. It is important to reemphasize that the bound hormone is in chemical equilibrium with the free hormone. Furthermore, it is the free hormone that is important for biologic activity. Binding of thyroid hormones to plasma proteins not only provides a transport system, but protects thyroid hormones from either being metabolized (conjugated with a glucuronide moiety) by the liver or excreted by the kidney. In addition, the bound hormone represents a storage depot that occurs because of the chemical equilibrium between the bound and free hormone.

Protein-bound iodide (PBI), a measure of the total amount of thyroid hormones bound to serum protein, has been used in the past to aid in assessing thyroid function clinically. Increases in PBI have been interpreted as being indicative of some forms of hyperthyroidism, whereas low values are indicative of hypothyroidism. Currently radioimmunoassay of T_3 and T_4 is used clinically to aid in the diagnosis of thyroid disorders (see Section 3-10).

Certain diseases and drugs are known to affect the transport and binding of thyroid hormone to plasma proteins. The simplest situation involves a drug or a disease known to alter the concentration of plasma protein. For example, in certain renal diseases plasma protein concentration is reduced because proteins are lost into urine. (Q. 3-2) *What would you expect the thyroid state of such patients to be?*

SECTION 3-5: POST-TEST QUESTIONS

1. Name three plasma proteins important in transporting thyroid hormones.
    a.
    b.
    c.
2. Why is it important for thyroid hormones to be transported by plasma proteins?

3. TBG is thyroglobulin released from the thyroid gland. (True/False)
4. The thyroid hormones bound to plasma proteins are in equilibrium with unbound or free thyroid hormones. (True/False)
5. The physiologically significant fraction of thyroid hormones in blood is the:
    a. bound fraction
    b. free fraction
    c. both fractions
6. What important physiologic benefits, besides transport, result from binding of thyroid hormones to plasma proteins?

7. PBI measures unbound T_4 and T_3. (True/False)
8. Increases in PBI are indicative of a. _____; decreases in PBI are indicative of b. _____.

SECTION 3-5: POST-TEST ANSWERS

1. a. thyroxine binding globulin (TBG)
   b. prealbumin
   c. albumin
2. Because they are poorly soluble at physiologic pH.
3. False
4. True
5. b
6. Protection from metabolism by liver and protection from excretion into urine.
7. False. PBI measures total bound thyroid hormones in plasma.
8. a. hyperthyroidism
   b. hypothyroidism

SECTION 3-6: METABOLISM OF THYROID HORMONES

OBJECTIVES:

The student should be able to:
1. State the half-lives of T_3 and T_4 and give reasons for differences in these values.
2. State the ways thyroid hormones are metabolized.
3. Give a brief description of the enterohepatic circulation for T_4 and T_3.
4. State an experimental method that can distinguish between hepatic conjugation and peripheral deiodination of thyroid hormones.
5. State the two proximate compounds to which T_4 is metabolized peripherally and their physiologic significance.

The biologic half-life of T_4 in the human is approximately 7 days, whereas that of T_3 is about 1.5 to 3 days. Thyroid hormones are metabolized by deiodination, by deamination, and by conjugation with a glucoronide moiety. Deiodination of T_4 and T_3 takes place presumably in all tissues of the body, but the kidney and the liver deaminate thyroid hormones. In addition, the liver conjugates T_4 and T_3 with a glucoronide moiety. This conjugate is then secreted via the bile duct into the small intestine (see step 8, Figure 3-4). Within the small intestines reside β-glucoronidase enzymes. These enzymes release the glucoronide moiety from the majority of the T_4 and T_3, which is then reabsorbed into the blood. This is called the enterohepatic circulation for thyroid hormones. In the normal human T_3 and T_4 are excreted mainly in feces, but a small amount of each appears in urine. If T_3 and T_4 are labeled with radioactive iodide and administered to humans, radioactivity in feces can be accounted for by the radioactive T_3 and T_4 found there. The radioactivity in urine is accounted for by radioactive iodide that was removed from the radioactive thyroid hormone. Thus, the radioactivity in feces is the result of hepatic conjugation, whereas the radioactivity in urine is the result of peripheral deiodination. These two processes can be affected both individually and simultaneously by such factors as drugs, pesticides, and exposure to cold.

All cells of the body appear to require thyroid hormone for their normal function. It now appears most likely that peripheral cells deiodinate T_4 to T_3, which is then taken up by the cell. Especially active in this regard are the cells of kidney and liver. It has been suggested that peripheral monodeiodination of T_4 to T_3 accounts for over 80% of the circulating T_3, the remainder being produced by the thyroid gland (see Figure 3-7). At the cellular level, it would appear that T_3 is "the" thyroid hormone.

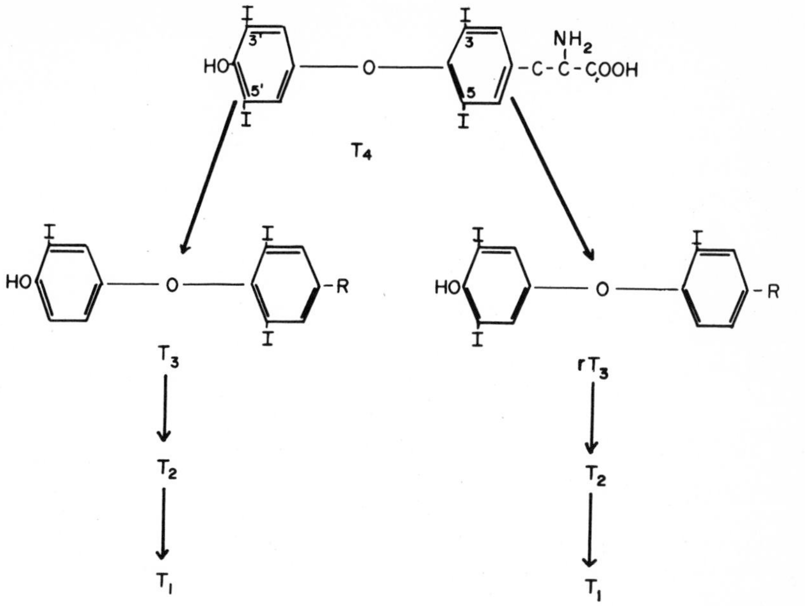

FIGURE 3-7: The pathways for the sequential deiodination of thyroxine. The only compound beyond T_4 with significant biologic activity is T_3.

There is also evidence that T_4 can be deiodinated to form reverse T_3 (rT_3) as shown in Figure 3-7. Notice the difference between T_3 and rT_3 with respect to the positions of the iodide atoms on the two molecules. The physiologic importance of rT_3, or any of the other metabolites of T_4 shown in Figure 3-7, is not known with certainty. rT_3 is present in the blood of humans (17–60 ng/dl) at about one-fifth the concentration of T_3 (80–200 ng/dl). Acute and chronic illness, caloric deprivation, and certain drugs such as cortico-steroids, propranolol (a β-adrenergic antagonist), and propylthiouracil (an antithyroid drug) increase the rate of peripheral conversion of T_4 to rT_3. When this happens, hypothyroidism could occur, depending on the relative amounts of T_3 and rT_3 formed per unit time and their rates of metabolism.

SECTION 3-6: POST-TEST QUESTIONS

1. The biologic half-life of T_3 is _____ days; that of T_4 is _____ days.

2. Name three ways in which thyroid hormones are metabolized.
   a.
   b.
   c.

3. Why is the enterohepatic circulation for thyroid hormones important physiologically?

4. What is reverse T_3?

5. In what organ does glucuronidation of thyroid hormones occur?

6. If radioactive T_4 or T_3 is administered, radioactivity is lost from the body via a. _____ and b. _____. The radioactivity in c. _____ _____ is the result of peripheral deiodination; that in d. _____ is the result of hepatic conjugation of the hormones.

SECTION 3-6: POST-TEST ANSWERS

1. a. 1.5 to 3.
   b. 7
2. a. Deiodination
   b. Deamination
   c. Glucuronidation
3. It is a method for recycling thyroid hormones that would otherwise be lost.
4. Reverse T_3 is a metabolite of T_4 possessing little known biologic activity.
5. Liver
6. a. urine
   b. feces
   c. urine
   d. feces

SECTION 3-7: CELLULAR MECHANISMS OF ACTION OF THYROID HORMONES

OBJECTIVES:

The student should be able to:
1. Discuss a theory to account for the mechanism by which T_3 increases the metabolic activity of the cell.
2. Explain why ouabain inhibits the metabolic response to T_3.
3. Discuss the latency of responsiveness to administered T_3.

In Section 3-6, it was mentioned briefly that T_4 is deiodinated to T_3 at the level of the peripheral cell. It was also pointed out that it is T_3 that appears to enter cells to induce the characteristic increase in metabolic activity accompanying administration of thyroid hormones to man or other mammals.

The actual mechanism by which T_3 affects cellular processes is not known with certainty. One theory is that after entering the cell, T_3 moves directly through the cytoplasm to the nucleus, where it is purported to stimulate a chain of events culminating in an increase either in the number or activity of the sodium pumps of the cell membrane. This is accompanied by increased metabolic activity (see Figure 3-8). It has been shown experimentally that ouabain will inhibit the metabolic response to administration of T_3. Ouabain, of course, inhibits Na^+/K^+-ATPase and thereby inhibits the sodium pump.

When either T_4 or T_3 is administered to man or other animals, there is a long latent period before physiologic effects are seen. For most responses, there is a latent period of 3 to 5 days before the expected response *just begins*. In some cases, as much as 10 days

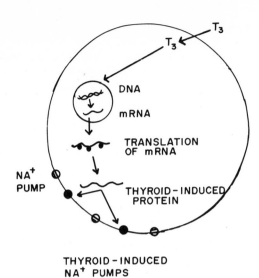

FIGURE 3-8: Speculative model of thyroidal control of sodium pump activity via induction of RNA and protein. (*Source:* Edelman, 1974.)

are required to reach a *maximal response* (e.g., basal metabolic rate). The reason for the latent period before a response to administered T_4 and T_3 occurs is not completely understood, but the induction of intracellular enzymes undoubtedly accounts for some of the latency.

It also appears at present that T_3 may interact in an interesting way with the cyclic adenosine monophosphate (cAMP) system at the cellular level. T_3 has been shown to inhibit the phosphodiesterase enzyme in certain tissues and thereby increase the half-life of cAMP, which normally is inactivated by this enzyme. The net effect of such an action is the same as that resulting from activation of a greater number of membrane receptors, since it is the cAMP that mediates the cellular response. This aspect is covered in greater detail in Section 4-2. Both induction of sodium pumps and interaction with the cAMP system constitute mechanisms by which T_3 may affect cellular metabolic activity.

SECTION 3-7: POST-TEST QUESTIONS

1. A proposed mechanism by which T_3 stimulates an increase in metabolic activity is by activation of cellular sodium pumps. (True/False)
2. T_3 exerts its effect on cells by activating the cyclic AMP system. (True/False)
3. Ouabain, an inhibitor of a sodium/potassium-activated ATPase, can inhibit the metabolic responsiveness to T_3 and T_4. (True/False)
4. The long latency for administered thyroid hormones to manifest an effect may be related to _____.

SECTION 3-7: POST-TEST ANSWERS

1. True
2. False
3. True
4. induction of intracellular enzymes.

SECTION 3-8: FEEDBACK CONTROL OF THE SECRETION OF THYROID HORMONES

OBJECTIVES:

The student should be able to:
1. State the anatomic site of origin of TSH, and this hormone's mechanisms of action.
2. State the anatomic site of origin of TRH, and the action of the hormone.
3. State the anatomic site at which thyroid hormones feedback to monitor their serum concentration.
4. State the chemical nature of TRH.

Thyroid stimulating hormone (TSH) is a trophic hormone produced by the anterior pituitary gland. It acts on the follicular cells of the thyroid gland to promote all phases of thyroid hormone synthesis including iodide uptake, iodide oxidation, iodination of tyrosyl residues, coupling reactions, and proteolytic release of thyroid hormones.

Histologic evidence for an increased rate of secretion of TSH includes an increase in height of the cells of thyroid follicles (from flat or cuboidal to columnar cells), a decrease in the amount of colloid contained in the follicles, and an increase in the vascularity of the gland. As mentioned in Section 3-4, the presence of colloid droplets in the cytoplasm of the follicular cell is thought to represent the movement of thyroglobulin from storage back into the follicular cell for degradation to T_4 and T_3. This occurs when the rate of TSH secretion increases.

Physiologic evidence for an increased rate of secretion of TSH includes an increase in rate of uptake of iodide into the thyroid gland, and an increase in rate of release of T_4 and T_3 from the thyroid gland into blood. TSH exerts its effect on the thyroid gland by way of the cAMP system. If the anterior pituitary gland, the source of TSH, is removed, thyroid secretory activity falls to a low, basal level. Thus, it is clear that in normal individuals TSH is responsible for modulating thyroid activity at levels considerably above the basal level observed in hypophysectomized patients or animals. The effect of an excess and deficient rate of secretion of TSH on the rate of uptake and release of radioactivity by the thyroid gland is shown in Figure 3-9. The uptake phase of the graph represents rate of uptake of radioiodide by the thyroid gland, and the release phase represents rate of loss of radioactive T_4 and T_3 from the thyroid gland. Excess TSH, as could occur in one form of hyperthyroidism, increases both rate of uptake and rate of release. The opposite occurs when the organism is deficient in TSH. Notice that as the rate of secretion of TSH increases, the rate of uptake of radioactivity by the thyroid gland increases. The rate of secretion of TSH is controlled by a negative feedback system. As the concentrations of free T_3 and T_4 in blood rise, the rate of secretion of TSH by the anterior pituitary is reduced until the concentrations of T_3 and T_4 in blood are decreased. This is negative feedback. In contrast, if the concentrations of free T_3 and T_4 in blood decrease, the rate of secretion of TSH by the anterior pituitary is increased.

As shown in Figure 3-10, TSH secretion is also controlled by another hormone, thyrotropin releasing hormone (TRH), produced in the hypothalamus and certain other regions of the brain. TRH is a tripeptide, pyroglutamyl-histidyl-proline amide (see Figure 7-13). TRH is secreted at nerve endings, where it diffuses into the capillary networks that form the hypophyseal portal vessels (see Figure 2-6). These vessels carry the hormone to the anterior pituitary, where it stimulates this gland to activity by way of the cAMP system. If the pituitary stalk is severed, or the hypophyseal portal vessels are destroyed by electrolytic lesions, the rate of secretion of TSH by the anterior pituitary falls to a low level. This, in turn, reduces thyroid activity.

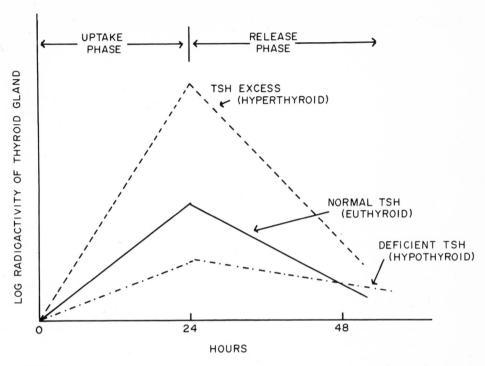

FIGURE 3-9: Uptake of radioiodide by thyroid gland and release of radioactive T_4 under normal, deficient, and excessive TSH states.

The principal site of feedback inhibition by T_4 and T_3 is at the level of the pituitary gland. Experiments have shown that T_3 and T_4 stimulate production in the pituitary of an inhibitory protein that is responsible for blocking the responsiveness of the TSH-producing cells to TRH. These studies suggest that the rate of production of the inhibitory protein intermediate is a direct function of blood concentration of T_3 and T_4. Supporting experimental evidence for this includes the variety of inhibitors of protein synthesis (e.g., actinomycin D, puromycin, and cycloheximide) that will prevent the feedback inhibition of high blood levels of T_3 and T_4 on TSH secretion (see Figure 3-10). The protein inhibitors, however, do not affect the response of the pituitary to adminis-

FIGURE 3-10: Effects of TRH, T_4 and T_3, and various RNA (actinomycin D) and protein synthesis inhibitors (puromycin and cycloheximide) on TSH secretion.

ANTERIOR PITUITARY GLAND

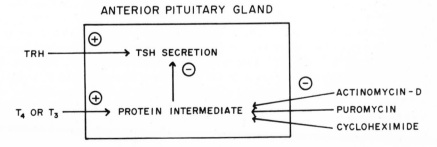

tration of TRH. (*Q. 3-3*) *What does this suggest regarding the mechanism of action of TRH at the level of the anterior pituitary gland?* Other studies have shown that thyroid hormones may also reduce the effectiveness of TRH by inducing a loss of receptors for TRH on the membranes of the thyrotropes (i.e., down-regulation and/or internalization of receptors). A relationship between these findings and the inhibitory protein discussed previously has not been established.

The feedback mechanism is very important clinically in establishing the level of dysfunction of the hypothalamopituitary-thyroid axis. In certain cases of hypothyroidism, it may be important to establish the level of dysfunction. (*Q. 3-4*) *How could this be done clinically?* (*Q. 3-5*) *Once you have established the level of dysfunction, how would you choose to treat the disease?*

The release of TRH in the hypothalamus appears to be mediated by catecholaminergic neurotransmitters. The most likely candidate in the rat is norepinephrine, but this issue is unsettled for man.

It is always somewhat surprising to find that hypophysiotropic hormones such as TRH and somatostatin are found outside the hypothalamus, and sometimes outside the central nervous system. In the case of TRH, more than 75% of the total amount in the entire brain is found outside the hypothalamus. It has also been found in the spinal cord. This suggests that TRH may act as a neurotransmitter in these areas. Indeed, administration of TRH has been shown to induce certain behavioral changes in experimental animals and man. It is also known that TRH can stimulate the release of prolactin from the anterior pituitary gland. Its role as both a prolactin releasing hormone and a thyrotrophin releasing hormone is discussed in more detail in Section 7-5C.

SECTION 3-8: POST-TEST QUESTIONS

1. Draw a schema to illustrate the feedback mechanism controlling the rate of secretion of thyroid hormones.

2. Name four histologic effects of an increase in the rate of secretion of TSH.
   a.
   b.
   c.
3. Name two physiologic effects of an increase in the rate of secretion of TSH.
   a.
   b.
4. Does secretion of thyroid hormones cease in hypophysectomized animals?
5. The rate of secretion of thyroid hormones is controlled by a (negative/positive) feedback system. Why?

6. The phase representing uptake of radioactivity by the thyroid gland reflects its ability to a. _____. The release phase reflects its ability to b. _____.

7. TSH excess (hyperthyroidism) a. (increases/decreases) rate of uptake and b. (increases/decreases) rate of release of thyroidal radioactivity.

8. According to Figure 3-9, an increase in the rate of secretion of TSH increases the rate of secretion of thyroid hormones. To produce a chronic hyperthyroidism by this means, what change in the feedback mechanism would be necessary?

9. TRH is produced by the anterior pituitary. (True/False)

10. The site of feedback inhibition by T_3 and T_4 is at the level of the:
    a. hypothalamus
    b. thyroid gland
    c. anterior pituitary gland

11. TRH is a:
    a. steroid
    b. protein
    c. tripeptide

12. Experimental evidence suggests that formation of a _____ is required for feedback inhibition by T_3 and T_4.

13. Evidence for this is that high blood concentrations of T_3 and T_4 no longer inhibit TSH secretion in the presence of a. _____, b. _____, and c. _____, all of which are inhibitors of RNA or d. _____ synthesis.

14. TSH initiates an increase in the rate of secretion of thyroid hormones by way of the cAMP system. (True/False)

SECTION 3-8: POST-TEST ANSWERS

1. See Figure 3-9.

2. a. Increase in height of follicular cells
   b. Decrease in amount of colloid in follicles
   c. Increase in vascularity of the gland
   d. Appearance of colloid droplets in cytoplasm of follicular cell

3. a. Increased rate of uptake of iodide from plasma into thyroid
   b. Increased rate of release of T_4 and T_3 from thyroid into plasma

4. No

5. Negative. See Figure 3-9. As the concentrations of free T_3 and T_4 rise in blood, the rate of secretion of TSH by the adenohypophysis is reduced until the concentrations of T_3 and T_4 in blood are reduced. The opposite situation arises when the concentrations of free T_3 and T_4 in blood decrease.

6. a. concentrate iodide
   b. release thyroid hormones

7. a. increases
   b. increases

8. A change in the set point for feedback inhibition at the level of the anterior pituitary gland.

9. False

10. c

11. c

12. protein intermediate
13. a. actinomycin D
    b. puromycin
    c. cycloheximide
    d. protein
14. True

SECTION 3-9: THE PHYSIOLOGIC EFFECTS OF THYROID HORMONES

OBJECTIVES:

The student should be able to:
  1. List five physiologic effects of thyroid hormones.
  2. List some distinguishing features of the hypothyroid state.
  3. List some distinguishing features of the hyperthyroid state.
  4. Indicate which of the physiologic effects of thyroid hormones may involve an interaction with catecholamines.

Thyroid hormones affect nearly every tissue of the body, and induce a variety of physiologic and biochemical effects. These effects are exaggerated in states of thyroid excess (hyperthyroidism) or deficiency (hypothyroidism) and result in the clinical and biochemical manifestations of these disorders. The effects of administration of T_4 and T_3 to patients are identical, although T_3 is two- or three-fold more potent on a weight basis than T_4 and its action is more rapid and shorter-lived than that of T_4.

The cardinal effects of thyroid hormones are manifested on the following: calorigenesis, growth and development, the cardiovascular system, the neuromuscular system, and intermediary metabolism.

A. CALORIGENESIS

The classic effect of thyroid hormones is stimulation of energy metabolism and heat production. These effects are reflected in an increased basal rate of oxygen consumption both in the whole organism and in most isolated tissues, a notable exception being the brain. A possible mechanism of the calorigenic effect was discussed briefly in Section 3-7 and may involve synthesis and/or activation of cellular sodium pumps. In a clinical setting, increased calorigenesis resulting from hyperthyroidism manifests itself as an increased appetite, poor weight gain, and heat intolerance. In hypothyroidism, a decreased appetite, weight gain, and cold intolerance are frequently found. (*Q. 3-6*) *Why would you expect hyperthyroid patients to manifest heat intolerance and hypothyroid patients to manifest cold intolerance?*

B. GROWTH AND DEVELOPMENT

Thyroid hormones are essential for normal development of the central nervous system and for maturation of the skeleton. A deficiency of thyroid hormones in early life leads to a delay in the development of the brain and if not corrected within 3 months after birth, to mental retardation. Thyroid hormone deficiency also leads to an abnormal stippled appearance of epiphyseal centers of ossification, with resulting impairment of linear growth (cretinism).

Perhaps the classic animal model illustrating the requirement of thyroid hormones for growth and development is the tadpole, which requires these hormones for metamorphosis to an adult frog.

C. CARDIOVASCULAR EFFECTS

The effects of an excess or deficiency of thyroid hormone are seen on the rate and strength of heart beat, on cardiac output and blood flow, and on arterial pressure. Accompanying an excess of thyroid hormones is an increase in the rate and strength of the heart beat. The mechanism by which this occurs is debated. It may be related indirectly to a hypersensitivity of catecholamine actions on the heart (see Section 3.7) induced by excess thyroid hormone, or it may be related directly to an effect of thyroid hormones on cardiac muscle. This effect of thyroid hormones is important clinically because it provides the physician with an important diagnostic sign of thyroid activity.

The amount of blood pumped by the heart per minute (cardiac output) is increased in hyperthyroidism and decreased in hypothyroidism. This is related in part to the increased heart rate and contractility and in part to the increased rate of metabolism of peripheral tissues induced by thyroid hormones. The latter results in vasodilation of blood vessels in peripheral tissue.

In hyperthyroidism induced by thyrotoxicosis, these effects are exaggerated and one observes increased cardiac output, increased systolic blood pressure, decreased diastolic blood pressure, widened pulse pressure, tachycardia (increased heart rate), shortened circulation time, and increased tissue perfusion. These hemodynamic alterations are responsible for the warm, moist, erythematous (red) skin seen in this condition. The converse changes occur in hypothyroidism.

D. NEUROMUSCULAR EFFECTS

In hyperthyroidism induced by thyrotoxicosis, a fine tremor of the hand and fingers is often observed when the arm is extended. There is also an eyelid retraction that produces stare and lid-lag. In addition, the net protein catabolism in this disorder leads to muscle wasting and weakness, especially of the limb musculature. In hypothyroidism, the rate of muscle contraction appears to be normal but the rate of muscle relaxation is lengthened considerably (e.g., the knee jerk reflex). The mechanism by which thyroid hormones interact in the neuromuscular system is poorly understood.

E. EFFECTS ON INTERMEDIARY METABOLISM

1. *Protein.* Synthesis of proteins is increased at the levels of both transcription and translation by thyroid hormone, and degradation of proteins is also enhanced. In hyperthyroidism, *net* catabolism results. This contributes to the weight loss and muscle wasting, and weakness observed. It is of interest that this effect occurs in spite of an increased caloric intake. In certain tissues thyroid hormones have recently been suggested to increase the synthesis of specific proteins (e.g., the β-adrenergic receptor in cardiac tissue; see Section 4-2) in addition to their more general effects on the turnover of other cellular proteins.

2. *Carbohydrate.* Thyroid hormones can increase glycogenolysis in both liver and muscle. Gluconeogenesis from lactate and glycerol is also enhanced by thyroid hormones. The glycogenolytic effect appears to be mediated by increased cAMP resulting

from an enhanced sensitivity of tissue adenylate cyclase to catecholamines induced by thyroid hormone (see Section 3.7). In thyrotoxicosis, liver glycogen is reduced, liver glucose output is increased, and pancreatic insulin reserve is challenged (see Section 9-4). The converse changes occur in hypothyroidism. The absorption of hexoses and pentoses across the gut wall is also affected by thyroid hormone. With a reduction in blood concentration of thyroid hormone, the rate of absorption of hexoses and pentoses is reduced. (*Q. 3-7*) *What significance would this have for the glucose tolerance test (see Section 9-5) in a hypothyroid patient?*

3. *Fat.* Thyroid hormones increase both the synthesis and the degradation of triglyceride and cholesterol. Free fatty acid oxidation is also enhanced under the influence of thyroid hormones, and this may contribute to the effect of these hormones on heat production. The lipolytic effect is related to an increased sensitivity of adipose tissue adenylate cyclase to catecholamines, which is induced by thyroid hormones (possibly through an increase in the synthesis of β-adrenergic receptors and inhibition phosphodiesterase; see Sections 3.7 and 4-2). The increased sensitivity of adipose tissue adenylate cyclase results in an increase in cAMP, which activates the lipase enzymes. In hyperthyroidism *net* lipid degradation occurs with increased plasma free fatty acid and decreased cholesterol concentration. In hypothyroidism, *net* synthesis occurs with decreased plasma free fatty acid and increased cholesterol concentrations.

4. *Mucopolysaccharides.* Thyroid hormones affect both the synthesis and the degradation of hyaluronic acid in ground substance of connective tissue. In hypothyroidism, degradation is slowed disproportionately. This results in an accumulation of hyaluronic acid in interstitial spaces. The hydrophilic property of hyaluronic acid leads to fluid retention and to a condition known as myxedema. It must be mentioned, although it is confusing, that in thyrotoxicosis (hyperthyroidism) an accumulation of hyaluronic acid frequently occurs in the orbits of the eye to produce exophthalmos (popping of the eyes) and over the skin to produce pretibial myxedema. Why an accumulation of hyaluronic acid occurs in both hypo- and hyperthyroidism is unknown. Why it is highly localized in hyperthyroidism is also poorly understood.

SECTION 3-9: POST-TEST QUESTIONS

1. On what do thyroid hormones manifest their major effects?
   a.
   b.
   c.
   d.
   e.

2. The calorigenic effect of thyroid hormones is reflected in the a. _____ _____, b. _____, and c. _____ of the patient. Hyperthyroid patients would be expected to have d. _____ _____, e. _____, and f. _____.

3. Thyroid hormones are necessary for normal development of the a. _____ _____ and for maturation of the b. _____.

4. A deficiency of thyroid hormones within the first 3 months of life may lead to _____.

5. Cardiovascular effects of either an excess or deficiency of thyroid hormones are seen on a. rate and strength of _____, b. _____, c. _____, and d. _____.

6. Some of the effects of excess thyroid hormones on the heart may be related to a change in the sensitivity of heart to _____, induced by hyperthyroidism.
7. Describe another situation in which thyroid hormones and catecholamines interact.

8. In hypothyroidism, the contraction time during the knee jerk reflex is increased and the relaxation time is normal. (True/False)
9. In hypothyroidism, the accumulation of hyaluronic acid in interstitial spaces results in _____.

SECTION 3-9: POST-TEST ANSWERS

1. a. Calorigenesis
   b. Growth and development
   c. Cardiovascular system
   d. Neuromuscular system
   e. Intermediary metabolism
2. a. heat production, energy metabolism, or oxygen consumption
   b. body weight
   c. food intake
   d. increased heat production, energy metabolism, or oxygen consumption
   e. weight loss
   f. increased food intake
3. a. central nervous system
   b. skeleton
4. mental retardation
5. a. heart beat
   b. cardiac output
   c. blood flow
   d. arterial pressure
6. catecholamines
7. In the glycogenolytic effect of thyroid hormone as well as in the lipolytic effect.
8. False. Contraction time is normal; relaxation time is increased.
9. myxedema

SECTION 3-10: TESTS OF UPTAKE, PRODUCTION, AND BINDING OF THYROID HORMONES

OBJECTIVES:

The student should be able to:
1. Describe a test used clinically to measure uptake of iodide by the thyroid gland.
2. State how an enzyme defect in the thyroid gland can be determined clinically.
3. Describe two tests for measurement of thyroid "suppressibility."
4. Describe how to determine the anatomic site of origin of hypothyroidism in a patient.
5. Describe the difference in the measurements of PBI, BEI, T_3, and T_4.
6. Describe a test used clinically to determine availability of binding sites for thyroid hormones on plasma protein.
7. Describe the measurement of basal metabolic rate and its significance.

Both hypothyroidism and hyperthyroidism can be induced in a number of ways. (Q. 3-8). *After reviewing Section 3-3, and particularly Figure 3-4, can you suggest at least eight ways these two conditions may occur?*

In assessing thyroid function clinically, it is important first to determine the state of thyroid activity and second, to find the level of the iodide-thyroxine cycle at which the problem exists. The tests described below should help you to do this.

Perhaps one of the most commonly used tests of thyroid function is the measurement of rate of uptake of radioactive iodide by the thyroid gland. You will recall that the thyroid gland is unable to distinguish between stable and radioactive iodide and will incorporate whichever is available into T_4 and T_3 molecules. Since the level of secretory activity of the thyroid gland is dependent on the rate of secretion of TSH by the anterior pituitary gland, measurement of rate of uptake of radioactive iodide by the thyroid gland reflects directly the rate of secretion of TSH.

Radioactive iodide is generally given by mouth (in water), and the radioactivity of the thyroid gland is measured 24 hours later by means of specially constructed scintillation detectors placed over the area of the thyroid gland in the neck. The radioactivity accumulated is expressed as a percentage of the administered dose per 24 hours. Depending on the thyroid state, the uptake within a 24 hour period may vary from 10% to 45% of the injected dose. Thus, the percentage of the injected dose of radioactivity measured in the thyroid gland at this time approximates the percentage of the iodide intake accumulated in the thyroid gland and is a function of the relative magnitudes of the thyroid and renal clearance rates (see Section 3-3). (Q. 3-9) *What effect would you expect an increased rate of iodide clearance by the kidney to have on 24-hour uptake of radiolabeled iodide by the thyroid gland?* (Q. 3-10) *Would you be concerned about doing an uptake measurement on a hypertensive patient who has been given a natriuretic diuretic agent for his disease?* (Q. 3-11) *What is the relationship among TSH, T_4, T_3, and iodide concentrations in blood?*

It is possible that the thyroid gland may be able to take up iodide normally but be unable to incorporate it into thyroid hormones because of certain enzymatic defects. In such a patient, the radioactivity within the thyroid represents unbound iodide, which may be discharged rapidly from the thyroid gland by acute administration of either perchlorate or thiocyanate salts. This discharge occurs *only* if the iodide is unbound. It may be monitored by measuring thyroidal radioactivity continuously after acute administration of perchlorate or thiocyanate. This is a technique commonly used clinically to detect an organification defect within the thyroid gland. (Q. 3-12) *What enzyme in the thyroid follicular cell is important for organification of iodide (placing iodide on a tyrosine moiety in thyroglobulin)?*

Experimentally, both the rate of uptake and the rate of release of radioactivity from the thyroid gland have been used to assess thyroid function. The half-life of thyroidal radioactivity is determined from the release phase of the curve (see Figure 3-9). In addition, an estimation of the rate of secretion of thyroid hormone can be measured indirectly by administering T_4 daily at increasing doses until the rate of release of radioactivity by the thyroid gland approaches zero. The dose of T_4 that inhibits completely the release of radioactivity from the thyroid gland is considered to be an estimate of the daily thyroid hormone secretion rate. (Q. 3-13) *By means of the feedback diagram in Figure 3-9, can you suggest why this measurement is an indirect estimate of the rate of thyroid hormone secretion?*

The concentration of thyroid hormones in circulating blood varies directly with the rate of secretion of thyroid hormones into blood, their rate of peripheral metabolism, and the quantity and binding avidity of thyroxine binding globulin (TBG) and, less critically, prealbumin and albumin concentrations in plasma. The quantities of both T_4 and T_3 in serum are often measured by chemical methods for determination of iodine. Hence, these methods are influenced by the presence in serum of exogenous iodine.

Protein-bound iodine (PBI, normal range 4–8 μg %) measures T_4 and T_3 bound to TBG iodoproteins, excess iodide, and any iodinated dyes in serum. The latter are used for x-ray visualization of gall bladder and other organs. Heavy metals (Hg, Au) also interfere and give falsely low values. The butanol-extractable iodine (BEI, 2.6–7.2 μg %) test is also a measure of total thyroid hormone concentration in blood. Acid-butanol extracts of serum remove T_4, T_3, iodide, and iodinated dyes, if present. An alkaline wash will remove iodide, leaving T_4, T_3, and any iodinated dyes. Thus, BEI is a more specific measure of total thyroid hormones than PBI.

Most clinical laboratories now have the capability for measuring serum T_4 and T_3 concentrations by radioimmunoassay. This technique is not influenced by iodide concentration of serum. Serum T_4 by this technique varies from 4 to 11 μg % and may be reported as T_4I, which is derived by multiplying serum T_4 concentration by 0.65, the molar fraction of T_4 that is present as iodine. Serum T_3 concentration is approximately 150 ng % (note that the concentration is in the nanogram range for T_3 and in the microgram range for T_4). Some clinical laboratories also measure reverse T_3 concentration in serum (60–100 ng %). The significance of this is discussed later.

The interaction between the hormone and the binding protein can be determined both directly and indirectly. A direct determination by electrophoretic analysis of individual binding proteins can be carried out by adding $[^{131}I]T_4$ to serum. (*Q. 3-14*) *What would you expect this test to show for serum from a hypothyroid patient?* An indirect determination can be carried out in vitro by means of a sponge-resin technique. The sponge contains a resin whose binding avidity for T_3 is less than that of plasma proteins. When serum is placed in a test tube containing the sponge and resin and a small amount of radioactive T_3 is added, the T_3 will be bound primarily to plasma protein if binding sites are available. If binding sites are unavailable, the resin will bind the T_3. At first glance the results of the test seem to be opposite of expectation because serum proteins from hypothyroid patients bind more T_3 whereas proteins from hyperthyroid patients bind less T_3. This means that hypothyroid patients not only may have lower free T_4 and T_3 concentrations in their serum but their thyroid hormone binding proteins may also have a larger number of available binding sites. In contrast, the hyperthyroid patient has a higher concentration of free T_4 and T_3, but the thyroid hormone binding proteins have fewer available binding sites.

Additional tests are available clinically to assess pituitary-thyroid interrelations. One of these is the thyroid suppression test, which consists of exogenous administration of either T_4 or T_3 daily for 2 to 3 weeks, followed by measurement of uptake of radioactive iodide by the thyroid gland. (*Q. 3-15*) *Why would this procedure be expected to suppress the activity of the thyroid gland?* (*Q. 3-16*) *Would this test reduce serum PBI?*

Many clinical laboratories now measure serum concentration of TSH. Measurement of serum TSH both before and after exogenous administration of either T_3 or T_4 can also be considered to be a "suppression test." This test may be more helpful in diagnosis than that involving measurement of uptake of radioactive iodide. (*Q. 3-17*) *Why?*

In hypothyroid patients, one may wish to know whether the origin of the disease is at the level of the thyroid gland (primary) or the pituitary (secondary). This can be determined by exogenous administration of TSH, which is commercially available. Subsequent measurement of serum PBI, T_4, or T_3 concentrations will indicate whether the thyroid gland is capable of responding. If a response occurs and one then wished to know whether the defect was pituitary (secondary) or hypothalamic (tertiary) in origin, TRH could be administered and the same measurements made. A positive response would suggest that the defect is at the level of the hypothalamus. TRH is also available commercially. (*Q. 3-18*) *If the defect were at the pituitary level, how would you choose to treat the patient?* (*Q. 3-19*) *If the defect were at the hypothalamic level, how would you choose to treat the patient?* (*Q. 3-20*) *Why?*

Other tests of thyroid dysfunction are also used. A classic method, not used commonly at present, is measurement of basal metabolic rate. This is measured as the rate of oxygen consumption (from which rate of metabolism can be calculated by multiplying by the caloric equivalent for oxygen) in a resting, supine subject who has fasted overnight. (*Q. 3-21*) *What would the hyperthyroid patient show?*

Thyroid antibodies in serum have also been measured. There are a variety of circulating antibodies to various fractions of the thyroid gland, and all are usually elevated markedly in autoimmune thyroidities (Hashimoto's disease). There may also be an elevation in serum thyroid antibodies in Graves' disease (hyperthyroidism) and nontoxic nodular goiter.

Tissue unresponsiveness to T_3 has not been described as a cause of hypothyroidism, and all cases of hypothyroidism seen clinically are correctable with T_3. It has recently become clearer, however, that a number of conditions may interfere with the deiodination of T_4 to T_3. One of these is starvation; another is chronic illness, and a third is chronic high blood levels of glucocorticoid hormones. All these factors appear to shift the deiodination of T_4 from T_3 to rT_3 (see Section 3-6). In these conditions serum concentration of T_3 decreases while rT_3 increases. The significance of this shift in the metabolic pathway is not clearly understood, but it would be expected to result in a reduction of metabolic rate. (*Q. 3-22*) *Why?* This shift in the metabolic pathway for deiodination of T_4 is regarded by some investigators as a physiologic adaptation to a hypometabolic state that may enhance survival under the conditions that initiated the shift. As measurements of rT_3 are made under other clinical and experimental conditions, it is likely that we will gain a better understanding of its physiologic significance.

SECTION 3-10: POST-TEST QUESTIONS

1. Hypothyroidism may be tentatively diagnosed if the 24-hour uptake of an administered dose of radioactive iodide by the thyroid gland is (increased/decreased) from normal values.

2. To determine whether the defect is at the level of the thyroid gland, a. _____ _____ could be administered with subsequent measurement of b. _____ _____ or c. _____. If the defect is *not* at the level of the thyroid gland, the test would show d. _____ _____.

3. To determine whether the defect is at the level of the pituitary gland, a. _____ _____ could be administered with subsequent measurement of b. _____ _____ or c. _____. If the defect is *not* at the level of the pituitary gland, is there another test that could be performed to localize it? d.

4. If the thyroid gland takes up radioactive iodide normally but you suspect that it has an organification defect related to an enzyme deficit, what test could be done to check your suspicion?

5. Describe a "suppression test" of thyroid function. What measurements would you make to assess suppressibility?

6. What is basal metabolic rate? How is it measured?

7. a. What factors alter the route of metabolism of T_4 from T_3 to rT_3?

   b. What physiologic significance has this?

SECTION 3-10: POST-TEST ANSWERS

1. Decreased
2. a. TSH
   b. PBI, T_4, T_3, BEI
   c. uptake of radioactive iodide
   d. Increased PBI, T_4, T_3, and BEI as well as an increased rate of uptake of radioactive iodide
3. a. TRH
   b. plasma TSH
   c. T_4, T_3, BEI, or PBI
   d. No
4. Perchlorate or thiocyanate discharge test
5. Administration of T_4 or T_3 will suppress TSH production in normal individuals. To assess suppressibility, it would be best to measure serum concentration of TSH following administration of T_4 or T_3. this illustrates an important use of the feedback mechanism in clinical medicine.
6. Basal metabolic rate is determined by measuring the rate of oxygen consumption (and therefore metabolism) in a resting, supine subject who has fasted overnight. This measurement represents the minimal metabolic rate of the subject. In hyperthyroidism the minimal or basal metabolic rate is elevated 25% or more above that of a euthyroid subject. In hypothyroidism it is reduced by 25% or more.
7. a. Starvation (fasting), chronic illness, and chronic administration of high doses of glucocorticoids.
   b. It suggests either that there are two separate deiodinase enzymes that deiodinate T_4 or that a single deiodinase normally exists whose usual activity can be changed by the circumstances listed in (a). If two separate enzymes exist for deiodination, it is likely that one is activated preferentially over the other by the circumstance listed in (a).

SELECTED REFERENCES

Baxter, J. D., Eberhardt, N. L., Apriletti, J. W., Johnson, L. K., Ivarie, R. D., Schachter, B. S., Morris, J. A., Seeburg, P. H., Goodman, H. M., Latham, K. R., Polansky, J. R., and Martial, J. A., 1979, Thyroid hormone receptors and responses, *Recent Progress In Hormone Research* 35: 97.

Chopra, I. J., Solomon, D. H., Chopra, U., Wu, S. Y., Fisher, D. A., and Nakamura, Y., 1978, Pathways of metabolism of thyroid hormones, *Recent Progress in Hormone Research* 34, 521.

De Visscher, M. (Ed.), 1980, *The Thyroid Gland*, New York: Raven Press.

Edelman, I. S., 1979, Effect of thyroid hormones on biochemical processes, *Progress In Clinical And Biological Research* 31: 685.

Oppenheimer, J. H., Dillman, W. H., Schwartz, H. L., and Towle, H. C., 1979, Nuclear receptors and thyroid hormone action: a progress report, *Federation Proceedings* 38: 2154.

4

THE AUTONOMIC NERVOUS SYSTEM AND THE ADRENAL MEDULLA

SECTION 4-1: THE AUTONOMIC NERVOUS SYSTEM

OBJECTIVES:

The student should be able to:
1. Describe the differences between the two major peripheral divisions of the nervous system.
2. Describe the differences in anatomic origin of the sympathetic and parasympathetic nerves.
3. Describe the differences in location of the synapse of preganglionic fibers in the sympathetic and parasympathetic divisions.
4. Describe some differences in the physiologic functions controlled by the sympathetic and parasympathetic divisions.
5. Describe the relationship between the sympathetic system and adrenal medullary secretion.

A. GENERAL FEATURES OF THE AUTONOMIC NERVOUS SYSTEM

There are a number of important differences between the two major peripheral divisions of the nervous system. The somatic or voluntary division is often thought of as the one enabling us to adjust to our external environment. It allows us to move our fingers, to run, to eat, and so on. In contrast, the autonomic or involuntary (vegetative) division is often thought of as the part of the peripheral nervous system that is somewhat removed from the direct control of the will. It is important in initiating appropriate physiologic responses to stimuli that arise outside the body as well as within it. The beating of the heart and the movements of the gastrointestinal tract are examples of functions controlled by the autonomic nervous system.

The two divisions of the peripheral nervous system are not independent of each other, but actually work together. For instance, during muscular exercise in which the somatic nervous system is active, the autonomic system is also active. Stimuli affecting the somatic nervous system generally affect the autonomic nervous system as well.

For the purpose of this chapter, the autonomic nervous system is defined as the efferent or output pathway to the viscera. This efferent system includes all nerve fibers and nerve cells involved in transmitting descending electrical impulses from the central nervous system to secretory glands, smooth muscles, and heart; that is, all efferent nerve fibers except those to the voluntary muscles. The definition above simplifies the under-

84

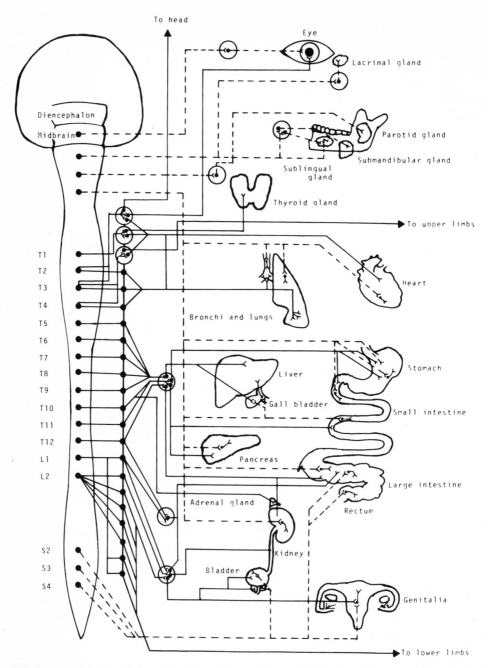

FIGURE 4-1: Schematic illustration of the autonomic nervous system: solid lines represent sympathetic nerves and dashed lines represent parasympathetic nerves; T designates thoracic segments; L and S designate lumbar and sacral segments, respectively, of the spinal cord.

standing of the material to be presented. It should be noted here that a more realistic, although more complicated, definition of the autonomic nervous system would include mention of its receptors and afferent pathways as well. In fact, many autonomic nerves such as the splanchnic, vagus, and chorda tympani contain both afferent and efferent fibers.

B. ANATOMY OF THE AUTONOMIC NERVOUS SYSTEM: GENERAL FEATURES

Anatomically, the autonomic nervous system may be divided into the craniosacral and thoracolumbar portions corresponding to the *parasympathetic* and *sympathetic* divisions, respectively (see Figure 4-1). Both these efferent divisions utilize a two-neuron series system composed of pre- and postganglionic neurons. The cell bodies of the *preganglionic* neurons are found in either the brain stem (i.e., the Edinger-Westphal nucleus of cranial nerve III, the oculomotor nerve, the dorsal efferent nucleus of cranial nerve X—the vagus nerve, the salivatory nucleus of cranial nerves VII and IX, the facial and glossopharyngeal nerves; see Table 4-1) or in the intermediolateral portion of the spinal cord (i.e., T_1–L_2 for the sympathetic and S_2–S_4 for the parasympathetic system, see Figures 4-1 and 4-2).

TABLE 4-1: Characteristics of the Parasympathetic and Sympathetic Divisions of the Autonomic Nervous System

	Parasympathetic Division	Sympathetic Division
Preganglionic cell loci	Tectal and medullary brain stem nuclei and intermediolateral regions of the sacral spinal cord	Intermediolateral regions of the thoracic and lumbar spinal cord
Preganglionic nerve loci	Cranial nerves III, VII, IX, and X; and pelvic nerves from sacral segments 2–4	White communicating rami and splanchnic nerves from thoracic segments 1–12 and lumbar segments 1–2.
Preganglionic axons	Long (myelinated)	Short (myelinated)
Preganglionic neurotransmitter	Acetylcholine	Acetylcholine
Ganglia	Terminal	Lateral and collateral
Postganglionic nerve distribution	Confined to restricted area	Widespread
Postganglionic axons	Short (unmyelinated)	Long (usually unmyelinated)
Postganglionic neurotransmitter	Acetylcholine	Norepinephrine (except in sweatglands—acetylcholine)
Ratio of pre- to postganglionic axons	May be 1 : 1 or 1 : 2	May be 1 : 20 or greater
Response to stimulation	Localized	Generalized
Response to cutting terminal axons	Loss of specific target organ stimulation	May lead a supersensitivity to circulating catecholamines in the specific target organ

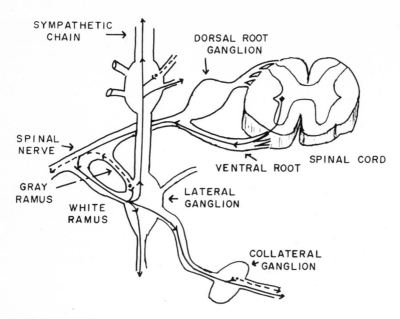

FIGURE 4-2: The passage of sympathetic nerves from the spinal cord to the lateral and collateral ganglia. The solid and dashed lines represent preganglionic and postganglionic fibers, respectively. The arrows indicate the direction of nerve impulses along the fiber.

The cell bodies of the *postganglionic* neurons are found in one of three types of ganglia: lateral (paravertebral), collateral (pervertebral), and terminal (intrinsic or peripheral) ganglia (see Figure 4-1). The lateral ganglia consist of two chains of ganglia that run parallel with, and on each side of the vertebral column (hence the term "vertebral" or "sympathetic chain"); the collateral ganglia are found some distance from the spinal cord but usually near the organ to be innervated. Both the lateral and collateral ganglia are used exclusively by the sympathetic neurons. The terminal ganglia lie on or within the tissue or organ innervated. These ganglia are used almost exclusively by the parasympathetic neurons. (*Q.* 4-1) *Can you think of a rather obvious exception to the last generalization?* Thus, the preganglionic axons of the sympathetic neurons are usually much shorter than those for the parasympathetic neurons, and the postganglionic axons of the sympathetic neurons are usually longer than those for the parasympathetic neurons (see Table 4-1).

C. ANATOMY OF THE AUTONOMIC NERVOUS SYSTEM: SYMPATHETIC DIVISION

The preganglionic axons of the sympathetic division emerge from the spinal cord through the nearest ventral route and enter adjacent lateral ganglia via the *white communicating rami* (see Figure 4-2). This bundle of axons is designated as white because each of the preganglionic axons of the sympathetic division is covered by a thin myelin sheath (produced by multiple layers of plasma membranes from the nonneural supportive glial elements called Schwann cells), which gives these axons a white appearance in living material. Within the lateral ganglion the preganglionic axon may form synaptic contacts with ganglion cells at the level it entered and pass rostrally or caudally several segments before synapsing, or it may leave the vertebral chain of lateral ganglia via a splanchnic nerve and synapse in one of the collateral ganglia (see Figure 4-1). Divergence of preganglionic axons of the sympathetic division is common, since each axon often synapses with several ganglion cells within several different ganglia. One estimate suggests that these axons may make synaptic contacts with as many as 32 postganglionic neurons. Convergence of the preganglionic input also occurs, since each lateral ganglion receives synaptic input from several segments.

In considering the destination of the postganglionic axons of the sympathetic neurons arising from the lateral ganglia, it is convenient to remember that the cervical and upper four thoracic ganglia send postganglionic axons to areas above the diaphragm (see Figure 4-1). These go to blood vessels in the skin and muscles of the head, neck, and arms, to the eyes, to the salivary, nasal, and lacrimal glands and the blood vessels in these glands, and to the visceral structures (heart, lungs, bronchi, and bronchial glands) in the thoracic cavity. As stated above, some of the preganglionic axons arising from thoracic segments below T_4 and the diaphragm pass through the lateral ganglia and make their initial synaptic contacts in the collateral ganglia further out in the abdominal cavity, and located anteriorly to the spinal column along the edge of the mesentery. Postganglionic fibers from the collateral ganglia go to the stomach and intestines, spleen, pancreas, and liver, supplying smooth muscles and glands in these structures.

The unmyelinated sympathetic postganglionic axons emerge from the lateral ganglia either via a *gray communicating ramus* or via one or more *splanchnic nerves*. The gray appearance of these axon bundles is due to their lack of a myelin sheath. Postganglionic axons in the gray communicating rami join spinal sensory nerves and supply innervation to blood vessels in the skin and muscles of the head, neck, arms, legs, and body wall. They also supply innervation to the sweat glands and the piloerector muscles around the hair shafts of the skin. Each lateral chain ganglion produces one or more gray communicating rami so that every spinal nerve receives a gray communicating ramus (see Figure 4-2). As stated earlier, the unmyelinated postganglionic axons of the sympathetic neurons within the splanchnic nerves distribute to the various autonomic plexuses of the viscera. Thus, postganglionic axons from both the lateral and collateral ganglia, except those destined for skin and muscles, form plexuses or networks of fine fibers that run outward, usually along the blood vessels, to the organs they innervate.

Some preganglionic sympathetic axons emerge from the lower thoracic portions of the spinal cord and pass through both lateral and collateral ganglia before making their initial synaptic contacts within the adrenal medulla. Since these synapses are the first for these preganglionic axons, the adrenal medulla may be considered as a ganglion. This organ has also been shown to be embryologically homologous with the other sympathetic ganglia. Last, electrical impulses coursing through the preganglionic axons of the sympathetic nerves reaching the adrenal medulla initiate the secretion of the catecholamines epinephrine (adrenaline) and norepinephrine by the chromaffin cells of this gland in much the same manner as catecholamines are released from the postganglionic axons of sympathetic nerves found in most other regions of the body. Greater detail regarding the mechanisms affecting the synthesis, secretion, and metabolism of these catecholamines is given later.

D. ANATOMY OF THE AUTONOMIC NERVOUS SYSTEM: PARASYMPATHETIC DIVISION

The preganglionic axons of the parasympathetic neurons are also myelinated, but in contrast to the preganglionic axons of the sympathetic neurons, the parasympathetic axons make their initial synaptic contacts in small isolated ganglia lying in or near their visceral target organs. The postganglionic fibers are, therefore, very short. (Q. 4-2) *Would you expect this anatomic arrangement to facilitate a more diffuse or more specific response to a stimulus than that displayed by the sympathetic neurons?* Within the parasympathetic division, the cranial outflow arises from the tectal (via cranial nerve III) and bulbar (via cranial nerves VII, IX, and X) areas of the brain and distributes to the upper portions of the body as well as the viscera, while the sacral outflow arises from the intermediolateral portions of the sacral spinal cord (S_2–S_4) and distributes to the remaining portions of the body below the level of the transverse colon within the abdomen (see Figure 4-1). In contrast to the sympathetic division, there is comparatively little convergence or divergence with the parasympathetic division, and there are smooth muscle tissues and visceral organs that are not innervated at all by the parasympathetic division.

The vagus nerve (i.e., cranial nerve X) forms the major component of the parasympathetic cranial outflow. Preganglionic axons within this nerve bundle distribute to terminal ganglia within the heart, lung, stomach, pancreas, intestine, upper colon, liver, and esophagus. Preganglionic axons from the parasympathetic neurons arising from the sacral portions of the spinal cord distribute to the descending colon, pelvic colon, bladder, rectum, uterus, and external genitalia. These axons emerge from the spinal cord via an adjacent sacral ventral route and unite to form the pelvic nerve without passing through the lateral chain ganglia. The pelvic nerve distributes to the terminal ganglia of the pelvic viscera and external genitalia via a network or plexus of axons usually associated with the blood vessels to the organs they innervate. (*Q. 4-3) How does this anatomic arrangement compare to that utilized by the postganglionic axons of the sympathetic division?*

E. CHEMICAL TRANSMISSION OF NERVE IMPULSES

The theory of chemical transmission of nervous impulses is based on experimental evidence for the presence of such chemical transmitters as acetylcholine (parasympathetic division) and catecholamines (epinephrine and norepinephrine; sympathetic division) at presynaptic axonal endings. The theory requires not only a chemical transmitter but also a postsynaptic receptor designed to interact with the transmitter. When the transmitter is liberated from the presynaptic nerve terminal, it interacts with the postsynaptic receptor to either depolarize or hyperpolarize the postsynaptic membrane. If the nerve terminal synapses on an effector cell of a gland, the later is stimulated to secrete when the proper transmitter interacts with its receptor. Under similar circumstances smooth muscle can be stimulated either to contract or relax by the proper transmitter. Thus, the response elicited by the combination of the transmitter with its receptor is not always one of stimulation but may also result in inhibition of the specific activities of the effector cells or organs. The receptor is a functional part of the effector cell and not a part of the nerve producing the chemical transmitter. Within the autonomic nervous system receptors are called cholinergic, adrenergic, or serotonergic, depending on their interaction with acetylcholine, catecholamines, or serotonin, respectively.

The chemical transmitters ordinarily are present in a stabilized (bound) form in the nerve terminals and become active after they have been released in a free or unbound form by a nervous (electrical) impulse reaching the nerve terminals. The bound transmitter is protected from enzymatic destruction. Once the transmitter is released and interacts with the receptor for a sufficient period of time, either inhibition or excitation of the effector cell may occur. When the transmitter becomes free of the receptor, it is inactivated very rapidly by hydrolytic, oxidative, reuptake, or conjugative mechanisms. Acetylcholine is inactivated by cholinesterase enzymes. Acetylcholinesterase, present in relatively high concentrations near nerve terminals of cholinergic nerve fibers, acts specifically on acetylcholine to hydrolyze it. (*Q. 4-4) What would be the probable effect*

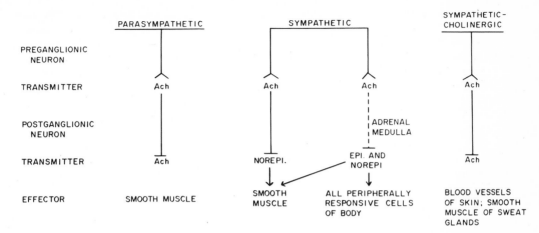

FIGURE 4-3: The neurotransmitters of the autonomic nervous system and effector tissues on which they act: Ach = acetylcholine, NOREPI = norepinephrine, EPI = epinephrine.

on a parasympathetic response of inhibiting acetylcholinesterase activity with a drug? The catecholamines are inactivated by the less specific enzymes monoamine oxidase and catechol-O-methyltransferase. In addition the secreted catecholamines are taken up by the same presynaptic neurons that secreted them. These mechanisms are discussed in greater detail in the next section.

It often seems surprising to learn that all the preganglionic neurons of both divisions of the autonomic nervous system secrete acetylcholine at their preganglionic terminals. The difference between the two divisions with respect to transmitters is at the terminal endings of the postganglionic neurons. Here the postganglionic parasympathetic fibers secrete acetylcholine, and the postganglionic sympathetic fibers usually secrete catecholamines. Since the preganglionic sympathetic fiber to the adrenal medulla terminates on secretory cells of this organ, both epinephrine and norepinephrine can be said to be the postganglionic transmitters. These two catecholamines are released by adrenal medullary cells when activated by acetylcholine. Since epinephrine and norepinephrine are released into blood, they are carried to all parts of the body where they may act directly on cells. An exception to this system seems to be the sympathetic fibers to smooth muscle of blood vessels in skin and to smooth muscle of sweat glands, which have acetylcholine as their transmitter at *both* pre- and postganglionic synapses (see Figure 4-3).

F. GENERAL FUNCTIONS OF THE AUTONOMIC NERVOUS SYSTEM

The two divisions of the autonomic nervous system differ not only anatomically, but usually in their functions as well. The sympathetic and parasympathetic divisions serve as a check and balance on each other, an important mechanism by which homeostasis is maintained. Most visceral organs are innervated by axons from both divisions, and stimulation of one division usually produces effects opposite those observed during stimulation of the other. Thus if one system inhibits a certain function, the other usually increases that function, although in some instances the two divisions may excite the same organ. For example, salivary gland secretion may be increased by both parasympathetic and sympathetic excitation; however, in this case the type of secretion varies with the division activating the secretion. In other instances only one division innervates a structure and may act unopposed by the other division. For example, the piloerector muscles receive only sympathetic fibers whose function is to stimulate muscle contraction, whereas the erectile tissue of the genitalia receive only parasympathetic fibers whose function is to stimulate vasodilation of the blood vessels in the penis (see Section 6-1). It should be noted, however, that these are not representative of the usual anatomic arrangement of innervation by the autonomic nervous system.

Clinical and experimental investigations have shown that when parasympathetic pathways are cut, the responses normally elicited by these pathways are eliminated, whereas cutting the sympathetic nerves to an organ may actually result in an increased response to circulating catecholamines (from the adrenal medulla). This phenomenon is known as denervation supersensitivity. Table 4-1 summarizes these and other differences between the parasympathetic and sympathetic divisions of the autonomic nervous system.

The general functions of the sympathetic division of the autonomic nervous system can be summarized as follows: a) ensuring reciprocity to counteract and balance the tonic effects of parasympathetic stimulation of visceral structures, b) assisting in the maintenance of the steady state functions of the body (digestion, secretion, vasomotor tone, etc.), and c) assisting in the mobilization of body reserves to meet unusual or emergency situations (fear, fright, injury, etc.). Dr. Walter Cannon, the great American physiologist, was the first to suggest that activation of the sympathetic nervous system prepares an animal for fright, fight, or flight.

The general functions of the parasympathetic division of the autonomic nervous system can be summarized as follows: a) ensuring reciprocity to counteract and balance the tonic effects of sympathetic stimulation of visceral structures, b) assisting in the maintenance of the responsiveness of visceral organs to natural, unharmful stimuli (e.g., secretory and motor activity in the gastrointestinal tract when food enters it), c) exerting an anabolic influence on certain organs and tissues, to conserve their energies and provide periods of comparative rest (e.g., slowing the heart rate), and d) initiating the evacuation of the rectum and bladder, as well as controlling the function of the accessory sexual organs.

G. SPECIFIC FUNCTIONS OF THE AUTONOMIC NERVOUS SYSTEM

Some specific functions of the *sympathetic division* of the autonomic system are listed below. This list is not complete and is intended only to illustrate the far-reaching physiologic responses to *stimulation of the sympathetic nervous system.*

Cervical Sympathetics:
    a. dilation of the pupil of the eye,
    b. constriction of blood vessels of the head (except the brain), face, salivary, and thyroid glands,
    c. vasodilation of mucous membrane of the nose, lip, and pharnyx,
    d. increase pilomotor activity of hairs of ears, between the eyes, and occiput,
    e. stimulate secretion of salivary, lacrimal, mucous, and sweat glands.
Cardiopulmonic Sympathetics:
    a. acceleration and augmentation of heart beat,
    b. bronchodilation,
    c. secretion of sweat glands located on the skin of the chest.
Splanchnic Sympathetics:
    a. contraction of the spleen in most animals except man,
    b. inhibition of motor activity of stomach, pyloric sphincter, and small intestine,

    c. secretion of liver, adrenal medulla, and pancreas (acinar cells),

    d. vasoconstriction of all abdominal visceral vessels.

Inferior Splanchnic:

    a. inhibition of motor activity of colon and wall of urinary bladder,

    b. contraction of vas deferens, uterus, Fallopian tubes, and trigone of bladder,

    c. ejaculation in the male.

The specific functions in *response to stimulation* of the *parasympathetic division* of the autonomic system are listed below.

Third Cranial Nerve (Edinger-Westphal nucleus):

    a. constriction of the pupil and ciliary muscle of the eye.

Seventh Cranial Nerve (*chorda tympani*) (salivatory nucleus):

    a. vasodilation of nasopharynx, sublingual, and submaxillary (submandibular) glands,

    b. secretion by nasopharynx, sublingual and submaxillary glands.

Ninth Cranial Nerve (salivatory nucleus):

    a. secretion and vasodilation in the parotid salivary gland.

Tenth Cranial Nerve (*vagus*) (dorsal efferent nucleus):

    a. inhibition of both rate and conduction of electrical impulses in the heart,

    b. bronchoconstriction,

    c. increased motor activity of esophagus, stomach, small intestine, and gall bladder,

    d. inhibition of motor activity of pyloric sphincter and ileocecal valve,

    e. stimulation of secretion by stomach, liver, and pancreas,

    f. vasodilation of blood vessels of stomach and intestines.

(It has been estimated that about 75% of all parasympathetic fibers in the body are in the vagus nerve.)

Sacral Nerves:

    a. increased motor activity of the large intestine and rectum and vasodilation of genitalia (i.e., erection).

H. MODULATION OF THE AUTONOMIC NERVOUS SYSTEM BY THE CENTRAL NERVOUS SYSTEM

The hypothalamus is the highest level of the central nervous system at which there is modulation of the electric activity descending to the autonomic nervous system (see Section 2-1). The parasympathetic division is thought to be influenced primarily by neuronal activity in the rostral hypothalamus, whereas the sympathetic division is thought to be influenced primarily by the caudal hypothalamus. To a large extent, the maintenance of a homeostatic balance between the two divisions of the autonomic nervous system depends on the interactions of each of the hypothalamic nuclei with internal and external stimuli and with the interconnections between these various nuclei and with other regions of the brain. These complex interactions are thought to be involved in the homeostatic regulation of many integrated physiologic processes (regulation of body temperature, water balance, feeding, etc.) Some of these examples are discussed in other chapters (e.g., Chapter 9).

The major descending pathway involved in the regulation of parasympathetic activity is the dorsal longitudinal fasciculus (DLF). The DLF arises from several hypothalamic nuclei, descends through the periventricular gray of the midbrain, and terminates in several preganglionic parasympathetic nuclei including the Edinger-Westphal (cranial nerve III), salivatory (cranial nerves VII and IX), and dorsal efferent (cranial nerve X) nuclei. The major descending pathway involved in the regulation of sympathetic activity is the hypothalamotegmental system. This pathway also arises from several hypothalamic nuclei (including the ventromedial nucleus; see Figure 9-1); is composed of several more or less distinct tracts and descends to make numerous synaptic contacts with neurons in the gray matter tegmentum and brain stem. Long axons from these neurons descend the brain stem and spinal cord and eventually make synaptic contacts with the preganglionic sympathetic cells in the intermediolateral portion of the thoracic and lumbar regions of the spinal cord.

SECTION 4-1: POST-TEST QUESTIONS

1. Name the two divisions of the peripheral nervous system.
   a.
   b.
2. Describe the differences between the two divisions with respect to the functions they perform.
   a.

   b.

3. Name the two subdivisions of the autonomic nervous system.
   a.
   b.
4. Name the *spinal cord segments* that give rise to the preganglionic axons of each of these subdivisions of the autonomic nervous system.
   a.
   b.
5. Name the three *brain stem nuclei* that contain the preganglionic cell bodies of the parasympathetic neurons.
   a.
   b.
   c.
6. Name the four *cranial nerves* that contain the preganglionic axons of the parasympathetic neurons.
   a.
   b.
   c.
   d.
7. Name the region in the spinal cord that contains the cell bodies of the preganglionic neurons of the autonomic nervous system.

8. Name the three types of ganglia found in the peripheral autonomic nervous system.
   a.
   b.
   c.
9. Which of these ganglia is used exclusively by the sympathetic division and which is characteristic of the parasympathetic division?

10. Name the pre- and postganglionic neurotransmitters of the parasympathetic and sympathetic neurons.

11. Why is the adrenal medulla considered to be part of the autonomic nervous system?

12. Describe convergence and divergence in the sympathetic nervous system.

13. Describe the principal differences between the white and gray communicating rami.

14. Are there more gray communicating rami than white? Why?

15. When the adrenal medulla secretes epinephrine and norepinephrine into blood in response to a stimulus, these agents are carried to the various organs and tissues of the body, where they exert their effects and in this way amplify the response to the original stimulus. (True/False)

16. The parasympathetic nervous system is important in preparing the body for "fright, fight, and flight." (True/False)

17. A general function of the sympathetic nervous system is to counteract and balance in a homeostatic fashion the tonic effects of the parasympathetic nervous system. (True/False)

18. Which regions of the hypothalamus are thought to be involved in the modulation of parasympathetic and sympathetic nervous activity?

19. Name the principal descending pathways from the hypothalamus concerned with modulation of autonomic nervous system activity.

20. Cutting the parasympathetic input to a given target organ frequently results in a hypersensitization (i.e., denervation supersensitivity) of the organ to circulating catecholamines. (True/False)

SECTION 4-1: POST-TEST ANSWERS

1. a. Somatic
   b. Autonomic
2. a. The somatic division of the peripheral nervous system controls voluntary functions such as movement of skeletal muscles.
   b. The autonomic division regulates involuntary functions such as secretions and motility of the gastrointestinal tract and heart rate.
3. a. Parasympathetic
   b. Sympathetic
4. a. S_2-S_4 (parasympathetic)
   b. T_1-L_2 (sympathetic)
5. a. Edinger-Westphal
   b. Salivatory
   c. Dorsal efferent
6. a. Cranial nerve III (oculomotor)
   b. Cranial nerve VII (facial)
   c. Cranial nerve IX (glossopharyngeal)
   d. Cranial nerve X (vagus)
7. Intermediolateral portion of the gray matter
8. a. Lateral
   b. Collateral
   c. Terminal
9. Lateral and collateral ganglia are used exclusively by the sympathetic nerves; the terminal ganglia are characteristic of the parasympathetic nerves.
10. Parasympathetic pre- and postganglionic nerves utilize actylcholine as a primary neurotransmitter. Although sympathetic preganglionic nerves also utilize acetylcholine, the postganglionic nerves utilize norepinephrine except in sweat glands where the postganglionic axons of the sympathetic neurons secrete acetylcholine.
11. Because the preganglionic sympathetic axons make their initial synaptic contact within the gland, thus making it analogous to a collateral or terminal ganglion. Activation of the adrenal medulla results in the secretion of the catecholamines epinephrine and norepinephrine, the latter being the primary neurotransmitter of the postganglionic axons of the sympathetic neurons.
12. Convergence refers to the fact that each lateral chain ganglion may receive synaptic input from several spinal segments; divergence refers to the fact that each preganglionic axon from sympathetic nerves may divide within the lateral ganglia before synapsing with several ganglion cells. These collaterals may also pass rostrally or caudally for several segments before synapsing with lateral ganglion cells.
13. The white communicating rami contain the finely myelinated preganglionic sympathetic axons, which connect the thoracolumbar regions of the spinal cord with the

lateral chain ganglia. The gray communicating rami contain the unmyelinated postganglionic sympathetic axons, which connect the lateral chain ganglia with peripheral blood vessels, sweat glands, and piloerector muscles of the hair follicles. The sympathetic axons within the gray communicating rami travel to these peripheral targets via the spinal sensory nerves innervating each region.

14. Yes. There are many more gray communicating rami than white communicating rami because the white rami are found only between the T_1 and L_2 regions of the spinal cord, whereas the divergence of the sympathetic preganglionic fibers in the lateral chain ganglia causes the gray rami to emerge from these ganglia at all levels of the spinal cord (i.e., from the cervical to the coccygeal level).

15. True

16. False

17. True

18. Rostral hypothalamic nuclei are thought to be involved in the modulation of parasympathetic activity; nuclei situated in more caudal (and ventral) regions of the hypothalamus are thought to be involved in the modulation of sympathetic activity.

19. Axons of the dorsal longitudinal fasciculus are involved in parasympathetic regulation; axons in the hypothalamotegmental system are involved in sympathetic regulation.

20. False

SECTION 4-2: THE ADRENAL MEDULLA AND CATECHOLAMINES: SYNTHESIS, STORAGE, UPTAKE, RELEASE, METABOLISM, AND PHYSIOLOGICAL EFFECTS

OBJECTIVES:

The student should be able to:

1. Describe the three general functions of the sympathetic nervous system.
2. Describe the three naturally occurring catecholamines and their sites of production.
3. Describe the biosynthetic pathway for catecholamines, including the enzymes involved.
4. Compare and contrast similarities and differences in storage, uptake, and release of catecholamines by the adrenal medulla and sympathetic nerve endings.
5. Describe where the enzymes important in the metabolism of epinephrine and norepinephrine are located and how they inactivate these hormones.
6. Describe the ultimate fate of secreted epinephrine and norepinephrine.
7. Describe how catecholamines produce their physiologic responses at the tissue level.
8. Classify in general terms α- versus β-adrenergic receptors and the physiologic responses resulting from activation of them.

A. SOME GENERAL CHARACTERISTICS OF THE SYMPATHETIC NERVOUS SYSTEM

The adrenergic or sympathetic nervous system plays an important role in the control of both the cardiovascular and metabolic functions of the body. It provides an important mechanism for rapid cardiovascular adjustments to a variety of situations, such as exercise, exposure to heat and cold, emotional stress, and assumption of an upright posture. Many of these situations occur during the course of a normal day. During

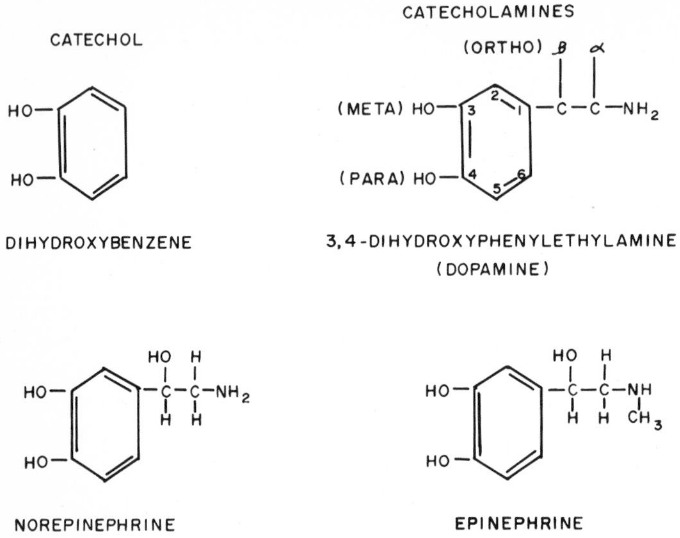

FIGURE 4-4: The biochemical structures of a catechol and of the endogenous catecholamines.

abnormal days, the sympathetic nervous system assumes even greater importance, particularly for such situations as fright, hemorrhage, and shock.

Catecholamines are the hormonal products of the sympathetic nervous system. They consist of an aromatic group—that is, the catechol (dihydroxybenzene) nucleus—and an aliphatic side chain (see Figure 4-4). The most prominent, naturally occurring members of this family are norepinephrine, epinephrine, and dopamine. Catecholamines are synthesized and stored in brain, in sympathetic nerve endings, and in cells of neural crest origin throughout the body (e.g., the adrenal medulla).

Epinephrine is secreted mainly by the adrenal medulla, but norepinephrine is secreted both by the adrenal medulla and sympathetic nerve endings. Adrenal medullary secretion normally contains a greater proportion of epinephrine (approximately 85%) than norepinephrine (approximately 15%). Norepinephrine is found wherever there are sympathetic nerve endings, as well as in the central nervous system. Dopamine is found in significant amounts mainly in the central nervous system. The adrenal medulla, hence epinephrine, does not appear to be essential for life. This may be because there is a certain amount of redundancy of physiologic action between norepinephrine and epinephrine, with norepinephrine appearing generally to play the more important role in cardiovascular adjustments, and epinephrine generally assuming the more important role in metabolic adjustments.

B. SYNTHESIS OF CATECHOLAMINES

Catecholamine synthesis takes place in brain, in sympathetic nerve endings, and in chromaffin tissue, such as the adrenal medulla. The most active functional unit in the adrenergic nervous system is the granular vesicle that is involved in the synthesis, storage, and release of the neurotransmitter norepinephrine. Granular vesicles are subcellular particles of 30 to 60 μm in diameter located in terminal adrenergic axons. These vesicles share some of the physical and biochemical properties of the larger, catecholamine storing granules found in chromaffin cells of the adrenal medulla. Just as the same steroid biosynthetic pathway is shared by all steroid hormone-secreting glands, the catecholamine biosynthetic pathway appears to be shared by all tissues that produce catecholamines. Again, as was the case with the steroid biosynthetic pathway, the difference in hormonal end products from tissue to tissue is related to the absence (or presence, if you wish) of one or two key enzymes.

The biosynthetic pathway for dopamine, norepinephrine, and epinephrine is shown in Figure 4-5. Just as cholesterol is the basic raw material from which steroid hormones are made, the amino acid tyrosine is the basic raw material of catecholamines. (*Q. 4-5*) *What other important hormone is formed from tyrosine?*

Three enzymatic steps are involved in the synthesis of norepinephrine, and four in the synthesis of epinephrine, from tyrosine.

1. *Tyrosine Hydroxylase.* The amino acid tyrosine, derived from food or by hydroxylation of phenylalanine in the liver, enters the cell, where it is converted by tyrosine hydroxylase, a mitochondrial enzyme, to dihydroxyphenylalanine (DOPA). Tyrosine hydroxylase has a high degree of substrate specificity but low substrate affinity. Thus, for optimal catecholamine synthesis, there must be both adequate quantities of tyrosine and active transport of tyrosine across cell membranes. The conversion of tyrosine to DOPA is the rate-limiting step in catecholamine synthesis. The pharmacologic agent α-methylparatyrosine, can inhibit tyrosine hydroxylase. There is evidence to suggest that norepinephrine may also inhibit this reaction, thus providing a negative feedback limb to regulate its own synthesis (see Figure 4-5).

2. *DOPA-Decarboxylase.* The second step in the synthesis of norepinephrine involves the conversion of DOPA to dopamine in the cytoplasmic fraction of the cell. This

FIGURE 4-5: Selected features of the biosynthetic pathway for the production of catecholamines. Epinephrine is produced in the adrenal medulla and chromaffin tissue; norepinephrine is produced mainly in sympathetic nerve endings but also in the adrenal medulla. Dopamine, norepinephrine, and epinephrine are also produced by neurons in the central nervous system. Increased blood concentrations of norepinephrine and dopamine form a portion of feedback limbs that regulate the enzyme tyrosine hydroxylase. (*Q. 4-6*) *Is this positive or negative feedback?*

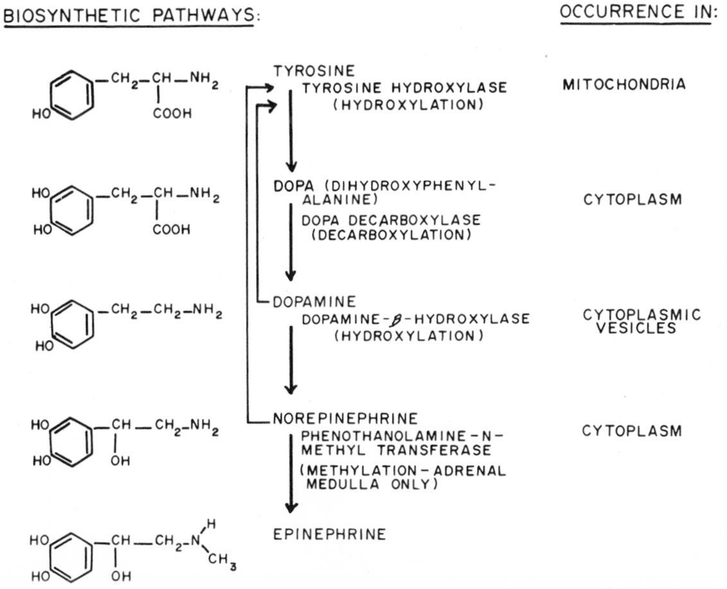

BIOSYNTHETIC PATHWAYS: OCCURRENCE IN:

TYROSINE
TYROSINE HYDROXYLASE
(HYDROXYLATION) MITOCHONDRIA

DOPA (DIHYDROXYPHENYL-ALANINE)
DOPA DECARBOXYLASE
(DECARBOXYLATION) CYTOPLASM

DOPAMINE
DOPAMINE-β-HYDROXYLASE
(HYDROXYLATION) CYTOPLASMIC VESICLES

NOREPINEPHRINE
PHENOTHANOLAMINE-N-METHYL TRANSFERASE
(METHYLATION-ADRENAL MEDULLA ONLY) CYTOPLASM

EPINEPHRINE

enzyme is relatively nonspecific, since it can also decarboxylate other aromatic amino acids, such as tyrosine, 5-hydroxytryptophan, and histidine to their corresponding amines (tyramine, serotonin, and histamine). The pharmacologic agent α-methyldopa can also serve as a substrate for this enzyme and can compete effectively with the natural substrate, DOPA. As a result, α-methyldopa enters the biosynthetic pathway and is ultimately converted to α-methylnorepinephrine, a false and less effective transmitter, which replaces norepinephrine in the nerve ending. α-Methyldopa has found clinical use as an antihypertensive agent.

3. Dopamine-β-Hydroxylase. Dopamine is actively transported from the cytoplasm into highly specialized granules that are localized in sympathetic neurons and the adrenal medulla. They contain the enzyme dopamine-β-hydroxylase (DBH), which hydroxylates dopamine to norepinephrine. Disulfiram, a drug used to produce an aversion to alcohol, inhibits dopamine-β-hydroxylase. Experimental evidence suggests that dopamine, like norepinephrine, can also inhibit tyrosine hydroxylase and can act as a negative feedback limb to regulate its own synthesis (see Figure 4-5).

4. Phenylethanolamine-N-Methyltransferase. The adrenal medulla, and other chromaffin tissue, contains phenylethanolamine-N-methyltransferase (PNMT), which is responsible for the conversion of norepinephrine to epinephrine. This process occurs in the cytoplasm of the cell.

C. STORAGE, UPTAKE, AND RELEASE OF CATECHOLAMINES

1. The Adrenal Medulla. In the adrenal medulla, catecholamines are stored in granules in a nonionic, nondiffusable form (bound to protein). The binding mechanism appears to be dependent on an ATP-Mg^{2+} complex. ATP is present in granules in a molar ratio to catecholamines of about $1:4$.

The adrenal medullary cells secreting catecholamines actually are modified nerve ganglion cells because they developed embryologically from the same cells as the sympathetic, postganglionic neurons. (*Q. 4-7*) *Do you recall the embryologic origin of these cells?* The adrenal medulla is therefore a ganglion, a postanglionic fiber, and an end organ all in one.

Catecholamine secretion by the adrenal medulla is activated when acetylcholine is released from preganglionic fibers during sympathetic nervous stimulation. This results in an increased influx of calcium ions from extracellular fluid into the cell and into the intracellular granules, where they trigger exocytosis. In this way, the contents of the granules, including catecholamines, ATP, and proteins, are discharged from the cell. (*Q. 4-8*) *What do you think happens to the dopamine-β-hydroxylase in the granules containing norepinephrine?*

2. The Sympathetic Nerve Ending. In the case of the sympathetic nerve endings, there appear to be two pools of norepinephrine. The smaller pool contains 10–20% of the total norepinephrine in the nerve ending. This is the *active pool*, with a norepinephrine half-life of approximately 2 hours. The remaining 80–90% of the total norepinephrine in the nerve ending appears to be in a relatively *inactive pool* with a norepinephrine half-life of approximately 24 hours. These pools are really conceptual ones that seem to have no actual or rigid anatomic location in the nerve ending. The entire concept is based on the turnover of the radioactive norepinephrine in the nerve endings as well as the failure of certain catecholamine depleting drugs, such as tyramine and reserpine, to deplete nerve endings of much more than 20% of their total norepinephrine content. Thus it is apparent that the physiologically important pool is the active one.

Electrical activity in sympathetic nerves initiates the release of norepinephrine from the active or smaller pool. When the sympathetic nerves are depolarized, the vesicles in the nerve terminals fuse with the neuronal membrane. An opening then occurs, making it possible for the soluble contents of the vesicle, including norepinephrine and the enzyme dopamine-β-hydroxylase, to be discharged into the synaptic cleft. This process of exocytosis is also dependent for its initiation on calcium ions. It is most likely that a similar process of release takes place in the adrenergic neurons of the brain.

In contrast to the adrenal medulla, the secretion process in sympathetic nerve endings is really a balance between release of norepinephrine from the vesicles and cells and reuptake by the same cells and vesicles. When norepinephrine is released, a small amount of it stimulates nearby effector sites (receptors) without ever getting into blood. It is estimated that 50% of the norepinephrine released reenters the neuron and is bound in the specialized vesicles (see Figure 4-6). Thus, the inactivation or modulation of the

FIGURE 4-6: The fate of norepinephrine (NE) at the peripheral adrenergic synapse. After release by sympathetic nerve impulses, the action of NE is terminated principally by reuptake into the sympathetic nerves, although some is O-methylated locally and some may escape into the circulation. NE in the circulation may be excreted unchanged or metabolized to normetanephrine (NMN) in liver or kidney. Storage NE is deaminated in the neuron by monoamine oxidase (MAO), which regulates the size of the storage pool. The dihydroxymandelic acid (DHMA) that results is O-methylated to vanillylmandelic acid (VMA), which is circled in the diagram to emphasize the large contribution to daily VMA excretion made by intraneuronal metabolism. The excretion of NE and NMN reflect release of active NE.

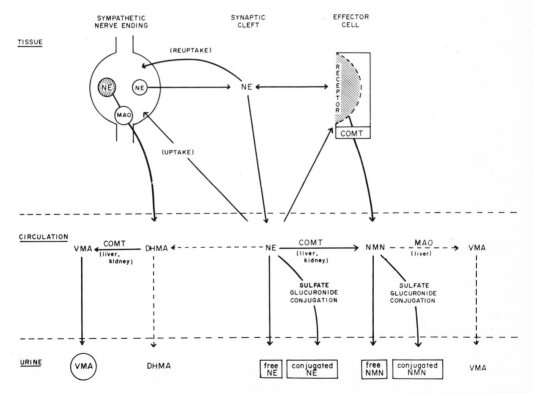

effects of released norepinephrine is accomplished without destruction of the molecule—an economic biologic recycling technique. If recycling of norepinephrine is prevented by drugs such as chlorpromazine or imipramine, or destruction of storage vesicles occurs with the use of reserpine or guanethidine, there is potentiation of the action of either endogenously released or exogenously administered catecholamines. (*Q. 4-9*) *What do you think happens to endogenous norepinephrine release during prolonged stimulation (e.g., during certain stressful situations), when norepinephrine reuptake is prevented?*

D. METABOLISM AND INACTIVATION

Circulating catecholamines are metabolized by the enzyme catechol-O-methyltransferase (COMT) found in plasma, liver, and kidneys. Inhibition of this enzyme in animals results in potentiation of the effects of both endogenously produced and exogenously administered catecholamines (see Figure 4-7).

A second enzyme, monoamine oxidase (MAO), also metabolizes catecholamines. It is found mainly in nerve endings and is primarily responsible for the intraneuronal metabolism of catecholamines after their release from storage vesicles and before they reach the circulation. MAO probably plays little, if any, role in the metabolism of circulating catecholamines. MAO deaminates norepinephrine, and the deaminated metabolites are released into the circulation, where they are O-methylated by COMT and finally excreted into urine as vanillyl-mandelic acid (VMA). The norepinephrine contained in the larger inactive pool in nerve endings plays little physiologic role

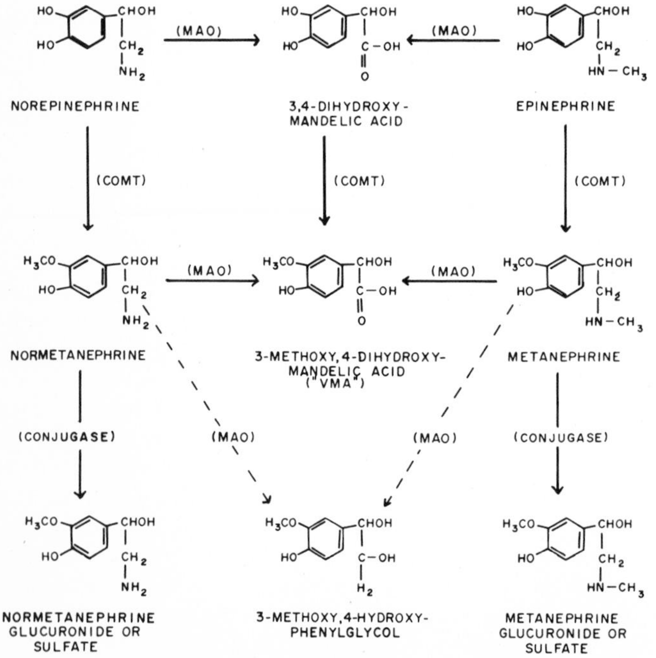

FIGURE 4-7: Steps in the metabolism of catecholamines. Initial deamination of norepinephrine and epinephrine to 3,4-hydroxymandelic acid by monoamine oxidase (MAO) occurs as the initial step in the metabolic process. Alternatively epinephrine and norepinephrine can be methylated by catechol-O-methyltransferase (COMT) to normetanephrine and metanephrine, respectively. Most of these metabolites are converted to 3-methoxy-4-dihydroxymandelic acid (VMA) and MAO. A small amount of the normetanephrine and metanephrine are reduced to 3-methoxy-4-hydroxyphenylglycol; another small amount is conjugated with glucuronides or sulfates. (*Adapted from:* Koelle, 1970.)

TABLE 4-2: Excretion of Catecholamines and Metabolites in Humans

	μg/day[a]	Source[b]
Epinephrine (free)	5	ADRENAL MEDULLA
Norepinephrine (free)	30	SYMPATHETIC NERVE ENDINGS Adrenal medulla
Conjugated catecholamines	100	SYMPATHETIC NERVE ENDINGS Dietary catecholamines Adrenal medulla
Metanephrine (total)	65	ADRENAL MEDULLA
Normetanephrine (total)	100	SYMPATHETIC NERVE ENDINGS Adrenal medulla
Vanillylmandelic acid	4000	SYMPATHETIC NERVE ENDINGS (Storage pool) ADRENAL MEDULLA, BRAIN
3-Methoxy-4-hydroxyphenylglycol	2000	BRAIN SYMPATHETIC NERVE ENDINGS (Storage pool) ADRENAL MEDULLA
Total	6300	

[a] Average daily excretion—not upper limit. [b] Major source names capitalized.

because it is not easily released by either physiologic or pharmacologic stimuli. Most of it is metabolized slowly in the nerve ending before ever reaching the circulation and is excreted eventually as VMA (see Figure 4-6). The average daily amounts of the catecholamines and their metabolites excreted by humans are shown in Table 4-2.

E. PHYSIOLOGIC EFFECTS OF CATECHOLAMINES

The regulatory actions of the sympathoadrenal system are exerted on three general physiologic functions: circulatory, metabolic, and visceral (see Table 4-3). Catecholamines are important in regulating the distribution of blood flow to metabolizing tissues in accordance with the needs of the organism. Thus, catecholamines contribute significantly to blood flow adjustments to the upright posture, to volume depletion (hemorrhage), to exercise, and to the postprandial state. They also influence the distribution of blood flow to the skin during exposure to heat and cold as well as influencing blood flow to the kidney. With regard to metabolic functions, catecholamines are important in the provision of adequate substrate to metabolizing tissues in accordance with the needs of the organism. They participate in the regulation of blood glucose and free fatty acid levels and in temperature regulation. Catecholamines are also important in the regulation of vegetative processes. Smooth muscle tone of the intestines and bladder is influenced by catecholamines, as is the control of sphincters in these organs. Ejaculation is also influenced by catecholamines (see Table 4-3).

Catecholamines produce their physiologic response by way of receptors. There are two general types of catecholamine receptor, α and β. These receptors were originally classified on the basis of their responsiveness to six sympathomimetic amines, includ-

TABLE 4-3: Functions of the Sympathoadrenal System

	Homeostatic Role	Physiologic Functions
Circulatory functions	The appropriate distribution of blood flow to metabolizing tissues in accordance with the needs of the organism	Blood flow adjustment to: Upright posture Volume depletion Exercise Postprandial state Renal blood flow Skin blood flow
Metabolic functions	The provision of adequate substrate to metabolizing tissues in accordance with the needs of the organism	Regulation of blood glucose: Postabsorptive fast Exercise Regulation of blood free fatty acids Temperature regulation
Visceral functions	The regulation of vegetative processes in accordance with the needs of the organism	Bowel tone and sphincter control Bladder tone and sphincter control Ejaculation Temperature regulation (sweating)

ing the naturally occurring catecholamines (epinephrine and norepinephrine) and the synthetic catecholamine isoproterenol, a "pure" β-adrenergic agonist. An additional basis for classification is the ability of certain pharmacologic agents to "block" the receptor. Thus, when epinephrine was the most potent and isoproterenol the least potent in eliciting a response, the receptor mediating the response was classified as an α-adrenergic receptor. The pharmacologic agents phentolamine and phenoxybenzamine, and certain ergot alkaloids, will block this response. These agents are classified as α-adrenergic antagonists. When isoproterenol was the most potent in eliciting a response and norepinephrine the least potent, the receptor was classified as a β-adrenergic receptor. The pharmacologic agent propranolol will block the effect of isoproterenol. Propanolol is classified as a β-adrenergic antagonist.

The cellular effects of catecholamines occur by way of the cAMP system. They were the first hormones shown to affect this system. As a generalization only, it is useful to think of β-adrenergic receptors as those that initiate an increase in the cAMP concentration of effector cells, whereas α-adrenergic receptors decrease the cAMP concentration.

The student should not be discouraged by exceptions to the generalizations outlined above. A careful perusal of Table 4-4 will reveal that the heart appears to have β-adrenergic receptors only, and these increase heart rate, conduction velocity, and contractility. This contrasts with other tissues such as skeletal muscle and stomach, and most other organs, in which activation of β-adrenergic receptors is accompanied by relaxation. This means that the bases on which we presently classify receptors do not include similarities in the physiologic effect of activation of the receptors.

Table 4-4 divides the effects of catecholamines into the same circulatory, metabolic, and visceral categories used in Table 4-3. Table 4-4, however, shows the predominant receptor types in that tissue or organ, the predominant physiologic or pharmacologic effects, and the predominant in vivo responses. Notice that there are some tissues, particularly in the gastrointestinal tract, whose response to either α- or β-adrenergic stimulation is the same. This represents another of those bothersome, sticky exceptions to the generalizations outlined above.

The contents of Table 4-4 are not to be memorized. They are provided to show the diversity of physiologic effects influenced by catecholamines. By the time you finish your formal education, you will have committed to memory most of these responses. For the present, the contents of Table 4-4 can be considered to be useful for reference only.

TABLE 4-4: Effects of Catecholamines (or Stimulation of Sympathetic Nerves)

Tissue	Receptor	Predominant Physiologic or Pharmacologic Effects	Predominant in vivo Response
CIRCULATORY EFFECTS			
Heart			
Sinus node	β	↑ Rate	↑ Cardiac Output
Junctional tissue	β	↑ Conduction velocity	
Myocardium	β	↑ Contractility	
Arteries			
Renal	α	Vasoconstriction	
Splanchnic	α	Vasoconstriction	↓ Local blood flow
Subcutaneous	α	Vasoconstriction	↑ Systematic blood pressure
Mucosa	α	Vasoconstriction	
Cerebral	*	Minimal direct effect	No change in cerebral flow
Coronary	*	Minimal direct effect	↑ Coronary flow (indirect effect)
Skeletal muscle	β	Vasodilation	↑ Local blood flow ↓ Systemic blood pressure
Veins	α	Vasoconstriction	↑ Venous return ↑ Cardiac output
Juxtaglomerular apparatus	β	↑ Renin secretion	↑ Na^+ reabsorption (via aldosterone) ↑ Blood pressure (via angiotensin II)
METABOLIC EFFECTS			
Liver	*	↑ Glycogenolysis	↑ Blood glucose
	*	↑ Gluconeogenesis	↑ Blood glucose
Muscle	β	↑ Glycogenolysis	↑ Blood glucose
	β	↓ Glucose utilization	↑ Blood glucose
Pancreas	α	↓ Insulin secretion	↑ Blood glucose
	β	↑ Insulin secretion	↓ Blood glucose
Adipose tissue	β	↑ Lipolysis	↑ Blood free fatty acids
VISCERAL EFFECTS			
Gastrointestinal tract			
Gastric glands	α,β	Decreases secretion	Decreases gastric acidity, volume
Gastric smooth muscle	β	Relaxation	

(continued)

TABLE 4-4: (*continued*)

Tissue	Receptor	Predominant Physiologic or Pharmacologic Effects	Predominant in vivo Response
		VISCERAL EFFECTS	
Intestinal smooth muscle	α,β	Relaxation	Decreases motility
Intestinal sphincter	α	Contraction	
Lung			
Bronchial smooth muscle	β	Relaxation	Bronchodilation
Urinary bladder			
Detrusor muscle	β	Relaxation	Inhibits micturition
Trigone, sphincter	α	Contraction	
Eye			
Iris, radial muscle	α	Contraction	Mydriasis
Ciliary muscle	β	Relaxation	Accommodation
Uterus			
Myometrium	α	Contraction	Depends on hormonal milieu
Skin			
Pilomotor muscle	α	Contraction	Piloerection
Sweat glands	α	↑ Secretion	"Adrenergic" sweating

* Characterization with regard to receptors not clearly defined (see text).

SECTION 4-2: POST-TEST QUESTIONS

1. The regulatory functions of the adrenergic nervous system are exerted on which three general physiologic functions.
    a.
    b.
    c.
2. What are the three naturally occurring catecholamines?
    a.
    b.
    c.
3. Respectively, where are these produced?
    a.
    b.
    c.
4. The biosynthetic pathway used by the body for synthesis of all catecholamines has as its basic precursor the amino acid tyrosine. (True/False)
5. In this sense it is similar to the steroid biosynthetic pathway, which uses _____ _____ as its common precursor.
6. A further similarity between the two biosynthetic pathways is that the different hormones produced are the result of the presence (or absence) of a few key enzymes. (True/False)
7. The chromaffin granules of the adrenal medulla take up epinephrine released into the circulation. (True/False)

8. A method by which the body attenuates or modulates the physiologic responses to secreted norepinephrine is _____ .

9. What enzymes are responsible for the metabolism of catecholamines?
   a.
   b.
10. Which enzyme is found mainly in nerve endings? _____
11. Where is the other enzyme mainly found? _____
12. What is the ultimate fate of the secreted epinephrine that does not activate tissue receptors?

13. What is the ultimate fate of the norepinephrine that does not activate tissue receptors and is not taken up again by the nerve ending?

14. In view of your answers to questions 12 and 13, what urinary metabolites would you measure if you wished to assess the rate of secretion of norepinephrine?

15. How do catecholamines produce their physiologic responses at the tissue level?

16. What are the two general types of adrenergic receptors?
    a.
    b.
17. How are they classified?
    a.

    b.

18. In general, what effect does stimulation of a β-adrenergic receptor have on generation of cellular cAMP?

SECTION 4-2: POST-TEST ANSWERS

1. a. Circulatory
   b. Metabolic
   c. Visceral
2. a. Norepinephrine
   b. Epinephrine
   c. Dopamine
3. a. Sympathetic nerve endings
   b. Adrenal medulla
   c. Nerve endings in central nervous system
4. True
5. cholesterol

6. True
7. False
8. the reuptake (recycling) of norepinephrine back into the vesicles of nerve endings.
9. a. Monoamine oxidase
   b. Catechol-O-methyltransferase
10. Monoamine oxidase
11. In the blood
12. Epinephrine is excreted into urine as metanephrine (free and conjugated), as vanillymandelic acid (VMA), as free epinephrine, and as 3-methoxy-4-hydroxyphenylglycol.
13. Norepinephrine is excreted into urine as normetanephrine (free and conjugated), as VMA, as free norepinephrine, and as 3-methoxy-4-hydroxyphenylglycol.
14. Urinary output of free norepinephrine and free and conjugated normetanephrine.
15. By effects on the enzyme adenylate cyclase.
16. a. α
    b. β
17. a. α-Adrenergic receptors have a greater responsiveness to norepinephrine and epinephrine than to isoproterenol, and the norepinephrine responses are blocked by α-adrenergic antagonists, such as phentolamine.
    b. β-Adrenergic receptors have a greater responsiveness to isoproterenol than to norepinephrine and epinephrine, and the isoproterenol responses are blocked by β-adrenergic antagonists, such as propranolol.
18. It increases it. Stimulation of α-receptors generally decreases cellular cAMP.

SELECTED REFERENCES

DeQuattro, V., Myers, M. R., and Campese, V. M., 1979, Anatomy and biochemistry of the sympathetic nervous system, in *Endocrinology*, L. J. DeGroot, G. F. Cahill, Jr., L. Martini, D. H. Nelsen, W. D. Odell, J. T. Potts, Jr., E. Steinberger, and A. I. Winegrad (Eds.), New York: Grune & Stratton, p. 1241.

Kunos, G., 1978, Adrenoceptors, *Annual Review Of Pharmacology And Toxicology* 18: 291.

Levitzki, A., 1978, Catecholamine receptors, *Review Of Physiology And Pharmacology* 82: 1.

Snell, R. S., 1980, *Clinical Neuroanatomy For Medical Students*, Boston: Little, Brown and Co., Ch. 25, p. 409.

Strosberg, A. D., Vaugquelin, G., Durieu-Trautmann, O., Delavier-Klutchko, C., Bottari, S., and Audre, C., 1980, Towards the chemical and functional characterization of the β-receptor, *Trends In Biochemical Sciences* 5: 11.

5

THE ADRENAL CORTEX

SECTION 5-1: ANATOMIC REVIEW OF THE ADRENAL GLAND

OBJECTIVES:

The student should be able to:
1. Name the embryonic origins of the adrenal cortex and medulla.
2. Name the three divisions of the adrenal cortex and identify their hormonal products.
3. Describe the similarities between the adrenal medulla and a postganglionic neuron.
4. Describe the adrenal blood supply.
5. Discuss the interrelation between adrenal cortical and medullary secretions.

The adrenal or suprarenal glands are two small, yellowish glands situated on the superior poles of the kidneys. Each weighs approximately 4 g in the human, with the weight in an adult being about one-thirtieth that of the kidney. During fetal development, this ratio is much larger due both to renal immaturity and to the presence of an enlarged fetal adrenal cortex.

Each adrenal gland is divided into two morphologically and functionally distinct regions (see Figure 5-1). The adrenal cortex, the more exterior region, is of mesodermal origin. At the cellular level it can be divided into three regions of variable distinctiveness. These are the zona glomerulosa (outermost zone), the zona fasciculata (intermediate zone), and the zona reticularis (innermost zone). The zona glomerulosa is responsible for the secretion of the *mineralocorticoid hormone aldosterone* (this hormone is discussed in detail in Section 5-8. The *glucocorticoid hormones cortisol* and *corticosterone* are both secreted by the inner two zones of the adrenal cortex, the fasciculata and reticularis. The same two zones have also been observed to secrete a significant amount of androgens, specifically dehydroepiandrosterone and androstenedione. The interior region, or medulla, of the adrenal gland is of neural crest origin. Likened to a large postganglionic neuron, the medulla secretes epinephrine and norepinephrine upon stimulation by preganglionic sympathetic fibers.

The adrenal glands, like all endocrine organs, are highly vascularized. The aorta, the renal arteries, and the phrenic arteries all supply numerous branches to each gland. These arterial branches enter the capsule to form a capsular plexus. From this plexus

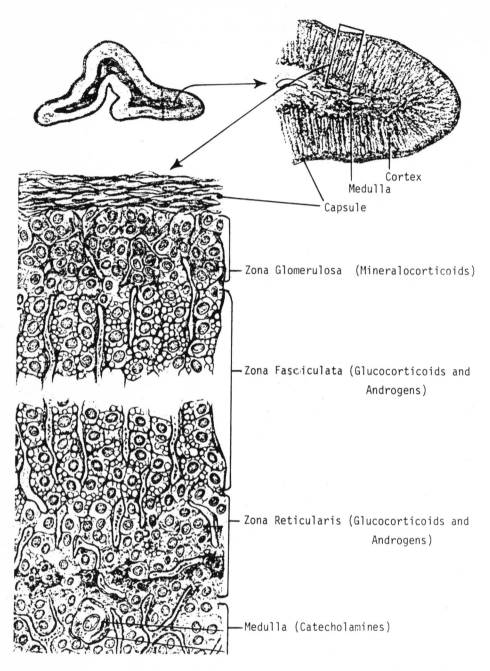

Cortex

Medulla

Capsule

Zona Glomerulosa (Mineralocorticoids)

Zona Fasciculata (Glucocorticoids and
Androgens)

Zona Reticularis (Glucocorticoids and
Androgens)

Medulla (Catecholamines)

FIGURE 5-1: Cross section through the adrenal, illustrating the major subdivisions and cell layers as well as their hormonal products. (*Adapted from:* Ham and Cormack, 1979.)

cortical arteries enter the anastomosing sinusoids of the cortex to drain eventually into the collecting veins at the corticomedullary junction. The capsular plexus also gives off medullary arteries, which pass through the cortex to form branching sinusoids in the medulla. Thus the medulla has a dual blood supply: from branches of the corticomedullary collecting veins and from the medullary arteries. The former vascular route to the medulla is of considerable physiologic interest. It seems that the activity of the enzyme that converts norepinephrine to epinephrine, phenylethanolamine-N-methyltransferase, is dependent on high concentrations of glucocorticoids. Blood from the corticomedullary collecting veins is rich in cortical steroids, and so is essential for the normal production of epinephrine. The medullary sinusoids eventually drain into the suprarenal vein, which empties into the inferior vena cava.

SECTION 5-1: POST-TEST QUESTIONS

1. Why are the adrenal glands often called the "suprarenal" glands?

2. Name the three zones of the adrenal cortex and their secretory products.
   a.
   b.
   c.
3. What are the embryonic origins of the adrenal cortex and medulla?

4. What type of stimulation causes the secretion of epinephrine and norepinephrine?

5. Why is the medulla considered to be a sympathetic postganglionic neuron?

6. How many vascular routes supply the medulla?

7. What is the special significance of one of these routes?

SECTION 5-1: POST-TEST ANSWERS

1. Because they are located anatomically on the superior poles of the kidneys.
2. a. Zona glomerulosa: aldosterone
   b. Zona fasciculata: cortisol, corticosterone, androgens
   c. Zona reticularis: cortisol, corticosterone, androgens
3. Adrenal cortex is derived from mesoderm. Adrenal medulla is of neural crest origin.
4. Preganglionic sympathetic (acetycholine)
5. Like a sympathetic postganglionic neuron, the medulla secretes catecholamines when stimulated by acetylcholine.
6. Two; one that bypasses the cortex and one that passes through the cortex.
7. The glucocorticoid hormones present in the second route activate the enzyme responsible for the conversion of norepinephrine to epinephrine.

SECTION 5-2: HORMONES OF THE ADRENAL CORTEX

OBJECTIVES:

The student should be able to:
1. Identify a steroid nucleus.
2. Be familiar with the sites on the steroid molecule that confer glucocorticoid, mineralocorticoid, estrogenic, and androgenic activity.
3. State in general terms the physiologic effects of glucocorticoid and mineralocorticoid hormones.

In Chapter 3, "The Thyroid Gland," you probably noticed that the chemical structures of the thyroid hormones could be characterized as amino acids. In contrast, the adrenal cortex is an endocrine organ that secretes steroid hormones. The structure of a steroid hormone with the standard numbering system used for exact identification is given in Figure 5-2.

Notice that the four rings of the structure are labeled A, B, C, and D. The numbering system begins on ring A. In many but not all steroids, there is a double bond in ring A between the 4 and 5 positions. We see later that notable exceptions to this are the naturally occurring estrogens, where ring A has a benzene (i.e., unsaturated) structure. We also see later that saturation of the double bond between the 4 and 5 positions is an important step in the metabolism of certain steroid compounds by the liver.

The adrenal cortex is generally considered to secrete three classes of steroids: glucocorticoids, mineralocorticoids, and androgens. Their generalized structures are shown in Figure 5-3, which also includes estrogenic-type compounds for comparison.

The compounds having a methyl group at the C-18 position and an unsaturated ring A are estrogens. The major source of these compounds is the ovary. The compounds having a methyl group at both the C-18 and C-19 positions are androgens. The major source of these compounds is the testis, although the adrenal gland also produces androgenic

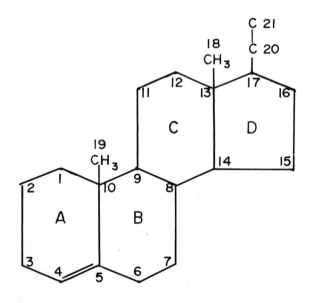

FIGURE 5-2: Steroid structure showing the numbering system used to identify specific steroid compounds.

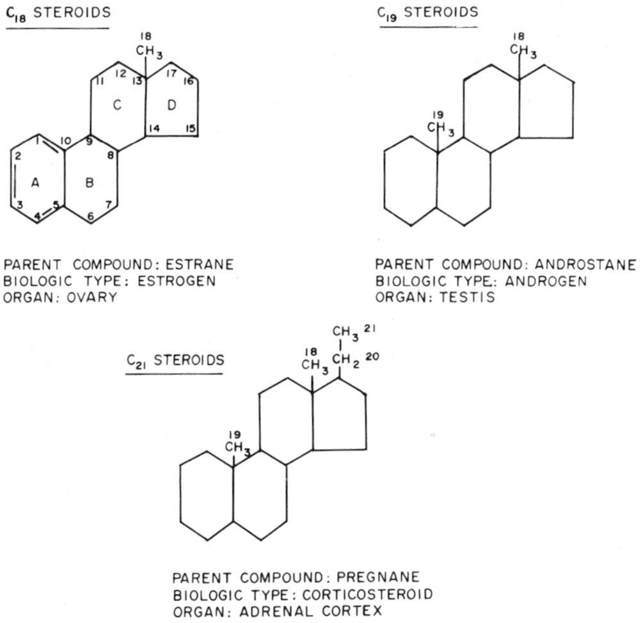

C_{18} STEROIDS

C_{19} STEROIDS

PARENT COMPOUND: ESTRANE
BIOLOGIC TYPE: ESTROGEN
ORGAN: OVARY

PARENT COMPOUND: ANDROSTANE
BIOLOGIC TYPE: ANDROGEN
ORGAN: TESTIS

FIGURE 5-3: Three classes of steroids produced by the body.

C_{21} STEROIDS

PARENT COMPOUND: PREGNANE
BIOLOGIC TYPE: CORTICOSTEROID
ORGAN: ADRENAL CORTEX

hormones. The compounds having methyl groups at C-18, C-19, C-20, and C-21 positions are corticosteroid compounds. These include both the glucocorticoid and mineralocorticoid steroids.

The mineralocorticoid hormone aldosterone promotes sodium reabsorption and increases the excretion of potassium and hydrogen ions by the kidney. The ratio of the concentrations in urine of sodium and potassium decreases when blood levels of aldosterone increase, and vice versa. In addition, an increase in the concentration of aldosterone in blood decreases the Na^+/K^+ ratio of saliva, sweat, and feces. All routes of loss of sodium and potassium from the body are controlled by aldosterone, which is the naturally occurring mineralocorticoid hormone. Other aspects of the physiology of aldosterone are discussed in Section 5-8.

The glucocorticoid hormone cortisol supports physiologic processes that supply glucose to the tissues. For example, during fasting, the body must supply its own glucose because critical organs such as the brain require glucose to continue functioning. Cortisol not only helps to get glucose into the blood, but may also help to direct it to the brain. The physiologic effects of cortisol are discussed in greater detail in Section 5-9.

The androgenic hormones (dehydroepiandrosterone and androstenedione) produced by the adrenal cortex have relatively weak androgenic activity. The physiologic importance of these hormones in normal individuals is unclear. We see in a later section that blocks in the biosynthetic pathway that result in an increased secretion of these hormones can produce pathologic consequences.

Table 5-1 shows the types of adrenal cortical hormones and their daily rates of secretion in normal humans.

It is clear from Table 5-1 that the major glucocorticoid hormone in humans is cortisol (also called hydrocortisone and compound F), and the major mineralocorticoid hormone is aldosterone. Although dehydroepiandrosterone (DHEA) is secreted at a rate equivalent to that of cortisol, its glucocorticoid potency is low. Present evidence sug-

TABLE 5-1: Adrenal Steroid Secretion in Normal Man

Group	Compounds	Mean 24 Hour Secretion in Adults
Glucocorticoids	Cortisol	15–30 mg[a]
	Corticosterone	2–5 mg[a]
Mineralocorticoids	Aldosterone	50–150 μg[a]
	11-Deoxycorticosterone	Normally only traces
Androgens	Dehydroepiandrosterone	15–30 mg[a]
	Androstenedione	0–10 mg
	11-β-Hydroxyandrostenedione	0–10 mg
Gestagens	Progesterone	0.4–0.8 mg
Estrogens	Estradiol	Trace

[a] Major secretory products in normal humans.

gests, however, that some of the adrenal androgens are converted to testosterone by peripheral tissues. In spite of the large production of androgenic hormones by the adrenal cortex and conversion to testosterone by peripheral tissues, the amounts are insufficient to maintain secondary sexual characteristics in castrated male humans or other animals. Several intermediate compounds in the biosynthetic pathway of the adrenal cortex can be found in adrenal cortical secretions. These include corticosterone, 11-deoxycorticosterone, dehydroepiandrosterone, and progesterone. It is not clear why and how this "leakage" occurs, but it is characteristic of steroid producing endocrine organs. Unlike the thyroid gland, the adrenal cortex appears to be unable to store appreciable amounts of its hormones.

SECTION 5-2: POST-TEST QUESTIONS

1. The steroid structure contains a. _____ six-carbon and b. _____ five-carbon rings.
2. The aromatic (i.e., benzenelike) ring in estrogens is called the D-ring. (True/False)
3. In the standard steroid numbering system the C-19 methyl group is found:
   a. Between the A and B rings
   b. Between the B and C rings
   c. Between the C and D rings
   d. Attached to the D ring only
4. The C-21 steroids have a. _____ and b. _____ activity.
5. A rise in blood concentration of aldosterone increases urine Na^+/K^+ concentration. (True/False)
6. The glucocorticoid hormone cortisol supports physiologic processes that _____ _____ .
7. The adrenal cortex normally produces a sufficient amount of androgenic hormones to compensate for castration in male animals. (True/False)
8. The adrenal gland, like the thyroid gland, has a sufficient store of hormones to last several weeks if production of hormones is suddenly stopped. (True/False)

SECTION 5-2: POST-TEST ANSWERS

1. a. three
   b. one
2. False
3. a
4. a. glucocorticoid
   b. mineralocorticoid
5. False
6. supply glucose to the tissues
7. False
8. False

SECTION 5-3: SYNTHESIS OF ADRENOCORTICAL HORMONES

OBJECTIVES:

The student should be able to:
1. Recite the biosynthetic pathways of the adrenal cortex.
2. Describe the cellular location of enzymes important in the biosynthetic pathways of the adrenal cortex.
3. State why the zona glomerulosa does not produce cortisol.

In Chapter 1, "Organization and Control of Endocrine Systems," the biosynthetic pathway for steroid secretion was discussed briefly. It is necessary in this chapter to consider the biosynthetic pathways in greater detail. An understanding of them, and the enzymes involved, is essential to an understanding of many clinical endocrinopathies.

Keep in mind as you study the steroid biosynthetic pathways that the same basic scheme for steroid synthesis can be seen in all the steroid hormone-producing endocrine glands of the body (e.g., adrenal cortex, testes, and ovaries). The small structural differences that are necessary to produce hormonal specificity are simply due to the presence or absence of a few key enzymes in the same basic biosynthetic pathway. As you observed in Fig. 5-3, the ovaries, testes, and adrenal cortex produce C-18, C-19, and C-21 steroids, respectively. These major structural differences, which are the result of the presence or absence of certain enzymes in these three endocrine organs, provide hormonal specificity. You will also see in this section that a single endocrine organ like the adrenal cortex may produce different steroid end products because the enzymatic complements of its three basic zones, the glomerulosa, fasciculata, and reticularis, are different.

A skeleton biosynthetic pathway for the adrenal cortex (with no chemical structures) is shown in Figure 5-4. This figure highlights the important adrenal cortical enzymes required for the production of mineralocorticoid, glucocorticoid, and androgenic hormones.

The chief precursor for all the steroid hormones is cholesterol, which the adrenal cortex, testes, and ovaries are capable of synthesizing de novo from acetate. The synthetic steps, which are identical up to the major branch points at progesterone for all three organs are as follows: a) cleavage of the cholesterol side chain at the C-21 and C-22 positions; this reaction involves a series of hydroxylations and is catalyzed by the

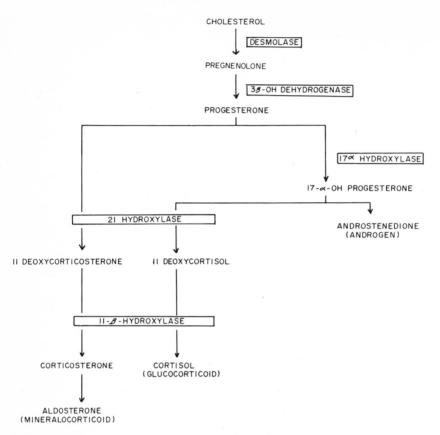

FIGURE 5-4: Five adrenal biosynthetic enzymes necessary for production of aldosterone, cortisol, and androstenedione.

desmolase enzyme complex apparently within the mitochondria, and b) conversion of the reaction product, pregnenolone, to progesterone by the enzymes 3β-hydroxy steroid dehydrogenase and 3-ketosteroid isomerase, which shift the double bond in ring A of the steroid structure from the 5-6 to the 4-5 position. These enzymes are localized in microsomal fractions of adrenal cortical cells.

In the zonae fasciculata and reticularis, progesterone is converted to 17α-OH-progesterone through the action of the cytoplasmic enzyme 17α-hydroxylase. 17β-OH-Progesterone is converted by a C-21 hydroxylase enzyme in cytoplasm to 11-deoxycortisol. An 11β-hydroxylase enzyme is present in mitochondria which converts 11-deoxycortisol to the finished glucocorticoid product, cortisol (see Figure 5-4). This conversion occurs in the zona fasciculata.

The cells of the zona reticularis are capable of cleaving the side chain from either 17α-OH-progesterone or 17α-OH-pregnenolone. This then shunts these compounds into the androgen pathway. In terms of physiologic significance in normal humans, this pathway is minor and the products secreted are largely the weak androgens, dehydroepiandrosterone and androstenedione, with only trace amounts of testosterone being produced (see Table 5-1). The zona reticularis is also potentially capable of producing estrogens, but neither these nor progesterone is secreted by the normal adrenal gland in more than trace amounts, the latter presumably because of its rapid conversion to other steroids. We see in Section 5-11 that the androgenic hormones produced by the adrenal cortex take on considerable significance when there is a genetically induced deficiency of the 11β-hydroxylase enzyme. (Q. 5-1) *After looking carefully at Figure 5-4, what hormones do you think would be secreted by the adrenal cortex if the 11β-hydroxylase enzyme were deficient?* We see later that a drug, metyrapone, inhibits specifically the 11β-hydroxylase enzyme in the adrenal glands and is used as a provocative diagnostic test in hypoadrenal humans.

In the zona glomerulosa the 17α-hydroxylase enzyme is absent, so progesterone is not converted to glucocorticoids, but it is hydroxylated at the C-21 position to form 11-deoxycorticosterone, a compound having potent mineralocorticoid activity. This steroid normally is not secreted, since it is converted rapidly to corticosterone by the 11β-hydroxylase enzymes of mitochondria. Aldosterone, the mineralocorticoid end product, is formed from corticosterone by C-18 hydroxylation and subsequent dehydrogenation (see Figure 5-4).

Figure 5-5 should help you visualize more clearly the "production-assembly" line for cortisol within a cell of the zona fasciculata of the adrenal cortex. Cholesterol may enter the cell from the plasma or be synthesized by the cells of the adrenal cortex. Cholesterol is converted to pregnenolone inside mitochondria. It then leaves the mitochondria and is converted to progesterone and 17α-OH-progesterone in the microsomal fraction. The

FIGURE 5-5: Schematic representation of the subcellular localization of biosynthesis in an adrenal cortical (fasciculata) cell.

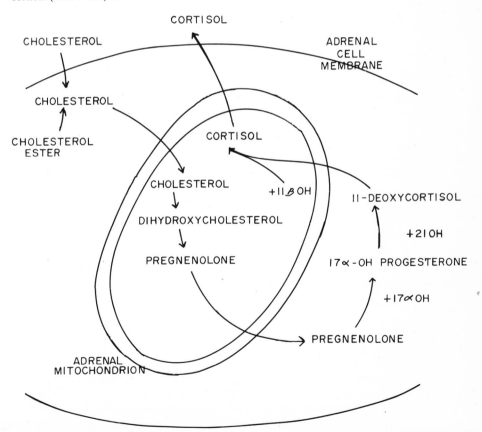

21-hydroxylase enzymes, also localized in the microsomes, convert 17α-OH-progesterone to 11-deoxycortisol. The 11β-hydroxylation of 11-deoxycortisol to cortisol occurs in the mitochondrion and the final product, cortisol, is released into plasma. All the hydroxylation steps, including the cholesterol hydroxylation, require reduced nicotinamide adenine dinucleotide phosphate (NADPH). A possible exception to this requirement may be the 11β-hydroxylase.

SECTION 5-3: POST-TEST QUESTIONS

1. The precursor of all steroid hormones is _____.
2. The biosynthetic pathway for all steroid hormones is identical up through the compound _____.
3. The differences in end product steroids by the various steroid producing endocrine glands are due to _____
_____.
4. Why does not the zona glomerulosa produce cortisol (hydrocortisone)?

5. The enzyme necessary for 17β-hydroxylation is found in the mitochondria. (True/False)
6. The enzyme necessary for 11β-hydroxylation is found in the microsomal fraction of the cytoplasm. (True/False)

SECTION 5-3: POST-TEST ANSWERS

1. cholesterol
2. progesterone
3. presence or absence of a few key enzymes
4. It lacks the 17α-hydroxylase enzyme
5. False. It is found in the microsomal fraction of the cytoplasm.
6. False. It is found in the mitochondria.

SECTION 5-4: TRANSPORT OF ADRENOCORTICAL HORMONES

OBJECTIVES:

The student should be able to:
1. State whether it is the free or the bound hormone that is important physiologically.
2. Describe how adrenocortical hormones are transported in blood.
3. Give the half-lives of cortisol and aldosterone in blood and tell why the biologic half-life of aldosterone is shorter than that of cortisol.

Cortisol, like T_4 and T_3, is poorly soluble in saline. This property is of no physiologic consequence normally, since cortisol is transported in blood bound to an α_2-globulin. At body temperature about 94% of blood cortisol is bound firmly to this *corticosteroid binding globulin* (CBG), also known as *transcortin*. The remaining 6% either is loosely bound to the albumin fraction of plasma or is free. Again, as with the thyroid hormones, it is the free hormone that is important for biologic activity. The binding not only

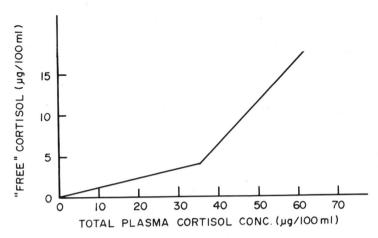

FIGURE 5-6: Effect of an acute increase in secretion of cortisol on concentrations of "free" cortisol in plasma.

provides a transport system, but it protects cortisol from being both metabolized (conjugated with a glucuronide moiety) by the liver and excreted by the kidneys. In addition, the bound hormone represents a storage depot, which releases more hormone as free hormone is removed from the circulation. This occurs because the bound hormone is in chemical equilibrium with the free hormone. Thus, the CBG acts to buffer changes in rates of secretion and metabolism of cortisol by providing a steady supply of the hormone.

Most of the binding sites on CBG or transcortin are saturated completely at normal concentrations of plasma cortisol. A sudden increase in secretion of cortisol by the adrenal cortex tends to "flood" the system and results in proportionately greater concentration of free hormone than is seen under normal conditions (see Figure 5-6). This occurs when total cortisol levels in plasma exceed 20 to 40 µg/100 ml. The beneficial consequence of the increase in concentration of free cortisol in plasma is that increased amounts of cortisol are available for use by the cells. However, the greater concentration of free hormone also means that proportionately more hormone will be lost in urine and conjugated by liver.

The concentration of CBG in blood is known to change under a number of conditions. Pregnancy and administration of oral contraceptive drugs or estrogenic agents increase production of CBG by the liver, as they are also known to do with thyroxine binding globulin. The concentration of CBG in blood is depressed by cirrhosis of the liver and by certain renal and other diseases.

Aldosterone, the mineralocorticoid hormone, is poorly bound and is mainly associated with albumin. Since aldosterone is so poorly bound to plasma proteins, it is readily available for metabolism by the liver. Nearly all the free aldosterone in blood is metabolized in one passage through the liver. This, of course, means that aldosterone would be ineffective if administered by mouth. This rapid metabolism by the liver also explains the short half-life of aldosterone in the circulation compared to cortisol. The half-lives for cortisol and aldosterone are 80 and 30 minutes, respectively. Because of the differences in binding, the turnover rate of aldosterone is estimated to be 10 times greater than that of cortisol in the human.

Measurement of the concentration of cortisol in plasma frequently is made by the Porter-Silber reaction and is reported as 17-hydroxycorticosteroid (17-OHCS) concen-

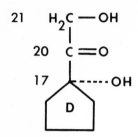

FIGURE 5-7: Ring D of the steroid nucleus illustrating the dihydroxyketone side chain (i.e., C-17 and C-21).

tration in plasma. The reaction measures all steroids with a dihydroxyketone side chain on ring D of the steroid nucleus (see Figure 5-7). The hormones measured by the Porter-Silber reaction primarily are cortisol and some of its metabolites, but this reaction will also measure some intermediates from the biosynthetic pathway that may appear under certain disease conditions. In normal individuals, 17-OHCSs circulate in plasma predominantly as:

> free "active" cortisol—about 5%
> protein bound cortisol—about 45%
> cortisol metabolites usually conjugated—about 50%

At present radioimmunosassay of cortisol is replacing the Porter-Silber reaction, and it is likely that this changeover will be complete within the next few years, although the radioimmunoassay is considerably more expensive now. (*Q. 5-2*) *Why does the development of a radioimmunoassay for a steroid hormone (as opposed to a peptide) present a problem?*

The concentration of aldosterone in blood has long been difficult to measure chemically because of its low concentration (approximately 0.001–0.0001 μg/100 ml plasma). Radioimmunoassay of aldosterone in blood has not yet developed into a sufficiently reliable technique for general use in a clinical laboratory. However, measurement of the concentration of aldosterone in urine can be made by several chemical techniques, but all are exacting and tedious, requiring several days for analysis. Radioimmunoassay of aldosterone is developing rapidly and should prove to be the method of choice for determinations of the concentration of this hormone in blood and urine in the near future.

SECTION 5-4: POST-TEST QUESTIONS

1. Cortisol is transported in blood almost completely bound to protein. (True/False)
2. The plasma protein to which cortisol is bound is called a. _____ _____ or b. _____.
3. Aldosterone is transported in blood almost completely bound to protein. (True/False)
4. In the case of both cortisol and aldosterone, it is the _____ hormone that is active biologically.
5. Why is the binding of hormones to plasma protein physiologically important?
   a.
   b.
   c.
   d.

6. Why does an increase in the rate of secretion of cortisol increase the percentage of free hormone in the circulation?

7. The concentration of corticosteroid binding globulin (transcortin) is quite constant. (True/False)

8. The Porter-Silber reaction measures _____.

9. The half-lives of cortisol and aldosterone are a. _____ and b. _____ _____ minutes, respectively.

10. Blood levels of aldosterone can be measured readily by most clinical laboratories. (True/False)

SECTION 5-4: POST-TEST ANSWERS

1. True
2. a. corticosteroid binding globulin (CBG)
   b. transcortin
3. False
4. free
5. a. It is a method of "solubilizing" otherwise insoluble hormones.
   b. It protects the hormone from metabolism by the liver.
   c. It protects the hormone from excretion by the kidney.
   d. It acts as a storage depot for the hormone, releasing it as needed by the tissues.
6. The binding sites on CBG for cortisol are nearly completely saturated at normal concentrations of cortisol. (Consider the advantages and disadvantages that result from this.)
7. False
8. 17-OHCS, and is a measure of circulating cortisol
9. a. 80
   b. 30
10. False

SECTION 5-5: METABOLISM OF ADRENOCORTICAL HORMONES

OBJECTIVES:

The student should be able to:

1. Name the organ primarily responsible for the metabolism of adrenocortical hormones.
2. State the rate-limiting enzymatic step in the metabolism of adrenocortical hormones.
3. State how the metabolites of adrenocortical hormones are solubilized to facilitate excretion into urine.

An understanding of the metabolites of all the major adrenocortical hormones is important for proper diagnosis of disorders of the adrenal cortex. Metabolism of adrenal steroid hormones occurs primarily in the liver. Here enzymatic transformations of free or unbound steroids occur. In the case of cortisol, which is in equilibrium in plasma with cortisone, ring A enzymatic reductions occur at both the 4-5 double bond and the C-3 keto group. These reductions appear to be the first, the rate-limiting, enzymatic reactions to occur. Following this, a reduction of the C-20 keto group occurs, after which the molecule is conjugated with glucuronic acid at the C-3 hydroxyl position (see Figure 5-8). Conjugation with glucuronic acid renders the steroid soluble in water. Since these metabolites are poorly bound to plasma proteins, they are excreted readily into urine. The urinary metabolites of cortisol are cortisol glucosiduronate, tetrahydrocortisol glucosiduronate, tetrahydrocortisone glucosiduronate, and cortolone glucosiduronate. During a 48-hour period, about 90% of a dose of radiocarbon-labeled cortisol is excreted into urine as metabolites of cortisol shown in Figure 5-8. The remaining 10% appears to be metabolized by side chain oxidation to 11β-hydroxy-17-ketosteroids.

Aldosterone appears to have two metabolic routes in the liver. It can be metabolized essentially by the same route as cortisol (i.e., ring A reduction with saturation of the C-20 keto group, followed by conjugation with glucuronic acid at the C-3 hydroxyl position). A second route of metabolism is conjugation with glucuronic acid at the C-18 position

FIGURE 5-8: Metabolism of cortisol in the liver. (*Adapted from:* Bethune, 1975.)

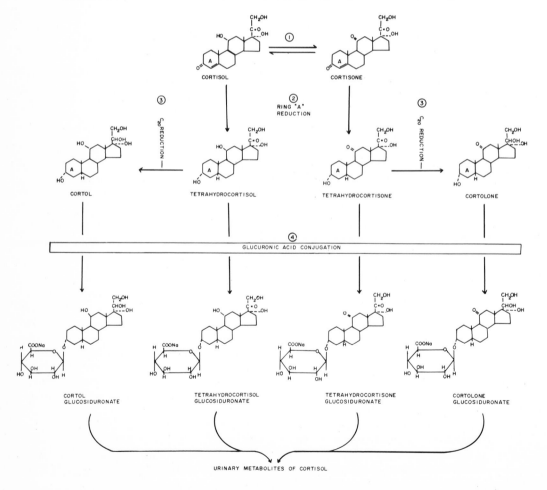

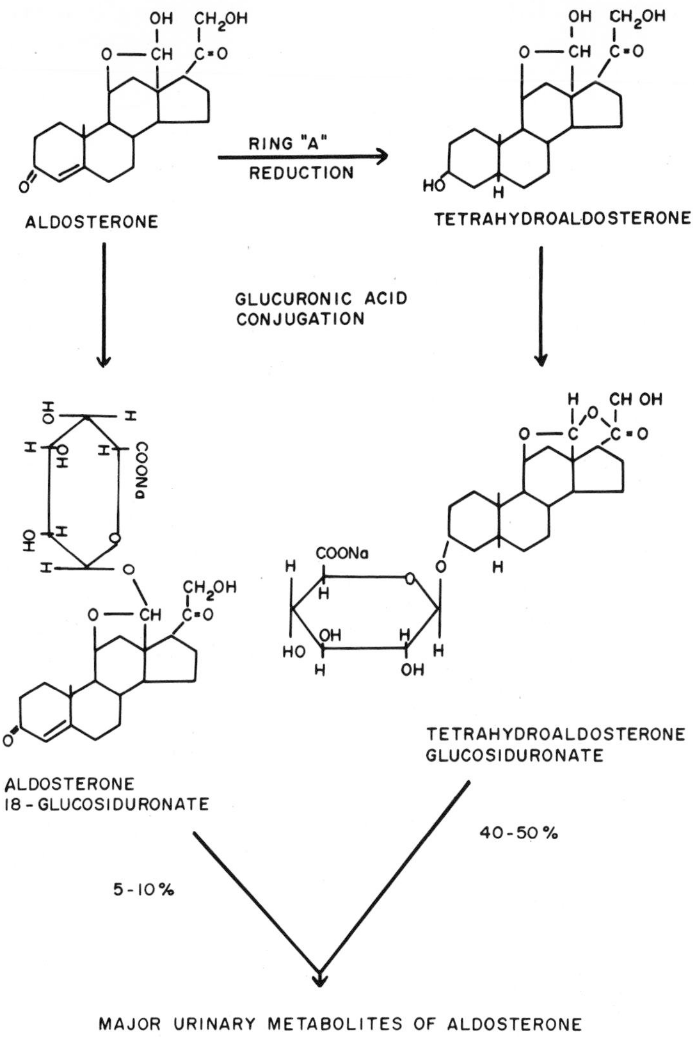

FIGURE 5-9: Metabolism of aldosterone in the liver. (*Adapted from:* Bethune, 1975.)

without reduction of ring A (see Figure 5-9). The importance of these different metabolites is that the enzyme β-glucuronidase can cleave the glucuronidate moiety from the C-3 position but not from the C-18 position. Reducing the urine pH to 1 will cleave the glucuronidate moiety from the C-18 position. The methods used most commonly to measure the concentration of aldosterone in urine use the enzyme β-glucuronidase, but not a low pH. In this case only a fraction of the total amount of aldosterone actually metabolized is measured. For this reason, plasma methods for measuring the concentration of aldosterone are likely to provide more meaningful information regarding function of the zona glomerulosa.

It was mentioned in Section 5-2 that certain of the adrenal androgens could be converted to testosterone by peripheral tissues. The adrenal androgens are secreted primarily as C-19 steroids containing a C-17 keto group. Ring A reduction of these steroids occurs in the same fashion as described for cortisol and aldosterone. However,

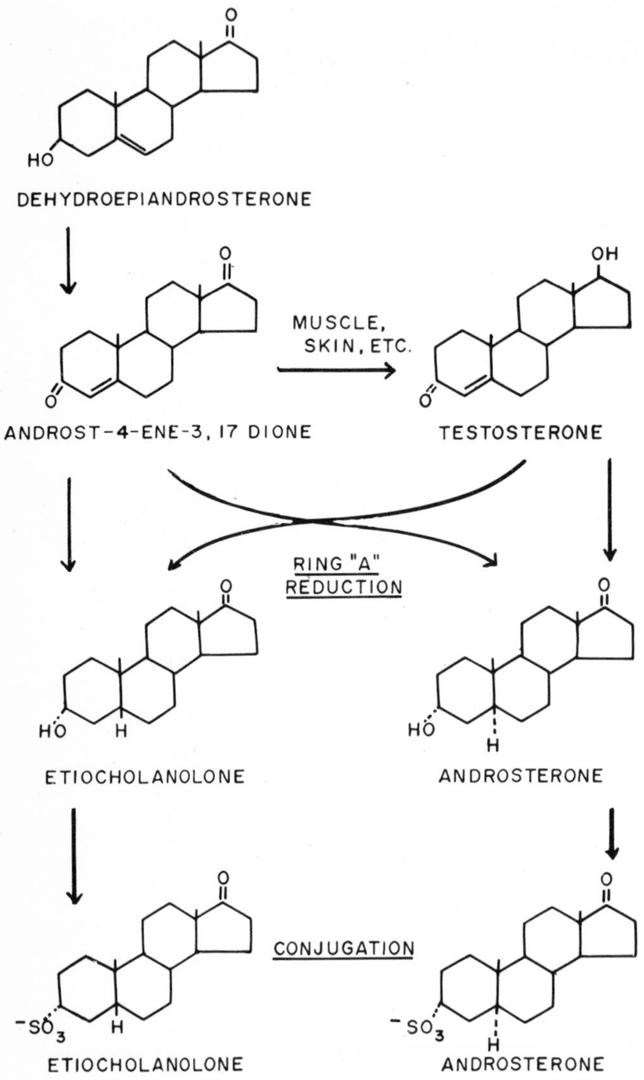

DEHYDROEPIANDROSTERONE

ANDROST-4-ENE-3, 17 DIONE   TESTOSTERONE

MUSCLE,
SKIN, ETC.

RING "A"
REDUCTION

ETIOCHOLANOLONE   ANDROSTERONE

CONJUGATION

ETIOCHOLANOLONE   ANDROSTERONE

FIGURE 5-10: Metabolism of adrenal androgens showing major urinary metabolites. (*Adapted from:* Bethune, 1975.)

instead of conjugation with glucuronic acid at position 3, conjugation with sulfate $(SO_3^=)$ occurs (see Figure 5-10). This conjugation also renders the steroids water soluble and facilitates their excretion into urine. These compounds are measured in urine by a chemical method that depends for its specificity on a C-17 keto group. This is called the Zimmerman reaction, and the compounds measured are called 17-ketosteroids. In the human male, about two-thirds of the urinary 17-ketosteroids excreted during the course of a day is contributed by androgens secreted by the adrenal cortex, the remaining third is contributed by androgens secreted by the testes. (*Q.* 5-3) *Which of the urinary metabolites of which adrenocortical steroids would be measured by the Porter-Silber (17-OHCS) reaction?*

The rate of metabolism of steroid compounds by the liver is a very important factor governing the biologic half-life of the compound in blood. A number of disorders that affect liver function can change the half-lives of steroids, and other compounds, in the circulation. For example, both hepatic congestion and cirrhosis of the liver can lengthen appreciably the half-lives of adrenocortical steroids. An increase in activity of the thyroid gland can shorten the half-lives of adrenocortical steroids, while the opposite is true in hypothyroidism. The state of liver function must be considered before administration of steroids, or other drugs, to patients. (*Q. 5-4*) *If a patient with serious liver congestion needed cortisol, would you prescribe more or less than the usual dose?*

SECTION 5-5: POST-TEST QUESTIONS

1. Metabolism of adrenocortical hormones takes place primarily in the _____ _____.

2. For most adrenocortical hormones, the first and rate-limiting enzymatic step in their metabolism is _____.

3. The metabolites are then a. _____ with glucuronic acid. Why is this step important?
   b.

4. From what you now know about the metabolism of cortisol, state why it is not given by mouth to patients who require it as part of their therapy.

5. Adrenal androgens are conjugated with _____ rather than glucuronic acid.

6. The Zimmerman reaction (for 17-ketosteroids) primarily measures metabolites of a. _____ in urine. In males, approximately b. _____ is contributed by the adrenal cortex and c. _____ by the testes.

7. The Porter-Silber reaction (for 17-OHCS) primarily measures metabolites of _____ in urine.

SECTION 5-5: POST-TEST ANSWERS

1. liver
2. reduction of ring A (see Figure 5-8)
3. a. conjugated
   b. It renders the metabolites water soluble and facilitates their excretion into urine.
4. After absorption from the gastrointestinal tract, cortisol would be carried directly to the liver, where it would be metabolized.
5. sulfate
6. a. androgens
   b. two-thirds
   c. one-third
7. cortisol

SECTION 5-6: CELLULAR MECHANISMS OF ADRENOCORTICAL HORMONE ACTION

OBJECTIVES:

The student should be able to:
1. Discuss a mechanism by which adrenocortical hormones are transported to target cell nuclei.
2. Discuss the difference between "fixed" and "mobile" receptors of target cells.
3. State the types of hormone that activate fixed and mobile receptors, respectively.

In Chapter 1, "Organization and Control of Endocrine System," it was mentioned briefly that the two major mechanisms by which hormones "communicate" with cellular elements are a) indirect, by way of the cAMP system (if they are catecholamines, proteins, or polypeptides) and b) by direct entrance into the cell (if they are lipid-soluble steroids). The receptors for these two systems have been designated "fixed" and "mobile," respectively. The receptors stimulating production of cAMP are fixed and are located in the membrane of the target cell. When these receptors are activated by certain proteins, peptides, catecholamines, and other compounds, the rate of formation of cAMP is increased, as is the rate of formation of phosphorylase A and the kinase enzymes. These, in turn, stimulate the target cell to perform certain functions including production and release of glucose, fatty acids, and hormones.

The mobile receptors are different in a number of respects (see Figure 5-11). These receptors are proteins and appear to be located in the cytoplasm (and nucleoplasm) of target cells where they couple with the steroid hormone (i.e., high-affinity, low-capacity, noncovalent, structure-specific binding) after it has moved through the plasma (and nuclear) membrane. This transmembrane movement is prevented if the steroid is bound

FIGURE 5-11: The mobile receptor model for the genomic actions of glucocorticoid hormones.

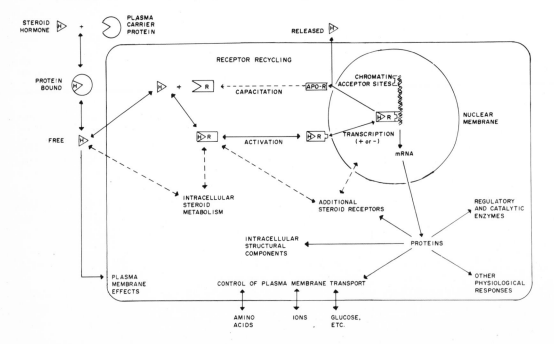

to a high-affinity transport protein in plasma (e.g., transcortin binding of cortisol), although it may not be precluded if the steroid is associated weakly with plasma albumin, which permits steroid-protein dissociation before transmembrane migration of the *free steroid*. This migration is thought to be mediated primarily by diffusion. Research with several systems suggests that the ability of the receptor to bind reversibly with the steroid (i.e., receptor capacitation-decapacitation) may be regulated (i.e., up/down regulation) in target cells by enzymatic mechanisms (possibly phosphorylation-dephosphorylation). The steroid-receptor complex undergoes a poorly understood "activation" process that facilitates its interaction with chromatin acceptors, but does not affect its transport through the nuclear membrane. Activation of the glucocorticoid-receptor complex also does not appear to undergo any major changes in size or molecular weight (as in the 4S to 5S aggregation-activation of the estrogen-receptor complex), but it does involve a conformational change such that more positively charged groups in the receptor are positioned nearer the outside of the protein, where they presumably can interact more efficiently with DNA and acceptor macromolecules. This interaction facilitates (or inhibits) the transcriptional production of specific mRNA species coding for proteins involved in the enzymatic, transport, or structural activities of the target cell.

It seems likely that this genomic mechanism of steroid hormone action is important in the process of gluconeogenesis, stimulated by glucocorticoid hormones, as well as in the reabsorption of sodium and the excretion of potassium, stimulated by mineralocorticoid hormones. Even the "catabolic" actions of glucocorticoid hormones on lymphoid tissues (see Section 5-9) appear to involve the production of specific proteins in response to steroid-stimulated genomic activity (which in this case may lead to cellular death). In spite of this nearly overwhelming support for the genomic mechanism of steroid hormone actions in target tissues, there are some exceptions, most notably the nearly instantaneous alterations in neuronal firing patterns when certain endogenous steroids (including cortisol) are allowed to contact specific neurons in the brain and spinal cord. The latter effects are thought to be mediated by membrane mechanisms as yet unknown.

SECTION 5-6: POST-TEST QUESTIONS

1. a. Why is the adrenocortical hormone cortisol freely permeable to cell membranes?

   b. Is this the case for all naturally occurring steroid hormones in their target and nontarget tissues? _____(Yes/No)_____
2. Steroid receptors within the cell are thought to require a. _____ before binding with the steroid and b. _____ before binding with chromatin acceptors.
3. The type of receptor to which steroid hormones bind in target cells is called a a. _____, as contrasted with the b. _____ receptor utilized by most protein and peptide hormones. The former receptor type is found in the c. _____ and d. _____; latter receptor type is found in the e. _____ of the target cell.
4. The molecular mechanism of steroid hormone action in most target cells involves the selective activation of adenylate cyclase production of cAMP. (True/ False)
5. Although there are some exceptions, steroid-receptor actions in target cell nuclei result in an alteration in the production of specific a. _____ that code for b. _____ involved in the regulation of target cell function.

SECTION 5-6: POST-TEST ANSWERS

1. a. It is a steroid and therefore soluble in the lipid-rich plasma membrane.
   b. Yes
2. a. capacitation
   b. activation
3. a. mobile receptor
   b. fixed
   c. cytoplasm
   d. nucleoplasm
   e. plasma membrane
4. False
5. a. mRNAs
   b. proteins

SECTION 5-7: REGULATION OF THE RATE OF GLUCOCORTICOID SECRETION

OBJECTIVES:

The student should be able to:
1. Describe the feedback control of glucocorticoid secretion.
2. Discuss how specific changes in the feedback mechanism would be expected to affect the rate of cortisol secretion.
3. Discuss the importance of hypothalamic control in the regulation of the rate of cortisol secretion.
4. Discuss some factors that influence hypothalamic control.
5. Discuss the diurnal variation in cortisol secretion and its significance.

Physiologic control of the rate of secretion of cortisol occurs by way of negative feedback, which is characteristic of most physiologic systems. The rate of secretion of cortisol is entirely under the control of adrenocorticotropic hormone (ACTH), which is produced by the anterior pituitary gland. ACTH stimulates the rate of secretion of cortisol by way of the cAMP system. Dibutyryl cAMP can mimic the effects of ACTH on the adrenal cortex, at least in vitro. The response of the adrenal cortex to changing blood levels of ACTH is very rapid in that the rate of cortisol secretion increases within seconds after injection of ACTH into the adrenal artery. In contrast, the rate of cortisol secretion decreases to one-twentieth of control level within 20 minutes after removal of the pituitary gland in rabbits. Studies such as these, and others, suggested some years ago that the feedback mechanism controlling the concentration of cortisol in blood was uncomplicated and readily understandable (see Figure 5-12).

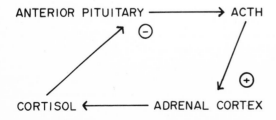

FIGURE 5-12: Simplified diagram of pituitary-adrenal negative feedback relationships.

Careful observation showed that ACTH not only was capable of stimulating the adrenal cortex to increase its rate of secretion of cortisol, but it also increased the size or weight of the adrenal cortex, as well as altering its histologic appearance. With an increase in the rate of secretion of ACTH, adrenal weight increases largely as a consequence of an increase in the size on the zonae fasciculata and reticularis. (*Q. 5-5*) *What significance do you attach to the fact that the zona glomerulosa is not increased?* Histologic staining techniques, as well as biochemical assays, showed that stimulation by ACTH was accompanied by depletion of both cholesterol and ascorbic acid in adrenal cortical cells of the zonae fasciculata and reticularis. Since cholesterol serves as the precursor of adrenal cortical hormones, its disappearance during stimulation by ACTH is understandable. However, there is still no adequate notion of why the adrenal gland contains such high concentrations of ascorbic acid and why it decreases during stimulation by ACTH. Before the availability of chemical analysis of plasma for glucocorticoid hormone concentration, these two tests served as bioassay procedures for estimating ACTH concentration in plasma.

With this background information, it is easy to explain why adrenal size and secretion rate decrease when either cortisol or a synthetic glucocorticoid is administered. (*Q. 5-6*) *Can you explain why this occurs, using your knowledge of feedback mechanisms?* (*It should also be easy to explain why the size of one adrenal increases when the other is removed.*) (*Q. 5-7*) *What do you think would happen to the concentration of cortisol in blood within a few minutes of removal of one adrenal gland, and at 24 hours afterward?*

The feedback mechanism described above is technically called a closed-loop, negative feedback system. For this system to work, the anterior pituitary gland would need to have a "set point," that is, a selected reference concentraton for cortisol against which it is constantly comparing the concentration of cortisol in blood. When the concentration of cortisol falls below the set point, the rate of ACTH secretion increases. This stimulates the rate of secretion of cortisol and thus brings the concentration of cortisol in blood back to the set-point. The opposite would occur if the concentration of cortisol in blood rose. Before the refinement of chemical methods sensitive enough to measure the concentration of cortisol in blood, it was known that infection, trauma, surgery, and many stressful situations increased the activity of the adrenal cortex. The explanation for this was that stressful situations increased the "utilization" of cortisol by peripheral tissues and thus decreased blood concentration of cortisol. As a consequence, the rate of secretion of ACTH increased.

As soon as the concentration of cortisol in blood could be measured chemically, it was shown that its concentration did not fall during stressful situations, and actually *increased without blocking ACTH secretion, suggesting that the set point had increased.*

It is now apparent that the central nervous system, and particularly the hypothalamus, plays an important role in the control of ACTH release. Thus, it is known that lesions in the anterior hypothalamus and median eminence block the increased rate of secretion of ACTH characteristically observed in stressful situations. In contrast, electrical stimulation of the same hypothalamic areas can provoke an increase in the rate of secretion of ACTH.

It now appears that a peptide called corticotropin releasing factor (CRF) is produced by neurons of the hypothalamus, which secrete CRF from their nerve endings in the vicinity of capillaries from the hypophyseal portal vessels. The peptide diffuses into the blood and is transported to the anterior pituitary gland. There it stimulates an increase in rate of secretion of ACTH. CRF has been isolated from hypothalamic tissue, but its structure has not been elucidated.

The present conception of the feedback mechanism controlling glucocorticoid concentration of the blood is illustrated in Figure 5-13. Plasma concentration of free cortisol is believed to be sensed at the level of both the anterior pituitary gland and the

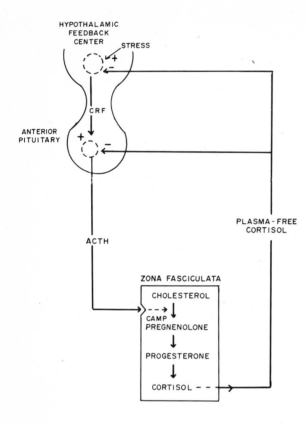

FIGURE 5-13: Regulation of cortisol secretion. (*Adapted from:* Catt, 1970.)

hypothalamus. As illustrated in Figure 5-13, stresses of various types can override the feedback effect of plasma cortisol concentration on the hypothalamus. During a severe stress, the amount of ACTH secreted actually exceeds the amount needed to produce maximal glucocorticoid secretion. Although it has always been clear that an animal without adrenal glands survives a stressful situation far less well than one with adrenals, the physiologic importance of the large outpouring of adrenocortical hormones during most stressful situations is less clear. Some investigators have argued that the physiologic benefit of the excess secretion of adrenocortical hormones under these conditions is that it allows or permits other hormones to act more effectively. This has been termed the "permissive" action of glucocorticoid hormones. For example, it is known that thyroxine, administered alone to hypothyroid animals, does not produce as good a metabolic response as occurs when the same dose is administered with a maintenance dose of glucocorticoid hormone. It should be added that the glucocorticoid hormone alone has no effect on the metabolic response of the hypothyroid animal.

It is well known that there is a diurnal variation in cortisol secretion in the human and that this is correlated with a corresponding diurnal variation in ACTH secretion (see Figure 5-14). In man, the maximal concentration of cortisol in blood occurs in the early morning (6–8 A.M.) with the minimal concentration occurring at 6–12 P.M. The concentration of ACTH in blood has a similar cyclicity. It is believed that input from the hypothalamus is responsible for cyclic increases in CRF which, in turn, stimulate secretion of ACTH and cortisol. Thus, the source of the factors controlling the diurnal secretory rhythm is in the brain.

The existence of this diurnal rhythm suggests that the regulation of glucocorticoid concentration of the blood is by no means constant. The diurnal variation in cortisol

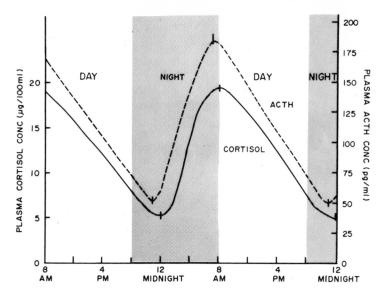

FIGURE 5-14: Fluctuations in plasma ACTH (dashed curve) and glucocorticoids (solid curve) throughout a 24-hour period in a normal human. Note the greater ACTH and glucocorticoid levels in the morning, before awakening from sleep, as contrasted with those at midnight. Note also that the cycle for plasma ACTH concentration precedes that for cortisol concentration.

concentration may range from four- to five-fold from the minimal to the maximal concentration. This complicates the discussion of feedback regulation in terms of the maintenance of a constant concentration of cortisol in blood. It is also of considerable significance to clinicians because the time of day at which cortisol (or plasma 11-OHCS) concentration is measured must be chosen with care. Thus, the cells of the body could be subjected to an increased amount of glucocorticoid hormone without a change in its maximal concentration in blood. This is essentially what happens in Cushing's syndrome, a disease characterized by hypersecretion of the adrenal cortex.

Some evidence is available regarding the central neural transmitter substances that influence the secretion of CRF (see Figure 5-15). For example, it appears that norepinephrine inhibits the secretion of CRF, whereas 5-hydroxytryptamine or serotonin stimulates it. It is possible that stress influences CRF secretion by way of 5HT pathways. It is not yet clear whether changes in the concentration of cortisol in blood can directly affect NE and 5HT pathways in the brain by increasing secretion of NE when the

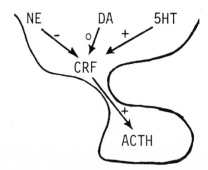

FIGURE 5-15: Neurotransmitter regulation of the secretion of corticotropin releasing factor (CRF). NE, norepinephrine; DA, dopamine; 5HT, 5-hydroxytryptamine; ACTH, adrenocorticotropic hormone.

concentration of cortisol in blood is high but increasing secretion of 5HT when the concentration of cortisol decreases.

ACTH has been characterized and synthesized. In contains 39 amino acids in linear sequence. The sequence has been determined for four species: cow, pig, sheep, and man. The porcine and human hormones have been synthesized completely. The first 24, and the last 6, amino acids are the same for all species. Amino acids 25 through 33 represent the region of species differences and immunologic specificity. The first 24 amino acids possess the full biologic activity of the entire 39, and a synthetic peptide containing this sequence is available and has been used clinically in adrenal stimulation tests. The sequence of the first 24 amino acids has been altered to produce a hormone with a more prolonged action in man than the native hormone.

The first 13 amino acids also have melanocyte stimulating hormone (MSH) properties in man. MSH appears to have only minor functions in man, but the hyperpigmentation that accompanies hypersecretion of ACTH may be related to this portion of the molecule. This possibility is debated, however, and some investigators believe that hypersecretion of MSH also occurs when ACTH is secreted in excessive amounts. In the rat MSH is secreted by the intermediate lobe of the pituitary gland.

ACTH has a circulating half-life of about 10 minutes in man. The site of its inactivation is uncertain, although a large part of an injected dose can be found in the kidneys. In spite of this, neither nephrectomy nor evisceration appears to increase its half-life in experimental animals.

SECTION 5-7: POST-TEST QUESTIONS

1. Biologic feedback systems are most frequently of the (negative/positive) type.
2. An advantage of this type of feedback system is that it promotes _____.
3. The rate of secretion of cortisol is entirely under the control of a. _____, which is produced by the b. _____.
4. The mechanism by which a. _____ stimulates production of cortisol is via the b. _____ system. Proof of this is that c. _____ can stimulate the secretion of cortisol in vitro.
5. In the adrenal glucocorticoid control system, it is the concentration of a. _____ in blood that is regulated. When it increases, b. _____ production is reduced.
6. ACTH not only increases rate of secretion of glucocorticoids but also increases adrenal a. _____ and decreases the concentration of b. _____ and c. _____ in adrenal cells.
7. Describe what would happen to the adrenal gland if the rate of ACTH secretion were decreased chronically.

8. ACTH secretion is controlled by a. _____ produced by neurons located in the b. _____. These can be stimulated to increase their rate of secretion of c. __(abbreviation)__ by stressful situations such as infection and trauma. Under these conditions the feedback inhibitory effect of cortisol on d. _____ and e. _____ is overridden and the concentration of cortisol in blood rises.
9. A diurnal cyclicity of the concentrations of ACTH and cortisol in blood is known in clinical medicine. The concentration of these two hormones in blood are

a. _____ at 8 A.M. and b. _____ at midnight. Why is this fact important in clinical medicine?

c.

10. ACTH can stimulate both the cells of the adrenal cortex and _____ in the skin.

11. ACTH has a circulating half-life of about _____ (minutes) in man.

SECTION 5-7: POST-TEST ANSWERS

1. negative
2. stability
3. a. ACTH
   b. anterior pituitary gland
4. a. ACTH
   b. cAMP
   c. dibutyryl cAMP
5. a. cortisol
   b. ACTH
6. a. size (weight)
   b. cholesterol
   c. ascorbic acid
7. The rate of secretion of cortisol would decrease; adrenal size (weight) would decrease; the zonae fasciculata and reticularis would be reduced in size.
8. a. corticotropin releasing factor (CRF)
   b. hypothalamus
   c. CRF
   d. hypothalamus
   e. anterior pituitary
9. a. highest
   b. lowest
   c. Interpretation of the clinical significance of a single plasma sample is hazardous unless the time at which the sample is drawn is carefully recorded or a number of samples are measured throughout a 24-hour period.
10. melanocytes
11. 10

SECTION 5-8: REGULATION OF THE RATE OF MINERALOCORTICOID SECRETION

OBJECTIVES:

The student should be able to:
1. Discuss four general types of stimuli that increase the release of renin from the juxtaglomerular cells of the kidney.
2. Describe the sequence of events occurring from the time of the release of renin to the secretion of aldosterone.
3. Describe the physiologic factors influencing feedback control of the rate of secretion of aldosterone.

4. State the role of the anterior pituitary gland in the secretion of aldosterone.
5. Describe the physiologic factors acting directly on the adrenal cortex to affect the rate of secretion of aldosterone.
6. Discuss the "escape phenomenon" and "third factor."
7. Describe the diurnal pattern of the secretion of aldosterone.
8. Describe the effect of aging on renin activity in plasma and the rate of excretion of aldosterone.

The control of the secretion of aldosterone and renin are interrelated. As you read on, you will recognize that this is still an emerging field of investigation in which there are many unanswered questions and many tentative answers.

Aldosterone controls sodium resorption and potassium loss by the kidney tubules. Hence, this hormone is responsible for maintaining body content of sodium, potassium, and water, since the reabsorption of sodium is accompanied by reabsorption of water to maintain isotonicity of body fluids. One would therefore expect that sodium depletion, potassium excess, or decreased intravascular volume would stimulate the secretion of aldosterone in an attempt to correct the disturbance. That is exactly what happens. How it happens remains somewhat controversial.

It seems most logical to begin where the physiologic stimuli that ultimately affect the secretion of aldosterone are sensed. This is at the level of the kidney and specifically at the juxtaglomerular apparatus where renin is secreted.

Renin is a highly specific proteolytic *enzyme* that has not yet been purified. It is synthesized, stored, and released mainly by the kidney, although reninlike enzymes have been extracted from the uterus, placenta, fetal membranes, amniotic fluid, brain, adrenal glands, and submaxillary glands. With the possible exception of brain, there is no convincing evidence that these extrarenal sources of enzyme either are identical with renin or play a physiologically important role in controlling blood pressure and the rate of secretion of aldosterone. They may, however, explain the occasional observation of plasma renin activity in anephric patients.

The juxtaglomerular (JG) cells, located in the kidney at the vascular pole of the afferent arteriole of the glomerulus, contain membrane-bound cytoplasmic granules that are the precursors of renin. The afferent arteriole, the efferent arteriole, and a group of specialized cells, called the macula densa and located at the origin of the distal tubule, form the structure known as the juxtaglomerular apparatus (JGA) (see Figure 5-16). A

FIGURE 5-16: The juxtaglomerular apparatus. (*Adapted from:* Davis, 1971.)

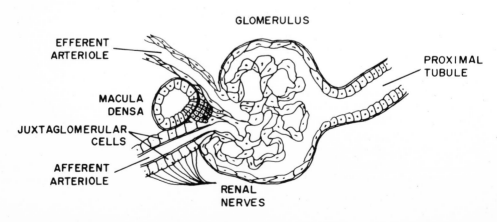

great deal of experimental effort has been expended to determine what stimuli initiate the release of renin from the JG cells. There are at least four stimuli that may influence the release of renin. These are related to 1) changes in transmural pressure sensed by receptors in the afferent arteriole of the JGA (baroreceptor hypothesis), 2) changes in delivery of sodium to the macula densa (receptor unknown) (macula densa hypothesis), 3) autonomic nervous control of the release of renin; and 4) humoral control of the release of renin. These are discussed briefly below.

It has been difficult to separate hypothesis 1 from hypothesis 2 because changes in renal arterial pressure change the delivery of sodium to the distal tubules of the kidney and to the macula densa. Recent experiments have used the denervated, nonfiltering kidney preparation in adrenalectomized dogs. In this experimental model there is no influence of the autonomic nervous system and no glomerular filtration; hence there can be no change in the delivery of sodium to the macula densa. In these animals, a decrease in renal arterial pressure increased the secretion of renin, and vice versa. This is strong evidence in support of the renal baroreceptor hypothesis.

A role for the macula densa was first postulated when changes in the release of renin were observed during studies in which the distal tubular sodium load was varied independently of a change in renal arterial pressure. Although it is clear that changes in the concentration of either sodium or potassium, not other ions, influence the macula densa, it is still unclear whether the rate of secretion of renin increases or decreases following the delivery of an increased load of sodium to the distal tubule and the macula densa.

The autonomic nervous system plays a role in the release of renin. The JGA is innervated by both adrenergic and cholinergic afferent nerve fibers (see Figure 5-16). These are found to be associated closely with both vascular and tubular components of the JGA. Electrical stimulation of the renal nerves results in both the release of renin and vasoconstriction. Renal sympathectomy decreases the basal rate of renin secretion and reduces the renin response to sodium depletion. Hence, it appears to be the adrenergic component of the autonomic nervous system that influences the release of renin.

The central nervous system appears to modulate the release of renin by way of the renal nerves. Electrical stimulation of several brain areas including the mesencephalic pressor area, or the medulla near the obex, pons, and posterior hypothalamus increased the release of renin in the dog. This effect was abolished by denervating the kidney. In contrast, electrical stimulation of the hypothalamus in conscious dogs resulted in a 50% reduction in plasma renin activity without altering renal blood flow. This response was also abolished by renal denervation. In addition, it has been shown that pharmacologic stimulation of central α-adrenergic neurons by the antihypertensive drug clonidine can inhibit the release of renin by way of the renal nerves. These experimental observations establish a role for the central nervous system in the modulation of the rate of secretion of renin.

Certain humoral substances may also influence the rate of renin secretion. Since electrical stimulation of the renal sympathetic nerves increases the secretion of renin, it is not surprising that an increase in the concentration of catecholamines in plasma can also increase the secretion of renin. Although there is still some disagreement, the weight of experimental evidence suggests that the receptors mediating the release of renin are of the β-adrenergic type. It is unlikely that the increase in the release of renin induced by β-adrenergic catecholamines is related either to changes in pressure in the afferent arteriole or to delivery of sodium to the distal tubule, since the effect occurs in slices of renal tissue in vitro.

Other humoral substances may also influence the rate of renin secretion. These include changes in the plasma concentrations of potassium, sodium, antidiuretic hormone (ADH), and angiotensin II.

An increase in the concentration of potassium in blood is accompanied by a reduction in renin activity in plasma and *an increase* in the rate aldosterone secretion. This is surprising at first glance because the rate of secretion of renin generally is considered to affect the rate of secretion of aldosterone. We see later that this apparent paradox can be explained by the fact that an increase in the concentration of potassium in plasma can act directly on the adrenal cortex to increase the rate of aldosterone secretion. Reduction in the concentration of potassium in blood results in the opposite response. The mechanism by which potassium affects either the release of renin by the kidney or the secretion of aldosterone by the adrenal cortex is not well understood. In the case of renin, a renal tubular mechanism (probably macula densa) is suspected, since the release of renin is unchanged in the nonfiltering kidney model when the concentration of potassium in plasma increases.

An increase in the concentration of sodium in blood is accompanied by reductions in the rate of secretion of *both* renin and aldosterone. Studies carried out in dogs in which hypertonic saline was infused into the renal arteries revealed a suppression in the rate of secretion of renin without an observable hemodynamic effect. The same study carried out in dogs with nonfiltering kidneys revealed no effect on the rate of renin secretion. This suggests that a renal tubular mechanism mediates the action of sodium on the release of renin. This mechanism is most likely located in the macula densa.

ADH inhibits the relase of renin when infused in high physiologic concentrations into blood. Since blood levels of ADH are not elevated normally, ADH is unlikely to play a major role in the control of the secretion of renin in normal man. ADH inhibits the release of renin in the nonfiltering kidney model; thus it probably acts directly on the JG cells.

Increasing concentration of angiotensin II in blood inhibits the secretion of renin and serves as a feedback limb in the control of the secretion of aldosterone. This is discussed in detail below.

It is not now possible to state which of the stimuli above primarily controls the rate of secretion of renin and which is secondary. It turns out, in actual clinical situations, that certain stimuli that increase the secretion of renin may act through more than one of these mechanisms. For example, a decrease in effective blood volume induced by a sudden hemorrhage can be visualized to do the following:

1. Decrease renal arterial pressure (activate baroreceptors).
2. Decrease delivery of sodium to the distal tubule and macula densa.
3. Increase sympathetic (β-adrenergic) nervous activity to the kidney.

Any one of these changes alone can increase the rate of secretion of renin. As can be seen from this example, there appears to be a good deal of redundancy regarding the initiation of an increased rate of secretion of renin under these conditions. This suggests that this particular response to hemorrhage is physiologically significant.

Once renin is secreted into blood, a series of enzymatic reactions takes place leading to the formation of the physiologically active polypeptide hormone angiotensin II (see Figure 5-17). You recall that renin is a proteolytic *enzyme*. It acts in blood on its substrate, an α_2-globulin produced by the liver, to form the decapeptide angiotensin I. A second enzyme, called converting enzyme (dipeptidylcarboxypeptidase), then cleaves two amino acids from angiotensin I to form the octapeptide and hormone angiotensin II. Converting enzyme is found mainly in the vascular beds of the lung, although it can also be found in circulating plasma, kidney, and a variety of other organ vascular beds.

Angiotensin II is a potent vasoconstrictor agent and a stimulus for production and release of aldosterone by the adrenal cortex. Angiotensin II is inactivated rapidly in capillary beds by a number of enzymes called angiotensinases. One of the metabolic

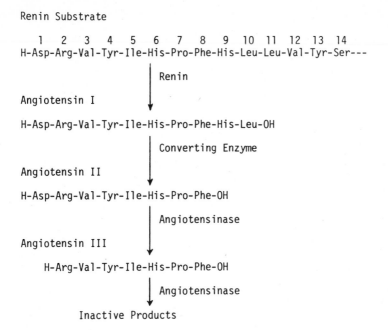

```
Renin Substrate

   1   2   3   4   5   6   7   8   9  10  11  12  13  14
H-Asp-Arg-Val-Tyr-Ile-His-Pro-Phe-His-Leu-Leu-Val-Tyr-Ser---
                          │   Renin
Angiotensin I             │
                          ↓
H-Asp-Arg-Val-Tyr-Ile-His-Pro-Phe-His-Leu-OH
                          │   Converting Enzyme
Angiotensin II            │
                          ↓
H-Asp-Arg-Val-Tyr-Ile-His-Pro-Phe-OH
                          │   Angiotensinase
Angiotensin III           │
                          ↓
    H-Arg-Val-Tyr-Ile-His-Pro-Phe-OH
                          │   Angiotensinase
                          ↓
        Inactive Products
```

FIGURE 5-17: Biochemistry of the renin-angiotensin system.

products of this inactivation is the hepapeptide des-Asp^1-Ile^3-angiotensin II, now commonly called angiotensin III. Angiotensin III appears to be as potent in stimulating the secretion of aldosterone (and in inhibiting the release of renin) as angiotensin II but to have a less pronounced effect on blood pressure than does angiotensin II. No other metabolites resulting from the inactivation of angiotensin II appear to have physiologic activity.

Angiotensin III does appear to be important physiologically, since a radioimmunoassay of the angiotensins present in arterial plasma of sodium replete rats revealed a mean of 33% of the immunoreactive material to be angiotensin II, 58% to be angiotensin III, and 9% other angiotensins. A similar analysis for man apparently is not available at present.

Figure 5-18 schematically represents some of the factors affecting the rate of secretion of aldosterone. The physiologic variable initiating an increase in the rate of aldosterone secretion usually begins at the level of the kidney. Using a sudden hemorrhage as the initiating factor, the consequent decrease in blood volume is probably sensed as a decrease in pressure by the renal baroreceptors. The rate of glomerular filtration probably also decreases, with a consequent decrease in delivery of sodium to the macula densa. The sympathetic (β-adrenergic) nervous stimuli to the kidney also increase, leading to the release of renin from the JG cells of the kidney into blood. Here the renin reacts with renin substrate to form angiotensin I. Estrogenic agents, including oral contraceptives, are known to stimulate, whereas adrenalectomy is known to reduce, the production of renin substrate by the liver. Conversion of angiotensin I to angiotensin II occurs mainly in the blood vessels of the lungs by a converting enzyme.

Angiotensin II performs a number of functions. It stimulates the zona glomerulosa of the adrenal cortex, via the cAMP system, to produce aldosterone, the hormone responsible for sodium reabsorption and potassium loss in renal tubules, salivary glands, intestines, and sweat glands. Rising concentrations of angiotensin II in blood also feed

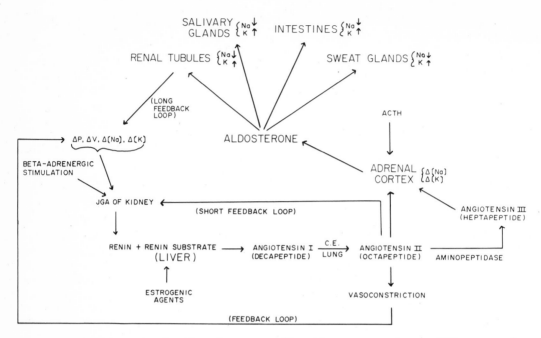

FIGURE 5-18: The physiologic factors controlling aldosterone secretion rate (C.E. = converting enzyme).

back on the JG cells of the kidney to inhibit further secretion of renin (via the short feedback loop). Angiotensin II also constricts the resistance vessels of the body to increase blood pressure and decrease vascular capacity. If a sudden fall in arterial pressure initiated the increased secretion of renin, the rise in blood pressure and decrease in vascular capacity induced by angiotensin II would act as a second feedback limb to decrease the secretion of renin (cardiovascular feedback loop). A third way that angiotensin II acts as part of feedback loop is by way of its effect on secretion of aldosterone (long feedback loop). If a decrease in blood volume initiated the increase in secretion of renin, the subsequent increase in the secretion of aldosterone would increase sodium and water resorption via the kidney in an attempt to return blood volume to normal. An additional effect of angiotensin II that is important under these conditions is its ability to stimulate thirst. This is believed to occur by a direct effect of angiotensin II on thirst receptors in the central nervous system.

Early experiments designed to localize the site of the control system for secretion of aldosterone used numerous ablation studies. Neither hypophysectomy, nor even total decapitation, destroyed the ability of the animal to increase its secretion of aldosterone in response to a sudden hemorrhage. However, bilateral nephrectomy did eliminate responsiveness, and the kidneys have come to be recognized as the ultimate initiators of aldosterone secretion. Although the rate of secretion of aldosterone may be increased independently of the anterior pituitary gland, its removal reduces the basal rate of aldosterone secretion. Furthermore, administration of ACTH to either hypophysectomized or intact animals increases the rate of secretion of aldosterone. However, this effect appears to be transient. When the secretion of ACTH is elevated chronically, the secretion of aldosterone increases initially but begins to decline within a day or two. This suggests, but does not prove, that the effect of ACTH on the secretion of aldosterone is more important acutely than chronically. In the situation of a hemorrhage, discussed above, the secretion of ACTH would increase, thus assuring an increase in the secretion of aldosterone in the event the kidney could not respond. This is an additional example of redundancy of function.

In addition to the direct effect of ACTH in stimulating the secretion of aldosterone, a rise in the concentration of potassium or a fall in the concentration of sodium in plasma may also increase the secretion of aldosterone *directly*. There is controversy regarding both the mechanism by which changes in the concentration of these electrolytes directly affect the adrenal cortex and the change in concentration required.

Studies have been carried out in humans that point up the relationship between the rate of excretion of sodium in urine and the concentration of angiotensin II, renin, and aldosterone in blood (see Figure 5-19). As the body becomes depleted of sodium, the excretion of sodium into urine decreases and the concentrations of renin, angiotensin, and aldosterone in blood increase sharply. With an excess of sodium in the body and an increased excretion of sodium in urine, there is a marked reduction in the concentrations of renin, angiotensin, and aldosterone in blood.

A change in posture from supine to upright position affects the rate of secretion of aldosterone via the renin-angiotensin system. An example of this is shown in Table 5-2, which illustrates the effects of changes in posture and dietary sodium content. Thus, both sodium depletion and moving from a supine to an upright posture (which causes pooling of fluid in the legs and a decrease in plasma volume) result in parallel increases in renin, angiotensin II, and aldosterone. These are both used commonly as clinical tests to assess the responsiveness of the renin-angiotensin-aldosterone system.

It has been known for more than 20 years that continued administration of either aldosterone or deoxycorticosterone to humans will induce the retention of sodium for only 5 to 8 days. Since water is reabsorbed with sodium to maintain isotonicity of body fluids, extracellular fluid volume increases. When the expansion of extracellular fluid volume passes a certain point, the excretion of sodium usually is increased in spite of continued administration of the mineralocorticoid hormone. This "escape phenome-

FIGURE 5-19: Correlation between urinary sodium excretion rate and plasma concentrations of renin, angiotensin II, and aldosterone, in normal human subjects. (*Adapted from:* Laragh et al., 1973.)

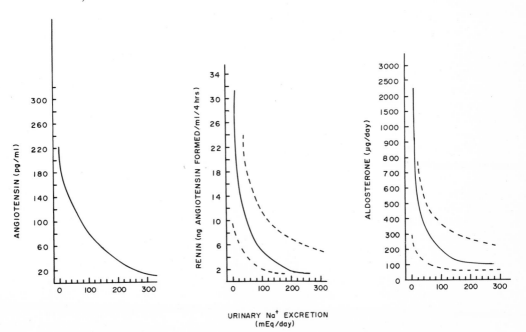

URINARY Na⁺ EXCRETION
(mEq/day)

TABLE 5-2: Effects of Changes in Posture and Dietary Sodium on the Renin-Angiostensin-Aldosterone System

Posture and Dietary Sodium	Plasma Renin Activity (ng/ml/hr)	Angiotensin II Concentration (pg/ml)	Aldosterone Concentration (ng/dl)
Supine (normal Na diet)	0.7	100	7
Upright (normal Na diet)	1.7	230	15
Supine (Na-restricted diet)	3.0	200	20
Upright (Na-restricted diet)	7.0	400	60

non" is due to decreased reabsorption of sodium by the kidneys and is thought to be mediated by a blood-borne substance called *third factor*. The name "third factor" was given to this substance because only two other factors are known to affect renal sodium loss; namely, the rate of glomerular filtration and the concentration of aldosterone in blood. Third factor has never been isolated or identified chemically. The site of production of third factor is still speculative. The escape phenomenon is important physiologically and most likely accounts for the failure of patients with excessive rates of secretion of aldosterone to become edematous.

There appears to be a diurnal pattern to the concentration of aldosterone in plasma that corresponds precisely with the diurnal pattern of renin activity in plasma (see

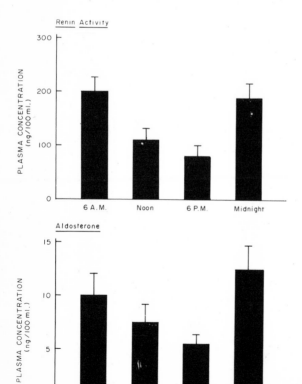

FIGURE 5-20: Diurnal pattern of plasma renin activity and plasma aldosterone concentration in man. (*Adapted from:* Bethune, 1975.)

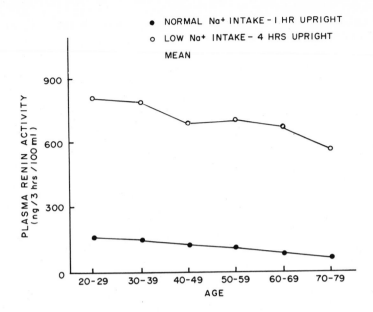

FIGURE 5-21: Plasma renin activity of normal subjects on unrestricted sodium intake plus less than 1 hour of ambulation and after sodium restriction and standing. (*Adapted from:* Sambhi, 1973.)

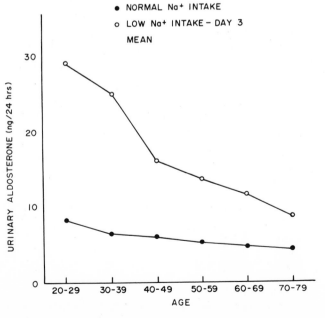

FIGURE 5-22: Rates of excretion of aldosterone in urine of normal persons in different age groups on unrestricted sodium intake and on day 3 of sodium restriction. (*Adapted from:* Sambhi, 1973.)

Figure 5-20). The concentration of aldosterone and renin activity in plasma are maximal from midnight to 6 A.M. and then decrease, reaching a nadir at about 6 P.M. The mechanism responsible for the diurnal pattern of these two substances is not well understood. (*Q. 5-8*) *Is this the same diurnal pattern as that observed for cortisol?*

Aging has a marked and significant effect on both aldosterone excretion (and secretion) and plasma renin activity (see Figures 5-21 and 5-22). From the twentieth to the seventieth years of life, renin activity in plasma declines approximately 25% whereas the excretion of aldosterone in urine declines approximately 40%. This suggests that the clinical assessment of the secretion of aldosterone on the basis of either or both plasma renin activity and the rate of excretion of aldosterone should take into account the age of the patient.

SECTION 5-8: POST-TEST QUESTIONS

1. Renin is released from the cells of the:
   a. glomerulus
   b. distal tubules of the kidney
   c. macula densa
   d. juxtaglomerular apparatus
2. Stimuli currently known to initiate release of renin may be placed into what four broad categories?
   a.
   b.
   c.
   d.
3. What comprises the juxtaglomerular apparatus?
   a.
   b.
   c.
4. Renin is a polypeptide hormone. (True/False)
5. The juxtaglomerular cells, which contain the precursors of renin, are located in the
   _____ .
6. Electrical stimulation of the renal nerves increases the release of renin. How can one determine whether the release of renin is related to cholinergic or adrenergic stimulation?

7. What are the humoral substances that may affect renin release?
   a.
   b.
   c.
   d.
   e.
8. The denervated, nonfiltering kidney model has been important in studies of factors affecting the release of renin. Why?

9. The mineralocorticoid hormone aldosterone, is:
   a. an intermediate in the biosynthetic pathway from progesterone to corticosterone

    b. a hormone that induces retention of potassium and elimination of sodium at the level of the kidney

    c. a hormone that induces retention of sodium and elimination of potassium

10. When renin is secreted into blood, a series of reactions occurs. Name these reactions in order.

11. Renin substrate is produced by the a. _____ . Production of substrate is known to be influenced by b. _____ and c. _____ _____ .

12. What are the functions of angiotensin II in the control of the rate of secretion of aldosterone?

13. Through what mechanism does angiotensin II stimulate the secretion of aldosterone?

14. On what zone of the adrenal cortex does angiotensin II act?

15. If an animal or a human is hypophysectomized, what would you expect the histologic appearance of the adrenal cortex to be?

16. Aldosterone affects electrolyte handling not only by the renal tubules but also by the a. _____ , b. _____ , and c. _____ _____ .

17. Hypophysectomy prevents the increase in secretion of aldosterone which occurs in response to hemorrhage. (True/False)

18. Movement from a supine to an upright position (increases/decreases) the renin activity and the concentrations of angiotensin II and aldosterone in plasma.

19. Ingestion of a sodium-restricted diet for 4 to 5 days (increases/decreases) the renin activity in plasma.

20. The "escape phenomenon" occurs when humans are treated chronically with mineralocorticoid hormones. It is preceded by a. _____ _____ . It is thought to be induced by a blood-borne substance called b. _____ _____ . The escape phenomenon is characterized by c. _____ _____ .

21. There appears to be a diurnal pattern of the concentration of aldosterone in blood. It appears to be maximal from a. _____ and minimal at b. _____ . c. How does this compare with the diurnal cycle of cortisol?

22. How does aging affect the secretion of aldosterone?

SECTION 5-8: POST-TEST ANSWERS

1. d
2. a. Changes in transmural pressure sensed by receptors in the afferent arteriole of the JGA
   b. Changes in the delivery of sodium to the macula densa
   c. Autonomic (β-adrenergic) control
   d. Humoral control
3. a. Afferent arteriole
   b. Efferent arteriole
   c. Macula densa
4. False. Renin is an enzyme.
5. afferent arterioles of the JGA.
6. Renal sympathectomy abolishes the response.
7. a. Circulating β-catecholamines
   b. Sodium concentration of plasma
   c. Potassium concentration of plasma
   d. Angiotensin II concentration of plasma
   e. Antidiuretic hormone concentration of plasma
8. It eliminates any autonomic influence on the release of renin as well as any influence from the macula densa.
9. c
10. Renin acts on renin substrate to release a decapeptide, angiotensin I, which in turn is converted to angiotensin II by a converting enzyme located mainly in the vascular beds of the lung. Angiotensin II can be converted to angiotensin III, a heptapeptide, by angiotensinase enzymes. Both angiotensins II and III stimulate the secretion of aldosterone by the adrenal cortex.
11. a. liver
    b. estrogenic steroids, including oral contraceptive agents that contain estrogens
    c. adrenalectomy
12. Angiotensin II stimulates secretion of aldosterone and also acts as a feedback limb to reduce release of renin.
13. cAMP system
14. Zona glomerulosa
15. Atrophied zonae fasciculata and reticularis; no change in the zona glomerulosa.
16. a. salivary glands
    b. intestines
    c. sweat glands
17. False
18. increases
19. increases
20. a. an increase in extracellular fluid volume
    b. third factor
    c. decreased renal tubular reabsorption of sodium in spite of continued administration of mineralocorticoid hormones.
21. a. midnight to 6 A.M.
    b. 6 P.M.
    c. Maximal concentration in blood occurs at 6–8 A.M.; minimal concentration occurs at midnight (see Section 5-7).
22. There is approximately a 40% decline from the twentieth to the seventieth year of life.

SECTION 5-9: PHYSIOLOGIC EFFECTS OF ADRENOCORTICAL HORMONES

OBJECTIVES:

The student should be able to:

1. Recite 11 physiologic actions of glucocorticoid hormones.
2. Describe the mechanisms by which glucocorticoid hormones affect carbohydrate metabolism.
3. Discuss why increased loss of urinary nitrogen (urea) occurs during administration of cortisol.
4. Describe the effect of administration of cortisol on fat distribution.
5. Describe the effect of administration of cortisol on water metabolism.
6. Describe the hematologic effects of administration of cortisol.
7. Describe the effects of administration of cortisol on the central nervous system.
8. Describe the effects of administration of cortisol on the gastrointestinal system.
9. Describe the effects of administration of cortisol on bone metabolism.
10. Describe the effects of administration of cortisol on the cardiovascular system.
11. Describe the antiinflammatory action and immunologic effects of administration of cortisol.
12. Describe the physiologic actions of mineralocorticoid hormones.

The hormones produced by the adrenal cortex are essential for life. As you now know, these are classed in general terms as glucocorticoid and mineralocorticoid types. It should be recognized at this point that these "types" are not pure. The glucocorticoids, secreted physiologically, have some mineralocorticoid activity and mineralocorticoids have some glucocorticoid activity. The categorization of the physiologically available hormones as mineralocorticoids or glucocorticoids is based on their relative potencies in each category. The clinical need for one hormone with high potency as both a glucocorticoid and a mineralocorticoid hormone has been met by the pharmaceutical industry. A synthetic hormone, 9α-fluorocortisol, is available and has two-thirds the sodium-retaining activity of aldosterone and 10 to 20 times the glucocorticoid activity of cortisol. Others are available with somewhat different potencies. In addition to synthetic hormones, with both glucocorticoid and mineralocorticoid activities, other synthetic hormones, such as dexamethasone, have been produced with relatively pure glucocorticoid activity. Dexamethasone should be kept in mind because of its use in clinical tests of adrenocortical function, which is discussed in the next section. These steroids clearly appear to represent a situation in which the pharmaceutical industry outdid mother nature. Not only do these compounds have greater biologic activity than their native counterparts, but they are effective when taken by mouth. These compounds incorporate a fluoride atom in ring B or have an otherwise altered molecular structure that is metabolized more slowly by the liver than the native compound.

It was mentioned in Section 5-2 that the glucocorticoid cortisol seemed to support the processes that supply glucose to the tissues of the body. Although this is an important physiologic function, it is not the only one performed and may not even be the most important one. This point is debated by a number of investigators. Table 5-3 lists the known peripheral actions of the glucocorticoid hormones. These are discussed in more detail below.

TABLE 5-3: Physiologic Actions of Glucocorticoid Hormones

1. *Carbohydrate Metabolism:* stimulates gluconeogenesis; increases glycogen content in liver and glucose concentrations in blood; may also decrease peripheral utilization of glucose.

2. *Protein Metabolism:* induces marked losses of nitrogen in urine as protein is catabolized to form glucose.

3. *Fat Metabolism:* increases total body fat at the expense of protein; leads to centripetal redistribution of fat.

4. *Water Metabolism:* enhances water diuresis by preserving the rate of glomerular filtration.

5. *Hematologic Effects:* decreases lymphocytes, basophils, and eosinophils; increases neutrophils; total white blood cell count rises slightly; red blood cell count rises.

6. *Central Nervous System Effects:* may control threshold for electrical excitability of the brain; psychiatric disturbances are common with both lack and excess of cortisol.

7. *Gastrointestinal Effects:* production of gastric acid increases and pepsin decreases; the tendency for peptic ulcer formation increases with increasing concentration of cortisol in plasma.

8. *Bone Metabolism:* high levels inhibit formation of protein matrix of bone; this may lead to demineralization of the bone and osteoporosis.

9. *Cardiovascular System:* maintains sensitivity to pressor effects of catecholamines.

10. *Mesenchymal System:* alters connective tissue response to injury, namely, decreased hyperemia, exudation, and cellular infiltration. This illustrates the antiinflammatory action of glucocorticoid hormones.

11. *Immunologic Effects:* high concentrations of glucocorticoids in blood lyse fixed plasma cells and lymphocytes, thereby decreasing antibody production.

A. CARBOHYDRATE AND PROTEIN METABOLISM

Cortisol maintains the concentration of glucose in blood by the process of gluconeogenesis during fasting and starvation. Fasting induces, among other things, an increased release of glucose from the liver, to maintain a relatively constant concentration of glucose in blood. Stored liver glycogen is broken down (glycogenolysis) to form glucose, which is also released into blood. Glycogenolysis is induced by catecholamines and glucagon, which act via the cAMP system. However, cortisol seems to act permissively to enhance the abilities of catecholamines and glucagon to induce glycogenolysis. Since the glycogen stored in liver is estimated to last less than 24 hours when there is no source of caloric intake, the rate of secretion of glucocorticoids is increased to initiate the process of gluconeogenesis. Before the hepatic glycogen runs out, the liver begins to make more glucose. The raw materials from which the glucose is synthesized derive from the breakdown of the body's own tissues, especially skeletal muscle. Cortisol somehow enhances the release of amino acids from proteins in muscle and other tissues, including the protein matrix of bone. It may also decrease the synthesis of proteins. The amino acids released, particularly alanine (a "glucogenic" amino acid), are transported to the liver and are converted to glucose. The deamination of these amino acids increases the output of urea into urine.

Cortisol acts at the level of the liver to induce gluconeogenic enzymes either by direct action or indirectly by substrate induction. The effects of cortisol on the liver have been shown to include an increased conversion of amino acids to glucose precursors (e.g., alanine to pyruvate), an increased activity and synthesis of enzymes that convert amino acids to glucose precursors (e.g., aminotransferase), and an increased rate of conversion of glucose precursors to glucose (e.g., pyruvate to glucose). It is clear that cortisol is needed for optimal hepatic gluconeogenesis, but it is not clear which specific rate-limiting process or enzyme it affects.

Cortisol not only makes an additional source of energy available under conditions of fasting but it appears to initiate mechanisms to conserve energy. For example, it promotes a shift in energy sources in muscle from glucose to fatty acid metabolism and aids in mobilizing fatty acids from adipose tissue. The glycerol released from the fat cell with the fatty acids also serves as a substrate for gluconeogenesis. Cortisol-inhibited glycolysis in peripheral tissue is probably aided by a superimposed inhibition of key glycolytic enzymes by the increased concentration of free fatty acids in blood and perhaps by a decreased sensitivity of the tissues to insulin.

Hence, cortisol supports glucose supply when glucose is needed, principally by acting on muscle to supply amino acid substrate and on liver to convert the amino acids to glucose. Cortisol also indirectly tends to increase the availability of glucose to the central nervous system when glucose is in short supply by inhibiting (or at least by preventing an increase in) glucose uptake by several nonneural tissues. The central nervous system depends on glucose as its major energy substrate.

B. FAT METABOLISM

The overall effect of glucocorticoids on fat is to induce a redistribution and slight increase in body fat. As a result, patients with hypersecretion of cortisol (Cushing's syndrome) have a characteristic centripetal fat distribution to the head and trunk. The face may be moon shaped and the ears may be nearly hidden when the head is viewed from the front. Supraclavicular fat pads may form and produce a characteristic "buffalo hump." A pendulous abdomen, resulting from excessive fat distribution, is also characteristic. Chronic excess of cortisol leads to hyperlipemia and hypercholesterolemia. The mechanism responsible for fat redistribution under these conditions is unknown. It does appear, however, that the increase in total body fat occurs at the expense of body protein.

C. WATER METABOLISM

Both cortisol and cortisone enhance water diuresis when administered to hypoadrenal patients. This is probably due both to an increase in their rate of glomerular filtration and to antagonism of the effect of antidiuretic hormone at the level of the renal tubule. In the absence of glucocorticoid hormone (Addison's disease), ingestion of a liter of water is not accompanied by the usual diuresis and loss of the water load within 1 to 2 hours. In such patients, as much as 12 hours may be required to eliminate the water load. This effect has been used clinically as a test of adrenocortical function and is corrected by administration of cortisol but not by aldosterone.

D. HEMATOLOGIC EFFECTS

Glucocorticoids produce a striking suppression of lymphoid tissue activity and formation. This effect is seen most clearly in blood as lymphopenia and eosinopenia. Eosinophils are decreased so consistently by glucocorticoids that a low eosinophil count was once commonly used as an indicator of excess cortisol activity in man. This effect is not due to suppression of bone marrow but to increased sequestration in lungs and spleen and increased destruction in blood. In contrast, administration of cortisol is accompanied by an increase in circulating neutrophils so that total white blood cell count increases. Following administration of cortisol there may also be a rise in total red blood cell count and a rise in thrombocyte count. Lymphoid tissue such as the thymus and lymph nodes hypertrophy in the absence of cortisol and atrophy when cortisol is present in excess.

E. CENTRAL NERVOUS SYSTEM EFFECTS

Glucocorticoid hormones have unpredictable and profound effects on the central nervous system and the psyche. Adrenal insufficiency is often accompanied by a slowing of electrical discharges as seen in the electroencephalogram. Excessive cortisol lowers the threshold for electrical excitability and may account for the increased tendency for seizures when this steroid is administered to epileptic patients. Large doses of cortisol also lead to insomnia. In a considerable number of patients there is initial euphoria and in long-term therapy a number of psychotic manifestations may occur. A frequent problem is depression. It is worth noting here that one of Dr. Cushing's first patients was found in an insane asylum. A surprising fact is that behavioral and other disturbances are noted with both a lack and an excess of glucocorticoids. Cortisol also appears to be necessary for proper hearing, tasting, smelling, and drinking and for the maintenance of body temperature. Many parts of the brain have cortisol binding sites, but what happens beyond this is still largely unknown.

F. GASTROINTESTINAL EFFECTS

Administration of cortisol is accompanied by an increase in gastric acidity and a decrease in the production of pepsin. Cortisol appears to act indirectly by permitting other agents to stimulate the production of gastric acid more effectively. Chronic treatment with high doses of cortisol may lead to the formation of peptic ulcer.

G. BONE METABOLISM

Administration of large doses of cortisol impedes the development of cartilage and can reduce the protein matrix of bone. This may be considered to be an aspect of its gluconeogenic effect, leading to a loss of calcium from bone and to osteoporosis. Thus, bones may fracture easily. Cortisol is also reported to impair the absorption of calcium from the gastrointestinal tract, possibly by antagonizing the effect of vitamin D.

H. CARDIOVASCULAR SYSTEM

On occasion, a hypotensive state unresponsive to pressor agents such as norepinephrine will yield promptly to a large dose of cortisol. An immediate rise in blood pressure occurs even though the concentration of cortisol had been normal. Apparently the steroid is important in sensitization of the arterioles to the pressor effect of catecholamines. It is also known that chronic administration of cortisol in excess to experimental animals can result in the development of high blood pressure (hypertension).

I. MESENCHYMAL SYSTEM

Cortisol in pharmacologic doses decreases vascular permeability, increases capillary resistance, and enhances the vasoconstrictive effect of norepinephrine. It is possible that glucocorticoids suppress either the release or the action of histamine on cells surrounding the injured area. The migration of inflammatory cells from capillaries is depressed. These effects reduce swelling of inflammatory tissue by lessening the formation of edema, and they prevent swelling and distortion of cells by maintaining the integrity of the cell membrane to water. In addition, glucocorticoids are known to stabilize lysosomal membranes, thus preventing direct injury to the cell membrane by enzymes and toxins released by rupture of lysosomes. The mechanism of the stabilization of lysosomal membranes by glucocorticoids is not well understood.

J. IMMUNOLOGIC EFFECTS

The lymphocytolytic effect of glucocorticoid hormones mentioned above has been used to suppress the immune response in many disease states related to hyperimmunity. For example, they have found important use in human organ transplantation by either preventing or ameliorating the posttransplant response related to organ rejection by the host.

The antiallergic action of glucocorticoids seems to be mediated primarily through a suppression of the inflammatory response that results from antigen-antibody-induced injury. Steroids do not interfere with the antigen-antibody reaction in man, at least in doses used commonly in therapy. However, if very high doses are administered for a week or more, new antibody formation is depressed, probably as a result of lysing of lymphocytes and fixed plasma cells.

A large percentage of the cases of Cushing's syndrome seen clinically are physician induced (iatrogenic). This occurs because of the necessity to use pharmacologic doses of glucocorticoid hormones as antiallergens, in prevention of immunologic reactions, and in the treatment of certain rheumatic diseases. Physiologic doses generally do not produce these responses.

K. PHYSIOLOGIC ACTIONS OF MINERALOCORTICOID HORMONES

As the name implies, mineralocorticoid hormones maintain electrolyte equilibrium. Secondary to this is the maintenance of blood volume and blood pressure.

The major physiologic effect of aldosterone is its action in stimulating the active reabsorption of sodium and the active transport of sodium and potassium across the membranes of many epithelial tissues that are specialized for this particular function, including the distal tubules of the kidney, the tubules of the salivary glands, the sweat glands, and the intestinal mucosa. The major site of action is the cortical collecting ducts of the kidney, where aldosterone increases the reabsorption of sodium and chloride but promotes the loss of potassium, hydrogen, ammonium, and possibly magnesium ions. A test used commonly to assess the physiologic effect of aldosterone is the measurement of Na^+/K^+ ratio in urine. An increase in the concentration of aldosterone in blood decreases the ratio, while a decrease in concentration increases it. When aldosterone or another mineralocorticoid is given in excess, a retention of sodium and water and a loss of potassium occur for 6 to 8 days. After a sufficient expansion of extracellular fluid volume, the sodium retaining effect subsides but the excretion of potassium continues. This is the "escape" phenomenon described in Section 5-8. In this situation, the Na^+/K^+ ratio in both saliva and sweat would be expected to decrease on administration of aldosterone, but escape does not occur in these glands. Furthermore, present evidence suggests that third factor acts at a site different from that at which aldosterone acts to affect the reabsorption of sodium; namely, the loop of Henle in the kidney.

Aldosterone plays an important role in the exchange of sodium ions for potassium and hydrogen ions in the distal renal tubules. This exchange can lead to a hypokalemic alkalosis during iatrogenic administration of excess aldosterone and in diseases characterized by excessive secretion of aldosterone (e.g., Conn's syndrome). With retention of sodium there must be retention of water, with a resultant increase in plasma and extracellular fluid volume. This overexpansion of body fluid volume can lead to hypertension. This may not be the only factor involved, since excess aldosterone may also affect the arterioles themselves by sensitizing them to the effects of endogenous pressor agents such as norepinephrine and angiotensin II.

SECTION 5-9: POST-TEST QUESTIONS

1. Why is cortisol called a glucocorticoid hormone?

2. The important feedback element in the control of the secretion of cortisol is the concentration of glucose in blood. (True/False)
3. During a fast or starvation, cortisol maintains the concentration of glucose in blood by the process of _____ .
4. This begins just before hepatic _____ is depleted.
5. The raw materials from which glucose is synthesized during starvation are derived mainly from _____ .
6. The released amino acids are transported by blood to the a. _____ , where they are used to produce b. _____ .
7. As a result of this process, the nitrogen removed from the amino acids is excreted in urine as _____ .
8. Cortisol not only stimulates production of glucose by the liver, it also inhibits glycolysis in peripheral tissue. (True/False)
9. This has the important physiologic advantage of increasing the availability of glucose to the _____ , which requires glucose as a substrate for energy.
10. Patients with increased secretion of cortisol often have a round, moon-shaped face and a characteristic "buffalo hump." Why do these effects occur?

11. A patient with a reduced concentration of cortisol in blood requires 10 to 12 hours to excrete a 1-liter water load. Why?

12. Reductions in lymphocyte and eosinophil counts in blood occur on administration of ACTH. (True/False)
13. Administration of cortisol to an intact, normal laboratory animal for several days is accompanied by an increased concentration of glycogen in liver. (True/False)
14. Administration of excess cortisol results in atrophy of the thymus and lymph nodes. (True/False)
15. Administration of pharmacologic doses of cortisol to a patient with arthritis can often result in psychosis. (True/False)
16. Administration of pharmacologic doses of cortisol can induce calcium deposition in bones. (True/False)
17. How does cortisol relieve inflammation?

18. Glucocorticoids in very high doses are often used to suppress immune responses in some disease states as well as during human organ transplantation. If you were given a choice between cortisol and dexamethasone (the synthetic glucocorticoid), which would you use and why?

19. In the absence of mineralocorticoid hormones, the concentration of sodium in urine a. _____ while that of potassium b. _____. The concentration of sodium in blood c. _____ while that of potassium d. _____ _____ .

20. Patients suffering with Conn's syndrome in which an adrenal cortical tumor secretes excessive amounts of aldosterone do not become edematous. Why?

21. Aldosterone not only acts on renal tubules to influence electrolyte excretion, it acts on a. _____ , b. _____ , and c. _____ _____ as well.

22. Sodium escape also occurs in these organs when excessive amounts of aldosterone are secreted chronically. (True/False)

SECTION 5-9: POST-TEST ANSWERS

1. It plays an important role in maintaining blood glucose levels, particularly during periods of fasting, by the process of gluconeogenesis.
2. False
3. gluconeogenesis
4. glycogen
5. skeletal muscle
6. a. liver
   b. glucose
7. urea
8. True
9. brain
10. Cortisol induces a centripetal redistribution of body fat.
11. The rate of glomerular filtration and the antagonism of antidiuretic hormone are reduced in the absence of cortisol.
12. True
13. True
14. True
15. True
16. False
17. By suppressing either the release or the action of histamine on membrane permeability of cells surrounding the injured area. This reduces inflammatory tissue swelling by lessening formation of edema fluid. In addition, glucocorticoids are known to stabilize lysosomal membranes.
18. Dexamethasone. It has no residual mineralocorticoid activity. Administration of large doses of cortisol chronically would produce mineralocorticoid-like effects.
19. a. increases
    b. decreases
    c. decreases
    d. increases

20. Escape from the renal effects of aldosterone occurs.
21. a. salivary glands
    b. sweat glands
    c. intestines
22. False

SECTION 5-10: TESTS OF ADRENOCORTICAL FUNCTION

OBJECTIVES:

The student should be able to:
1. Discuss the concepts of "secretory reserve" capacity and "suppressibility" of secretory capacity as they apply to the adrenal cortex.
2. Discuss a clinical test of secretory reserve capacity used commonly for glucocorticoid hormones.
3. Discuss "primary" as opposed to "secondary" adrenal insufficiency.
4. Discuss the tests used to differentiate primary from secondary adrenal glucocorticoid insufficiency.
5. Discuss how pituitary secretory reserve capacity for the secretion of ACTH may be tested.
6. State the four recognized causes of Cushing's syndrome.
7. Discuss a clinical test used commonly to assess adrenocortical suppressibility.
8. Discuss the effect of withdrawal of chronic, high-dose therapy of glucocorticoid hormone on anterior pituitary and adrenal function.
9. Define primary versus secondary hyperaldosteronism.
10. Describe seven situations that may lead to secondary hyperaldosteronism.

Both the adrenal cortex and anterior pituitary gland, as well as other endocrine glands, secrete their hormones normally at a rate that permits them either to increase or decrease their secretory activity. The additional increase in the rate of secretion that each gland is capable of achieving is called its "secretory reserve" capacity. The maximal reduction in the rate of secretion that may be induced is termed "suppressibility" of secretory capacity. This concept is an extremely important and useful one and serves as the basis for the tests of adrenocortical function described in this section.

The adrenal cortex may be destroyed by certain infectious processes (e.g., tuberculosis), metastatic neoplasms, and idiopathic involution. When adrenal hypofunction is due to diseases originating in the adrenal gland, the hypofunction is classified as primary adrenal insufficiency or Addison's disease. In such patients both the concentration of cortisol in plasma and 17-OHCS in urine are reduced and there may be little or no circadian rhythm in the concentration of cortisol in plasma. (*Q. 5-9*) *What would you expect the concentration of ACTH in plasma to be in these patients?*

There are often gradations in the extent to which adrenal cortical tissue is destroyed in Addison's disease, and sometimes a near-normal concentration of cortisol in blood is maintained by an increased rate of secretion of ACTH. To establish the diagnosis of Addison's disease, it is often important to determine the secretory reserve of the gland. This can be accomplished by intravenous infusion of large doses of ACTH (e.g., 50 units over a period of 8 hours). Such infusion maintains the concentration of ACTH in plasma well in excess of the 3 mU/100 ml of plasma necessary for maximal adrenal activation.

Normal subjects respond to such infusions by increasing their concentrations of cortisol in plasma and 17-OHCS in urine to approximately 2 to 4 times their basal levels. The hallmark of Addison's disease is the absence of adrenocortical reserve. Even if there were remnants of adrenocortical tissue that were functional, they would be stimulated maximally under normal circumstances and administration of additional ACTH would have little effect on secretory capacity.

Reduced secretion of adrenal cortical hormones may also result from impaired ACTH secretion. This can occur as a result of adenomas arising within the anterior pituitary gland or, in women, by infarction of the gland during a postpartum hemorrhage (Sheehan's syndrome). Production of ACTH decreases under these conditions and, as a consequence, the normal adrenals produce less cortisol and adrenal atrophy may occur. Thus, secondary adrenocortical insufficiency is characterized by low concentrations of ACTH and cortisol in plasma and a reduced concentration of 17-OHCS in urine.

To distinguish between primary and secondary adrenocortical insufficiency, the infusion of ACTH should be continued for at least 3 successive days as described above. In patients with Addison's disease, ACTH will fail to stimulate the diseased adrenals regardless of the number of days of infusion of ACTH. Therefore, the concentration of 17-OHCS in urine and cortisol in plasma will be unchanged. On the other hand, the adrenals of patients with secondary adrenal insufficiency are intrinsically normal and have become atrophic only because stimulation by ACTH was lacking. Although the adrenals generally do not respond to the first 8-hour infusion of ACTH, successive 8-hour infusions generally result in production of cortisol and in regeneration of the atrophic adrenal gland. Stimulation of adrenocortical secretion under these conditions suggests that the anterior pituitary gland is not secreting ACTH at an optimal rate. The next question requiring an answer is whether the anterior pituitary gland is capable of secreting more than a certain minimal quantity of ACTH.

Certain patients with anterior pituitary disease secrete enough ACTH to prevent adrenal atrophy and to maintain responsiveness of the adrenal cortex to ACTH. The presence of a normal adrenocortical reserve, as suggested by a reasonable increase in the concentration of cortisol in plasma during the first 8 hours of infusion of ACTH, does not necessarily imply that the anterior pituitary gland is capable of secreting more than basal quantities of ACTH. Thus, it is possible that a patient could have a normal adrenocortical reserve with a limited pituitary reserve. Although these patients maintain normal baseline function, they are unable to increase endogenous ACTH production under conditions of increased demand such as surgery, trauma, and stresses of many kinds.

Metyrapone (Metopirone®), an 11β-hydroxylase enzyme inhibitor, may be used to test anterior pituitary reserve capacity for the secretion of ACTH. You recall from Section 5-3 that the 11β-hydroxylase enzyme is responsible for the conversion of 11-deoxycortisol to cortisol and 11-deoxycorticosterone to corticosterone. When metyrapone is administered to a normal individual, the concentration of cortisol in plasma decreases because the 11β-hydroxylase enzyme is inhibited. The fall in the concentration of cortisol in plasma is sensed at the levels of both the hypothalamus and the anterior pituitary, and the rate of secretion of ACTH is increased. The increasing concentration of ACTH in plasma drives the biosynthetic production of adrenal steroids at a more rapid rate, leading to the accumulation of 11-deoxycortisol. Since the blockage of the biosynthetic pathway is seldom complete, normal amounts of cortisol, but large amounts of 11-deoxycortisol, are released. Some of the urinary metabolites of 11-deoxycortisol, like those of cortisol, are measured as urinary 17-OHCS. Therefore, the normal response to metyrapone is an increase in urinary 17-OHCS. This sequence of events can occur only when the pituitary can increase its secretion of ACTH. The metyrapone test should be done only after the ACTH stimulation test has been performed. (*Q. 5-10*) Why?

Other tests of ACTH reserve have been devised that are less complicated to perform than the metyrapone test. One such test involves the induction of hypoglycemia by means of intravenous insulin. Hypoglycemia stimulates the secretion of ACTH and, secondarily, the production of cortisol. The change in the concentration of cortisol in plasma from its preinsulin level serves as the index of responsiveness of the pituitary-adrenal axis to hypoglycemia.

A second test involves the administration of vasopressin (pitressin or ADH), which also stimulates ACTH secretion. This probably occurs because vasopressin stimulates the same receptors in the anterior pituitary stimulated by CRF. This has lead some investigators to suggest that the chemical structure of vasopressin is similar to CRF. Once again, the concentration of cortisol in plasma serves as the index of responsiveness of the pituitary-adrenal axis. The insulin and vasopressin tests are used less commonly than the metyrapone test.

A chronic excess secretion of cortisol leads to the development of Cushing's syndrome. Apart from induction of the syndrome by the medicinal use of large doses of glucocorticoid hormones (iatrogenesis), there are now three recognized causes of Cushing's syndrome: inappropriately excessive secretion of ACTH by the pituitary, ectopic secretion of excess ACTH by a nonpituitary neoplasm, and excessive secretion of cortisol by an adrenocortical neoplasm. All are characterized by excessive production of cortisol and supernormal concentrations of cortisol in plasma and 17-OHCS in urine. Usually the diurnal rhythmicity of the secretion of cortisol is disturbed, so that the concentration of cortisol in plasma may be as high in the evening as it is in the morning. When cortisol is secreted in amounts large enough to induce this disease, it is clear that the rate of secretion is no longer under feedback control; that is, the secretion of cortisol has become relatively or absolutely nonsuppressible.

Suppressibility of the anterior pituitary secretion of ACTH is tested clinically by means of the potent glucocorticoid analogue dexamethasone, mentioned in Section 5-9. Dexamethasone is about 30 times more potent as a glucocorticoid than cortisol. For this reason it can be administered in small doses that do not interfere with the chemical measurement of cortisol and its metabolites. (Q. 5-11) *Could one use cortisol instead of dexamethasone in a test of pituitary suppressibility? Why?* The normal, nonstressed individual usually responds to small doses (0.5 mg every 6 hours) of dexamethasone with a profound decrease in the secretion of ACTH and cortisol. Patients with Cushing's syndrome have either a relative or an absolute resistance to suppression by dexamethasone. It is important to the differential diagnosis of Cushing's syndrome to determine whether the resistance is relative or absolute. The distinction can be achieved by using a somewhat larger dose of dexamethasone (2–8 mg every 6 hours). During treatment with the larger dose, adrenal function is reduced appreciably in patients with inappropriate secretion of ACTH by the anterior pituitary. In patients with Cushing's syndrome due to autonomously functioning adrenocortical neoplasms and in patients with an ectopic source of ACTH, adrenal function generally is not affected by the larger dose of dexamethasone.

The only way dexamethasone can suppress function is by suppressing the secretion of ACTH at the level of the pituitary or the secretion of CRF at the level of the hypothalamus. Hence, resistance to the suppressive effect of large doses of dexamethasone should suggest either that the patient has a nonpituitary source of ACTH that is responsible for adrenal overactivity, or that the adrenal overactivity is due to an adrenocortical neoplasm that is capable of secreting large amounts of cortisol, even in the absence of ACTH. These two neoplastic disorders can be distinguished from each other by measurement of the concentration of ACTH in plasma.

Long-term treatment with supraphysiologic doses of glucocorticoids for arthritis, immunosuppression, and allergy can suppress the secretion of ACTH and induce adrenocortical atrophy. If suppression of ACTH secretion has been continuous for more than a year, pituitary-adrenal recovery after withdrawal of the excess steroid follows a course in which there is an initial phase, lasting about a month, during which the concentration of ACTH in plasma remains subnormal and adrenocortical response is subnormal (see Figure 5-23). Such patients are likely to experience mild symptoms of adrenocortical deficiency. In the next phase, lasting several months, the anterior pituitary gradually recovers its ability to secrete ACTH, but the responsiveness to ACTH of the adrenal cortex is still subnormal. From 3 to 8 months after withdrawal of exogenous glucocorticoid therapy, the secretion of ACTH is supernormal. At this time the adrenal cortex increases its rate of secretion, and after 8 or more months, the normal feedback mechanism is again in operation (see Figure 5-23). Until pituitary-adrenal reserve can be demonstrated to be normal, it is wise to protect such patients during periods of severe stress by giving exogenous glucocorticoid therapy.

Primary aldosteronism (Conn's syndrome) is a curable cause of hypertension (high blood pressure). However, only about 1% of patients with hypertension have Conn's syndrome. It is due to a single adrenocortical adenoma (80% of cases) which secretes aldosterone at an excessive rate. This leads to retention of sodium and loss of potassium. Plasma volume expands until the escape mechanism occurs. The expanded volume may be responsible for the hypertension, but this is not yet clear. The patient usually has a low concentration of potassium in plasma (less than 3.5 mEq/liter) and is alkalotic, while the concentration of sodium in plasma may be unchanged. (*Q. 5-12*) *Why?* Measurement of the concentration of aldosterone in plasma is important in the diagnosis. (*Q. 5-13*) *What would you expect plasma renin activity to be?*

The conditions under which secondary hyperaldosteronism occurs include the following: a) a persistent decrease in intravascular volume, such as chronic diuretic

FIGURE 5-23: Patients recovering from prolonged pituitary-adrenal suppression. (*Adapted from:* Liddle, 1965.)

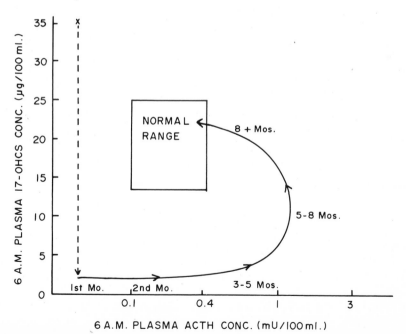

therapy and a number of edematous states (nephrosis, cirrhosis), b) a chronic inadequate cardiac output, such as congestive heart failure and valvular heart disease, c) a
persistent decrease in renal blood flow, such as renal artery stenosis, d) a decreased
perfusion of afferent arterioles, as in malignant hypertension, e) chronic hyperactivity
of the JG cells (Bartter's syndrome), f) an increase in renin substrate as in pregnancy and
during ingestion of oral contraceptives, and g) presence of another source of renin, as
may occur during pregnancy (uterine source). Under these conditions the secretion of
aldosterone increases because the activity of the renin-angiotensin system has increased. Thus, the increase in the secretion of aldosterone is secondary to an increase in
the activity of the renin-angiotensin system. Many, but not all, of the effects just listed
are accompanied by hypokalemic alkalosis; only a few are accompanied by hypertension. It is not clear why patients with primary aldosteronism have hypertension and
those with secondary aldosteronism generally do not.

Several tests of the secretory reserve capacity of the entire renin-angiotensin-aldosterone system were discussed in Section 5-8. These include administration of a
sodium-restricted diet and the movement from a supine to an upright position. These
should be reviewed in the context of tests of function of the renin-angiotensin-aldosterone system.

A screening test for adrenal hypofunction that has been introduced recently involves
measurement of the concentrations of aldosterone and cortisol before, and 30 to 60
minutes after, intramuscular administration of a pharmacologic dose of ACTH. This test
can distinguish the difference between primary and secondary adrenal hypofunction on
the basis of the assumption that in primary adrenal hypofunction, the rate of secretion
of neither cortisol nor aldosterone can be stimulated. Hence, 30 to 60 minutes after
administration of ACTH, the concentration of neither aldosterone nor cortisol in blood
increases above pre-ACTH levels (see Table 5-4). In the presence of secondary adrenal
hypofunction, both the concentration of aldosterone and cortisol increase, but the
cortisol response is subnormal whereas the aldosterone response is normal. In secondary adrenal hypofunction induced by chronic treatment with a glucocorticoid-type
hormone, the ACTH-stimulated aldosterone response is normal whereas that of cortisol
is unchanged. (Q. 5-14) *What does the differential responsiveness of the secretion of
aldosterone and cortisol to stimulation by ACTH during secondary adrenal hypofunction suggest?*

**TABLE 5-4: Summary of the Changes in the Concentrations of Aldosterone and
Cortisol Following the Administration of ACTH**

	n	Aldosterone (ng/dl)			Cortisol (μg/dl)		
		Pre-ACTH	30 min Post-ACTH	(%) Increase	Pre-ACTH	30 min Post-ACTH	(%) Increase
Normals	12	14	28	100	9	24	167
Primary adrenal hypofunction	5	2	2	0	1	1	0
Secondary adrenal hypofunction (hypopituitarism)	6	5	11	120	4	5	25
Secondary adrenal hypofunction (steroid treated)	6	18	44	144	4	4	0

Before chemical and immunoassays were available, several tests of adrenocortical function were used commonly. One of these, the eosinophil (Thorn) test, is based on the fact that an increasing rate of secretion of cortisol induces a progressive fall in the concentration of eosinophils in blood. If an injection of ACTH is followed by a marked decrease in the eosinophil count in blood, a responsive adrenal cortex is presumed to be present.

A second test is the water excretion test mentioned in Section 5-9. Subjects with adrenocortical insufficiency fail to excrete a water load as promptly as normal individuals. A normal individual can excrete a 1-liter water load within 1 to 2 hours; patients with adrenocortical insufficiency may take up to 12 hours to excrete the load. As discussed in Section 5-9, such patients have a low rate of glomerular filtration that may account for the delay in excretion of the water load.

The tests of adrenocortical function that have been covered here are based on the biologic feedback mechanisms discussed earlier. They illustrate the practical importance for an understanding of the biosynthetic pathway, the feedback mechanisms, and the physiologic effects of adrenocortical hormones.

SECTION 5-10: POST-TEST QUESTIONS

1. Exogenous glucocorticoid therapy inhibits endogenous adrenocortical activity by:
   a. inducing gluconeogenesis
   b. a direct inhibitory action on the adrenal cortex
   c. increasing extracellular fluid volume
   d. inhibiting secretion of ACTH

2. Discuss the concepts of secretory reserve capacity and suppressibility of secretory capacity as they apply to the adrenal cortex.

3. What is primary adrenocortical insufficiency?

4. What is secondary adrenocortical insufficiency?

5. How can primary adrenocortical insufficiency be distinguished clinically from secondary adrenocortical insufficiency?

6. Which of the following tests are useful in making a diagnosis of adrenal insufficiency?

   a. baseline urinary 17-OHCS
   b. morning and evening concentrations of cortisol in plasma
   c. basal metabolic rate
   d. eosinophil test

7. Which of the following is useful in testing the reserve capacity for secreting ACTH by the anterior pituitary gland?
   a. baseline urinary 17-OHCS
   b. ACTH stimulation test
   c. metyrapone test
   d. morning and evening concentrations of cortisol in plasma

8. What effect has metyrapone at the level of the adrenal cortex?

9. The normal response to administration of metyrapone is an (increase/decrease) in urinary 17-OHCS. Why?

10. Describe two other tests of anterior pituitary reserve.

11. State the four recognized causes of Cushing's syndrome.
   a.
   b.
   c.
   d.

12. Ectopic secretion of ACTH by a nonpituitary neoplasm generally is under the normal feedback control mechanisms. (True/False)

13. Dexamethasone is used to test suppressibility because it acts directly on the adrenal cortex to reduce secretion of cortisol. (True/False)

14. Dexamethasone is an intermediate in the biosynthetic pathway to corticosterone. (True/False)

15. The limiting factor in the recovery of the pituitary-adrenal axis after long-term, high-dosage glucocorticoid therapy is:
   a. restoration of adrenocortical production of cortisol
   b. restoration of secretion of ACTH
   c. restoration of biosynthesis of cholesterol
   d. reduction in the rate of hepatic metabolism of cortisol

16. Which of the following (is/are) true?
   The actions of glucocorticoid hormones include:
   a. increase in hepatic gluconeogenesis
   b. decrease in muscle protein synthesis
   c. increase in hepatic enzyme activity
   d. eosinopenia

    e. lymphopenia

    f. stabilization of lysosomal membranes

    g. inhibition of antibody production at high doses of steroid

17. What is primary hyperaldosteronism? How is it characterized clinically?

18. What is secondary hyperaldosteronism?

19. How could one distinguish between these two?

SECTION 5-10: POST-TEST ANSWERS

1. d
2. The adrenal cortex normally secretes at a rate that permits it either to increase or decrease its secretory activity. The additional increase in secretion rate which the adrenal cortex is capable of achieving is its secretory reserve capacity. The maximal reduction in secretory rate that may be induced is termed suppressibility of secretory capacity.
3. Addison's disease. It is characterized by adrenocortical hypofunction due to diseases originating in the adrenal gland.
4. Secondary adrenocortical insufficiency is characterized by adrenocortical hypofunction as a result of reduced secretion of ACTH.
5. To distinguish between primary and secondary adrenocortical insufficiency, infusions of ACTH should be administered on at least 3 successive days. (Q. 5-15) *Why is this important?*
6. a, b, d
7. c
8. Metyrapone is an 11β-hydroxylase enzyme inhibitor.
9. Increase. Metyrapone partially blocks production of cortisol by the adrenal cortex with a subsequent decrease in the concentration of cortisol in plasma. This is sensed at the levels of the pituitary and hypothalamus, which initiate an increase in the rate of secretion of ACTH. This drives the adrenal cortex, still under blockade by metyrapone. An increase in the concentration in blood of 11-deoxycortisol results. The metabolites of 11-deoxycortisol consist mainly of 17-OHCS. Therefore, the concentration of 17-OHCS in urine increases.
10. Administration of insulin and vasopressin.
11. a. Iatrogenic
    b. Excessive secretion of ACTH by the anterior pituitary gland
    c. Ectopic secretion of excessive ACTH by a nonpituitary neoplasm
    d. Excessive secretion of cortisol by an adrenocortical neoplasm
12. False
13. False. It acts at the level of the pituitary and hypothalamus.
14. False. It is a synthetic steroid, not a naturally occurring one.
15. a
16. All are true.

17. Conn's syndrome. It usually is due to an adrenocortical adenoma. It is characterized by sodium retention with expansion of extracellular fluid volume, hypokalemic alkalosis, and hypertension.
18. It is characterized by an increase in the secretion of aldosterone resulting from an increased activity of the renin-angiotensin system.
19. Plasma renin activity is low in primary hyperaldosteronism and high in secondary hyperaldosteronism.

SECTION 5-11: CONGENITAL ADRENAL HYPERPLASIA

OBJECTIVES:

The student should be able to:
1. Recite the five enzymatic defects that may occur in the biosynthetic pathways of the adrenal cortex.
2. Discuss the physiologic consequences of these blocks in terms of the biosynthetic pathways.
3. Discuss the rationale for treatment of patients with certain of these defects.
4. Demonstrate both an understanding and an appreciation of the probabilities of the hereditary transmission of a biosynthetic enzyme deficiency of the adrenal cortex.

Congenital adrenal hyperplasia may result from a genetic enzyme deficiency at any one of the five positions in the biosynthetic pathway shown in Figure 5-4.

A genetic deficiency of the desmolase enzyme is incompatible with life because no adrenal cortical hormones can be synthesized. At autopsy, infants with this enzyme deficiency have been found to have large amounts of cholesterol in their adrenal glands.

A genetic deficiency of the 3β-hydroxydehydrogenase enzyme is also incompatible with life. Infants with this genetic deficiency survive only a few months. A deficiency of this enzyme decreases the formation of both glucocorticoids and mineralocorticoids. The pregnenolone formed is shunted to 17α-OH-pregnenolone and dehydroepíandrosterone. The latter is produced in excess and is secreted into blood (see Figure 5-4) and carried to peripheral tissues, where it is converted to testosterone. All cases observed clinically have been associated with symptoms of excessive loss of sodium.

A genetic deficiency of the 17α-hydroxylase enzyme is compatible with life. A reduction in the synthesis of cortisol and androgenic hormones occurs while the aldosterone pathway is activated. However, the secretion of aldosterone does not appear to increase. Instead there are increases in corticosterone and 11-deoxycorticosterone, the precursor of aldosterone. The latter steroid has very good mineralocorticoid characteristics, and its excess results in a hyperaldosterone-like syndrome. Glucocorticoid deficiency is usually not serious because corticosterone is an active glucocorticoid. When the 17α-hydroxylase enzyme deficiency occurs, it affects not only the adrenal glands but the testes and ovaries as well. Hence, patients have a deficiency of both male and female sex hormones and both sexes are of the female phenotype, regardless of the genetic sex. Patients with this deficiency usually present at puberty because of lack of menarche. Hypertension and hypokalemic alkalosis are also found.

The most common form of congenital adrenal hyperplasia is represented by the adrenogenital syndrome. Most frequently found in females, this condition results from an hereditory congenital deficiency of the 21-hydroxylase enzyme. (*Q. 5-16*) *From this information and your knowledge of the pertinent biosynthetic pathways, can you describe the resulting clinical picture?*

The first direct result of the enzyme deficiency is a buildup of substrates and a depletion of products. Thus, in the 21-hydroxylase deficiency, the concentrations of progesterone and 17α-OH-progesterone increase and spill over into the blood. At the same time the concentrations of both cortisol and aldosterone are diminished. The hypothalamus and anterior pituitary gland sense this drop in cortisol as a simple lack in their activity and so the hypothalamus secretes large amounts of CRF, which in turn stimulates the secretion of large amounts of ACTH. The resulting overstimulation by ACTH puts the adrenal gland into a state of hyperplasia. In this instance, though, the adrenal's hyperactivity is shunted into pathways having no requirement for the 21-hydroxylase enzyme. The only pathway that meets this criterion leads to the synthesis of androgens. Large concentrations of dehydroepiandosterone and androstenedione are produced in plasma. These steroids are then converted to testosterone by peripheral tissues. Newborn females with adrenogenital syndrome therefore present with enlarged clitorises and high levels of testosterone in plasma. (*Q. 5-17*) *What hormonal metabolites would you expect to find in such a patient's urine?*

The extent of the enzymatic deficiency varies among patients. If the deficiency is only mild, a sufficient amount of aldosterone may be produced to meet physiologic need. In this case, the androgenic effects may appear only at puberty, manifesting themselves in poor breast development, hirsutism, and amenorrhea. If the enzymatic deficiency is severe, the production of aldosterone can be so inhibited that the patient loses sodium and becomes dehydrated, which can result in death.

Most cases are intermediate in severity. If a loss of sodium does not occur, treatment consists of replacement therapy with glucocorticoid to reduce the excessive secretion of ACTH and to supply the body with the necessary glucocorticoid hormone.

A genetic enzymatic deficiency of the 11β-hydroxylase enzyme can deprive the body the both glucocorticoids and mineralocorticoids. This leads to a syndrome similar to the 21-hydroxylase enzyme defect except that 11-deoxycorticosterone is produced in excess. Since this steroid has good mineralocorticoid properties, a hyperaldosterone-like syndrome coexists with virilization. Thus, one can differentiate the 11β-hydroxylase enzyme deficiency from the 21-hydroxylase deficiency by the presence of hypertension in the former. You recall from Section 5-10 that administration of metyrapone results in changes in adrenal function analogous to an 11β-hydroxylase deficiency.

Congenital adrenal hyperplasia illustrates the practical importance of an understanding of the adrenal biosynthetic pathways for diagnosis and treatment.

Congenital adrenal hyperplasia results when a child inherits two defective genes—one from each parent—for an adrenocortical enzyme (see Figure 5-24). The parents who carry a defective gene are normal because the normal gene of the pair is dominant, the

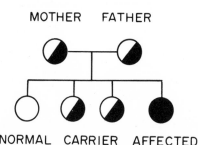

MOTHER FATHER

NORMAL CARRIER AFFECTED

FIGURE 5-24: Genetics of congenital adrenal hyperplasia.

defective gene is recessive. About one person in 50 carries this recessive gene. When such an individual marries another carrier, they have a 25% (1 in 4) chance of having one child inherit both the abnormal genes, and therefore having the condition.

Since congenital adrenal hyperplasia is a recessive trait, a carrier can have affected children only if he or she marries another carrier, a 1 in 50 chance; then, as indicated above, each of their children would have a 1 in 4 chance of inheriting both carrier parents' defective genes and having the condition. A brother or sister of a child with the condition has a 2 out of 3 chance of being a carrier; thus his or her risk is $\frac{2}{3} \times \frac{1}{50} \times \frac{1}{4}$, or 1 in 300, of having an affected child. Brothers and sisters of carriers, that is, the aunts and uncles of patients, have a 1 in 2 chance of themselves being carriers. They too have a 1 in 50 chance of marrying carriers, and then a 1 in 4 chance of having a child who is affected. Thus, the risk in first cousins of affected children is $\frac{1}{2} \times \frac{1}{50} \times \frac{1}{4}$, or 1 in 400.

As can be seen from this example, an understanding of the probabilities of the hereditary transmission of enzymatic defects is very important in genetic counseling.

SECTION 5-11: POST-TEST QUESTIONS

1. What are the five enzymatic defects that may occur in the biosynthetic pathways of the adrenal cortex?
   a.
   b.
   c.
   d.
   e.
2. Which two enzyme deficiencies are incompatible with life?
   a.
   b.
3. When a 21-hydroxylase enzyme deficiency occurs in the biosynthetic pathway, what compensatory physiologic response occurs?

4. What effect does this have on the adrenal cortex?

5. What treatment would you prescribe? Why?

6. What steroid metabolites would you expect to see in the urine of patients with a 21-hydroxylase enzyme deficiency?

7. The enzymatic deficiencies of the adrenal cortical biosynthetic pathway that are compatible with life can vary in the extent of their deficiency. (True/False)

8. The more complete the 21-hydroxylase deficiency, the more likely the patient is to have excessive _____ as well as virilization.

9. An 11β-hydroxylase deficiency can be induced by the drug a. _____. This drug is used clinically to test b. _____.

10. A patient with an 11β-hydroxylase deficiency differs from one with a 21-hydroxylase deficiency in that the former patient has an elevated a. _____ _____ and the latter does not. This is due to an excessive build up of b. _____ _____ ahead of the enzymatic deficiency.

11. In congenital adrenal hyperplasia, the probability of hereditary transmission in the family of an affected individual can be calculated. This information is used clinically in _____.

SECTION 5-11: POST-TEST ANSWERS

1. a. Desmolase enzyme
   b. 3β-Hydroxydehydrogenase enzyme
   c. 17α-Hydroxylase enzyme
   d. 21-Hydroxylase enzyme
   e. 11β-Hydroxylase enzyme
2. a. Desmolase enzyme
   b. 3β-Hydroxydehydrogenase enzyme
3. Secretion of ACTH increases.
4. ACTH increases the biosynthetic activity of the adrenal cortex. As a result there is a pileup of steroids ahead of the enzymatic block. If the block is only a mild one, enough cortisol and aldosterone may still be produced to meet physiologic requirements. However, the secretion of ACTH would still be elevated and an increase in the secretion of androgen by the adrenal cortex would still occur.
5. Administration of a glucocorticoid hormone. This would reduce the secretion of ACTH and the production of excess androgens by the adrenal cortex.
6. An increase in 17-ketosteroids, and in the hepatic metabolites of 17α-OH-progesterone and progesterone, which are pregnanetriol and pregnanediol, respectively.
7. True
8. sodium loss
9. a. metyrapone
   b. pituitary reserve
10. a. blood pressure
    b. deoxycorticosterone
11. genetic counseling

SELECTED REFERENCES

Baxter, J. D., 1976, Glucocorticoid hormone action, *Pharmaceutical Therapy B* 2: 605.

James, V. H. T. (Ed.), 1972, *The Adrenal Gland*, New York: Raven Press.

Kotchen, T. A. and Guthrie, G. P., Jr., 1980, Renin-angiotensin-aldosterone and hypertension, *Endocrine Reviews* 1: 78.

Krieger, D., Liotta, A. S., Brownstein, M. J., and Zimmerman, E. A., 1980, β-Lipotropin and rleated peptides in brain, pituitary and blood, *Recent Progress In Hormone Research* 36, 277.

Peach, M. J., 1977, Renin-angiotensin system: biochemistry and mechanisms of action, *Physiological Reviews* 57: 313.

6

MALE REPRODUCTIVE ENDOCRINOLOGY

SECTION 6.1: ANATOMY OF THE MALE REPRODUCTIVE TRACT

OBJECTIVES:

The student should be able to:
1. State why the testes of the human male are located outside the abdominal cavity.
2. State where spermatozoa are produced in the testes.
3. State where testosterone is produced in the testes.
4. Describe the anatomic organization of the testes, including the route by which spermatozoa leave the body.
5. Name three sex accessory organs of males and describe their function in reproduction.

The testes in man are paired organs located in the scrotum. Their location outside the abdominal cavity is essential for the process of spermatogenesis to occur. Being suspended within the scrotum maintains their temperature below internal body temperature and prevents the degeneration of certain cells of the seminiferous tubules. This degeneration is evident in males born with undescended testes (i.e., cryptorchidism) and is correlated with the inhibition of certain temperature-dependent enzymes essential for cellular vitality. A further demonstration of the importance of a reduced scrotal temperature was provided by a rather unusual clinical study in which a 75% reduction in sperm count was noted in men who voluntarily wore an insulated jockstrap for several weeks. This reduced fertility was reversible.

Although descent of the testis from the abdomen to the scrotum is essential for reproduction in man and certain other mammals, it does not occur in all mammals. For example, the whale, elephant, seal, and rhinoceros have no scrotum, and in many seasonally breeding mammals, the testes descend from the abdomen to the scrotum only during the breeding season. In certain other mammals (e.g., the rat) the testes can ascend to the abdomen or descend to the scrotum at any age, a process that may be influenced by stress and other factors. The differences among mammals undoubtedly are related to the different strategies for survival adopted by each species.

The human testes usually descend to the scrotum during the final month of fetal life and the inguinal canal, through which they descend, becomes sealed off shortly after birth. Each adult testis is contained within its own scrotal compartment, which is separated from the other compartment by a septum. The adult testis is ovoid and measures 4 to 5 cm in length and 2.5 to 3 cm in width. The weight range of each testis in the mature adult human is 10–45 g. Partially surrounding each testis is the tunica vaginalis, a remnant of its origin in the peritoneum (see Figure 6-1). Each testis is divided into a number of pyramidal septa (septate testis), which are separated by a connective tissue capsule called the tunica albuginea. Each septum contains a large number of tubules, the seminiferous tubules, which are convoluted such that they occupy a minimal amount of space within the septum. It has been estimated that if the seminiferous tubules of the adult male human were placed end to end, they would extend a mile or more.

The seminiferous tubules are composed of a tubular wall formed by peritubular cells resting on a basement membrane that encloses both Sertoli cells and spermatogenic cells. The latter are referred to as germinal epithelium because sperm cells are produced there. Interstitial cells of Leydig, lymphatics, blood vessels, and various connective tissue elements occupy the space between seminiferous tubules. This space is rich in extracellular fluid into which testosterone, produced by the interstitial cells of Leydig, is released. From the interstitial fluid, the hormone can diffuse into the seminiferous tubules to produce local effects on sperm production. Testosterone can also diffuse into nearby lymphatics and blood vessels to produce its systemic effects. Testicular steroidogenesis and spermatogenesis, as well as the systemic actions of testosterone, are discussed in upcoming sections of this chapter.

The seminiferous tubules empty their contents into the rete testis through which the contents move to the head of the epididymis (caput epididymidis) (see Figure 6-1). In the head of the epididymis, the smooth muscle lining the tube undergoes rhythmic peristalsis, independent of nerve stimulation, which serves to transport the sperm along the duct. From the head of the epididymis, a convoluted tubule runs caudally along the

FIGURE 6-1: Anatomy of the testis and locations of the sex accessory tissues of the human male. (*Source:* Ham and Cosmack, 1979.)

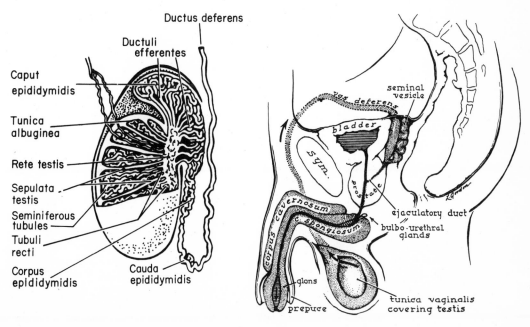

testis to form first the body (corpus epididymidis) and then the tail of the epididymis (cauda epididymidis). The tail of the epididymis demonstrates less peristalsis and acts as a storage area. Within this portion of the epididymis, 90% of the fluid containing the sperm is reabsorbed. Some sperm maturation occurs there, although final maturation, motility, and the ability to fertilize the egg occurs in the female reproductive tract, a process known as sperm capacitation (not to be confused with receptor capacitation as described in Section 5-6). It is interesting to note that sperm can remain viable in the female reproductive tract for about 48 hours, thus increasing the probability for fertilization even if copulation is infrequent.

Arising from the tail of the epididymis is the ductus deferens. This structure forms a component of the spermatic cord in the posterior portion of the scrotum (see Figure 6-1). Within the spermatic cord the ductus deferens is surrounded by an interweaving network of veins known as the pampiniform plexus. This plexus is thought to form a heat exchange mechanism in conjunction with the arterial supply to the testis, which is also within the cord. A transfer of heat from the warm arterial supply to the cooler venous blood in the plexus may be important in maintaining a cooler temperature within the scrotum. (Q. 6-1) *Why is this heat exchange important?* The ductus deferens contains a thick three-layered wall of smooth muscle that is highly innervated by sympathetic nerves. These smooth muscles, along with sympathetically innervated smooth muscles of the tail of the epididymis, serve as the main propulsive force for ejaculation. Distally, the ductus deferens widens and is known as the ampulla. The ductus enters the inguinal canal, passes through to enter the peritoneum, and then passes dorsally into the pelvis. Just before contacting the prostate, it is joined by the secretory duct of the seminal vesicles. The seminal vesicles are paired male sex accessory organs that secrete a pale yellow, viscous liquid, rich in fructose (a carbohydrate utilized by spermatozoa as an energy source). The secretions of the seminal vesicle, as well as spermatozoa from the testes, empty into the ejaculatory duct, which passes through the prostate, another single male sex accessory organ, to join the urethra at the prostatic utricle.

The prostate is surrounded by a fibroelastic capsule and is composed of about 40 tubuloalveolar glands. The glands are embedded in a connective tissue stroma containing elastic tissue and smooth muscle bundles. The glands open separately into the prostatic urethra, which passes through the prostate. The prostate contributes a milky, irridescent, slightly acid liquid. It is the source of various enzymes including acid phosphatase. Condensation of prostatic secretions may form concretions that calcify and lodge in the prostate. These concretions increase in number and size with age. The final male accessory organs are the bulbourethral (Cowpers) glands, which empty into the beginning of the penile urethra. They are typical mucus secreting tubuloalveolar glands that secrete a clear viscous lubricant early in erection.

The penis is composed of three major structural units, two corpora cavernosa and the corpus spongiosum. These three structures are bound together by several fascial layers to form the dependent penis. The cavernosa are divided by numerous trabeculae into a series of interconnected spaces. The filling of these spaces with blood during sexual arousal leads to erection of the penis. The corpus spongiosum lies in the ventral groove formed by the cavernosa. Its terminal portion, the glans penis, is enlarged and constitutes the distal end of the cavernosa.

Upon sexual arousal and ejaculation, semen or seminal fluid (spermatozoa and secretions from accessory glands) passes through the prostatic urethra (that portion of the urethra surrounded by the prostate gland) and then into the penile urethra contained within the corpus spongiosum. During normal ejaculation, 3 to 4 ml of semen containing approximately 80 million to 100 million sperm cells per milliliter (60%

motile forms) are expelled. If the sperm count falls below 10 million to 20 million per milliliter, infertility can be expected. Vasectomy (bilateral transection of the ductus deferens) produces infertility by preventing the transport of sperm from the epididymis to the ejaculatory duct. (*Q. 6-2*) *What effect would you expect this operation to have on testosterone production and secretion from the testis?*

SECTION 6-1: POST-TEST QUESTIONS

1. The testis is divided into many pyramidal compartments by a connective tissue capsule known as the a. _____ . Within these compartments are the b. _____ tubules. Within the structural components of the walls of these tubules are the c. _____ cells and the d. _____ _____ cells. Between these tubules are found the e. _____ cells of f. _____ , lymphatics, blood vessels, and various connective tissue elements.

2. The contents of the seminiferous tubules are emptied into the a. _____ from which the contents enter the head of the b. _____ . They wind their way through the body of the c. _____ to the tail of the d. _____ _____ , which serves as a e. _____ site for spermatozoa.

3. The vas deferens arises from the a. _____ of the epididymis to form part of the b. _____ plexus, which enters the peritoneum by way of the c. _____ .

4. Connecting with the vas deferens in the peritoneal cavity are ducts from the a. _____ , a pair of sex accessory organs in the abdominal cavity. These organs contribute b. _____ containing c. _____ , which is important for d. _____ .

5. The vas deferens passes through the a. _____ , which also contributes b. _____ to the contents of the vas deferens.

6. Name three male sex accessory organs.
   a.
   b.
   c.

7. The penis is composed of two a. _____ and the b. _____ _____ . The urethra passes through the c. _____ .

SECTION 6-1: POST-TEST ANSWERS

1. a. tunica albuginea
   b. seminiferous
   c. Sertoli cells
   d. sperm (germ) cells
   e. interstitial
   f. Leydig
2. a. rete testis
   b. epididymis
   c. epididymis
   d. epididymis
   e. storage

3. a. tail
   b. pampiniform
   c. inguinal canal
4. a. seminal vesicles
   b. fluid
   c. fructose
   d. nourishment of spermatozoa
5. a. prostate gland
   b. fluid
6. a. Seminal vesicles
   b. Prostate
   c. Bulbourethral (Cowpers) glands
7. a. corpora cavernosa
   b. corpus spongiosum
   c. corpus spongiosum

SECTION 6-2: ANDROGENS

OBJECTIVES:

The student should be able to:
   1. Describe the basic structural features of the androgens.
   2. Describe the biosynthetic pathways used for the production of testosterone.
   3. Describe how testosterone is transported in blood.
   4. Describe the physiologic effects of the naturally occurring androgenic steroid hormones.

A. STRUCTURE AND BIOSYNTHESIS OF ANDROGENS

The naturally occurring androgens are steroids of the C-19 group that are synthesized primarily in the testes, ovaries, and adrenal cortex. The basic structure and biosynthesis of these lipophilic-hydrophobic compounds were described in Sections 5-2 and 5-3 (see Figure 5-3). The cells of the testis responsible for biosynthesis of testosterone are called interstitial cells of Leydig or interstitial cells (see Figure 6-6). Cholesterol, the principal precursor for all steroid hormones, can enter the interstitial cells of Leydig by diffusion from the blood, or it can be synthesized from acetate within these cells. Both sources are used for the biosynthesis of testosterone. It is likely that the cholesterol found as cholesterol ester in lipid droplets within interstitial cells is also used for biosynthesis of testosterone. As is the case for all other steroid biosynthetic pathways, the principal step controlling the biosynthesis of testosterone is the conversion of cholesterol to pregnenolone (see Figures 6-2 and 6-3). The desmolase enzyme responsible for this conversion is located within the mitochondria.

There are two major biosynthetic routes for the conversion of pregnenolone to testosterone (see Figure 6-2). The 4-ene pathway involves the production of progesterone, its conversion to 17α-OH-progesterone, androstenedione, and finally testosterone. The second route, the 5-ene pathway, involves the production of 17α-OH-pregnenolone, its conversion to 17α-OH-progesterone, androstenedione, and finally testosterone. The enzymes responsible for both these pathways are found in the microsomal fraction (i.e., smooth endoplasmic reticulum) of the interstitial cells. There is still considerable debate over the relative importance of each of these pathways, but it is clear that both

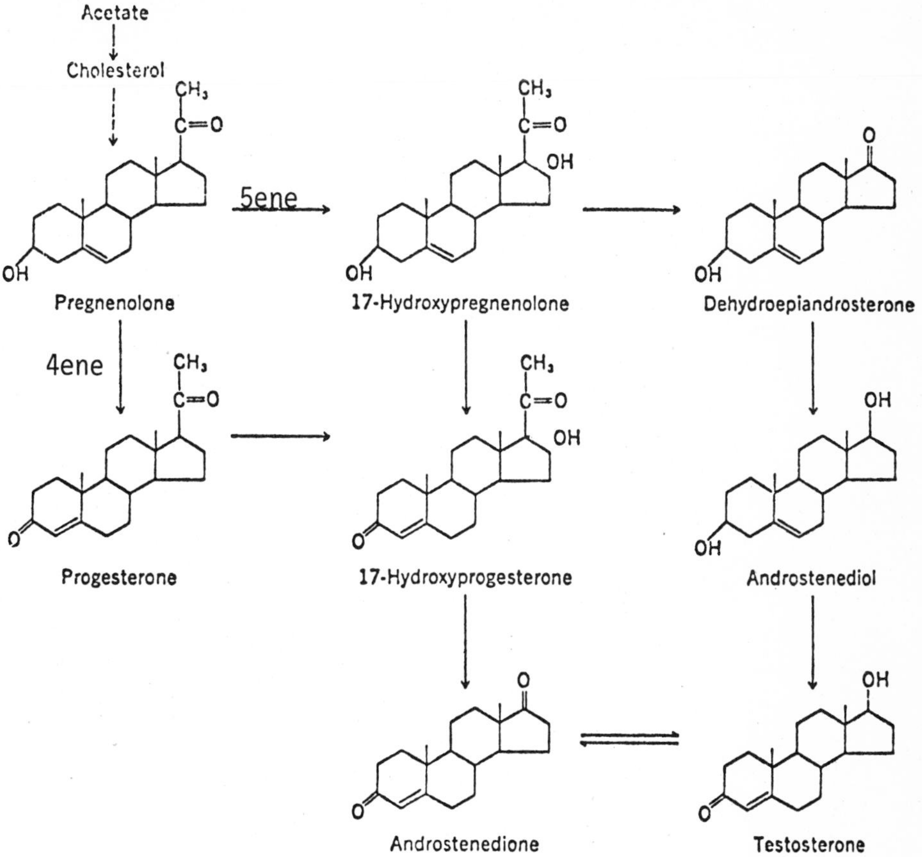

FIGURE 6-2: Androgen biosynthetic pathways in the interstitial cells of Leydig.

are involved in the biosynthesis of testosterone by the interstitial cells of Leydig. As described earlier in Section 5-3, the adrenal cortex can also synthesize androstenedione and testosterone in addition to its major secretory product, cortisol. (*Q. 6-3*) *Why are the interstitial cells of the testis unable to produce cortisol in addition to their major secretory product, testosterone?* (*Q. 6-4*) *Do the same cells in the adrenal cortex produce both cortisol and androstenedione?*

B. SECRETION, TRANSPORT IN BLOOD, AND PROTEIN BINDING OF TESTOSTERONE

Following its synthesis, testosterone is not stored in the testis but is secreted rapidly into the blood, where more than 97% of the circulating concentration of this hormone is bound to plasma proteins. As with the other steroid hormones, protein binding of testosterone serves several useful functions, including a) solubilizing the hydrophobic androgen for transport in an aqueous environment, b) protecting testosterone from catabolism and excretion by the liver and kidneys, and c) acting as a storage depot for testosterone. Testosterone bound to plasma proteins is in equilibrium with the free (i.e., unbound) testosterone. This small amount of free hormone (3%) is especially important

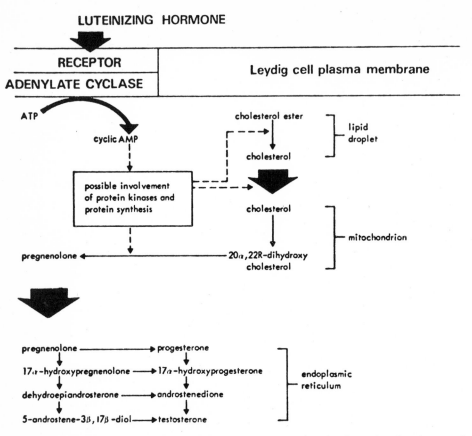

FIGURE 6-3: Biochemical actions of luteinizing hormone on, and subcellular distribution of, testosterone biosynthetic enzymes in the interstitial cells of Leydig. (*Source:* Cooke et al., 1973.)

because it is only the free hormone that can enter target cells and induce a biologic response (see Figure 5-11).

Testosterone is bound to three principal proteins: albumin (approximately 40% of the total bound), transcortin (approximately 2% of the total bound), and testosterone binding globulin (TeBG) (approximately 56% of the total bound). All three proteins are synthesized primarily in the liver. Although albumin has a low hormone specificity and binding affinity, more testosterone is bound to it than might be expected because it is the protein in highest concentration in the blood. Transcortin is used primarily by glucocorticoids for their transport in blood (see Section 5-4). It has a lower total capacity, but a slightly higher affinity for androgens than albumin. TeBG has a relatively high affinity and capacity for androgens. Estradiol (the principal estrogen in women, see Section 7-3) is also bound to TeBG, as is dihydrotestosterone, the active metabolite of testosterone in many target tissues (see below). The binding affinity of TeBG for estradiol is 75% of that for testosterone, whereas the binding affinity of TeBG for dihydrotestosterone is 200% of that for testosterone. However, since both estradiol and dihydrotestosterone concentrations are very low in the blood of normal human males, they do not represent a significant challenge for the binding of testosterone to TeBG.

TABLE 6-1: Alterations in TeBG Binding Capacity, Total Plasma Testosterone, and Free Plasma Testosterone

Age	Total TeBG Binding Capacity	Total Testosterone	Free Testosterone
Newborn	Low in both males and females	Males much greater than females	Males much greater than females ($5\times$)
Birth to 6 months	Increases in both males and females	Males much greater than females	Males much greater than females ($10\times$)
6 months to puberty	No change in both males and females	Decrease in males and no change in females	Decrease in males to a level equal to females
Puberty	Large decrease in males and small decrease in females	Large increase in males and no change in females	Very large increase in males and small increase in females
40–50 years and older	Variable increase in males and variable decrease or no change in females	Variable decrease in males and variable changes in females	Large decrease in males and variable changes in females

As shown in Table 6-1, the total binding capacity of TeBG changes during aging. An increase in TeBG concentration in plasma may occur in males in the age range 40–50 years compared with that observed in males at puberty. Since total testosterone concentration generally decreases in these middle-aged men, the free testosterone concentration of plasma may be reduced markedly. After perusal of Table 6-1, it should be clear that changes in total plasma binding capacity resulting from changes in plasma concentration of TeBG contribute to the overall regulation of androgenic activity. (Q. 6-5) *Assuming that the concentrations of the other two transport proteins remain constant, why do you think small changes in the plasma concentration of TeBG should have such important effects on plasma free testosterone concentration?* TeBG concentrations can also be altered by the administration of certain drugs, exogenous androgens, liver disease, and a variety of other natural and pathologic factors. (Q. 6-6) *Noting that ingestion of anabolic steroids may lead to a depression in the total binding capacity of plasma TeBG, what effect would you predict this to have on the virilizing potency of circulating androgens?* Diabetes mellitus in males may depress both TeBG and total testosterone concentrations in plasma, whereas the opposite situation may result during pregnancy in women. (Q. 6-7) *What effects might these alterations have on the concentration of free testosterone in plasma?* The actual hormonal regulation of total TeBG binding capacity is complex and not well understood. However, there does appear to be an inverse correlation between total TeBG binding capacity for testosterone and its metabolic clearance rate (MCR) (i.e., the rate of disappearance of testosterone from the plasma).

C. CATABOLISM AND METABOLIC CLEARANCE OF ANDROGENS

While the testis, adrenal cortex, and ovaries are involved primarily in steroid biosynthesis and secretion, the liver and kidney are involved primarily in steroid catabolism and excretion. Assuming negligible storage, the circulating plasma level of testosterone, and all other hormones, represents a balance between these two opposing metabolic processes. As might be expected, diseases that alter the capability of either the liver or kidneys to perform their catabolic functions will also alter the effective concentrations of biologically active steroids in the blood. The basic action of enzymes of the liver and kidneys is to reduce the double bonds in ring A of the steroid nucleus and to introduce hydroxyl groups, which can then serve as the loci for further introduction of hydrophilic groups, such as glucuronides. As a consequence, the steroids are rendered soluble in plasma and can then be excreted from the body into urine and feces. In man the principal urinary products of the metabolism of testosterone are the glucuronide conjugates of 5α- and 5β-androstanediol, which are in turn derived from 5α- and 5β-dihydrotestosterone (see Figure 6-10). Androstenedione, which is both a metabolite and precursor of testosterone, is excreted primarily as androsterone and etiocholanolone or as their sulfates (see Figures 5-10 and 6-2).

D. ACTIONS OF TESTOSTERONE IN TARGET TISSUES OTHER THAN BRAIN AND PITUITARY

You will recall from an earlier discussion in Chapter 5 on the adrenal cortical hormones that steroids cross cell membranes and exert their molecular actions primarily through high-affinity interactions with macromolecular protein receptors in target cell cytoplasm (and nucleoplasm). (Q. 6-8) *Why do naturally occurring steroids have so little difficulty crossing cell membranes?* The steroid-receptor complex then undergoes a still poorly understood activation process that facilitates the association of the mobile complex with nuclear chromatin. Activation of the complex formed by a receptor and testosterone (and dihydrotestosterone; see below) does not appear to involve any major changes in the size of the complex (as might occur following aggregation of the complex with other macromolecules), but there may be a change in conformation. The interaction of the steroid-receptor complex with its nuclear chromatin acceptors may lead to the increased synthesis of specific mRNA species coding for proteins involved in numerous essential cellular functions (e.g., androgen binding protein synthesized in the Sertoli cells; see Section 6-3). The details of the genomic process, together with the synthesis, activation, recycling, and degradation (or processing) of the receptors, are beyond the scope of this chapter.

Recent evidence has shown that the genetic locus of the mobile receptor for testosterone (i.e., the Tfm locus) is found on the X chromosome in humans. Mutations at this site lead to the situation known as testicular feminization. This genetic defect manifests itself as a phenotypic female with a genotypic XY male chromosomal pattern. Such individuals lack functional androgen receptors, hence do not display the typical masculine somatic and behavioral characteristics elicited by testosterone and its physiologically active metabolite dihydrotestosterone. (Q. 6-9) *Would you expect them to respond to estrogens?* The 5α-reduction of testosterone to dihydrotestosterone in target tissues appears to be essential for the elicitation of some, but not all, of the physiologic activity of testosterone (see Figure 6-10). Thus, the growth of the external genitalia at puberty is a testosterone-dependent process, whereas the growth and secretory capabilities of the internal sex accessory tissues such as the seminal vesicles and prostate utilize dihydrotestosterone and its 3α-hydroxylated metabolite. Lowering of the voice and the masculine pattern of development of skeletal muscle, and possibly libido, appear to be dependent on testosterone; acne, body and facial hair, and the recession of the scalp hairline appear to be dependent on dihydrotestosterone. A small population of people with a defective 5α-reductase enzyme resulting from a genetic mutation has been described recently. (Q. 6-10) *Would you expect XY genotypes with this mutation to be phenotypically male or female?*

SECTION 6-2: POST-TEST QUESTIONS

1. Steroid hormones are a. _____ -philic and b. _____ -phobic.
2. The principal control step in androgen biosynthesis is the conversion of a. _____ to b. _____.
3. Although the enzyme responsible for this initial metabolic step is located in the a. _____ fraction, the enzymes responsible for subsequent steps in testosterone biosynthesis are located in the b. _____ fraction.
4. Less than a. _____ % of the androgens in blood are in the free state, the rest are bound to one of the following three (source) b. _____ -synthesized proteins: c. _____, d. _____, and e. _____.
5. Name three functions or benefits of steroid-protein binding in blood plasma.
   a.
   b.
   c.
6. Alterations in the total binding capacity of plasma a. (name the carrier protein) _____ help regulate the concentrations of the active b. (free/bound) form of the hormone. For example, at puberty c. _____ concentration in males decreases, total testosterone concentration d. _____, thus producing e. (no change/increased/decrease) blood concentrations of f. (free/bound) testosterone.
7. The 5α-reduction of testosterone to a. _____ produces an extremely potent metabolite that appears to be required for the elicitation of certain androgenic actions in somatic target tissues such as the b. _____, whereas in other tissues such as the c. _____, testosterone appear to be the active androgen.
8. The a. _____ and b. _____ are the principal organs involved in androgen catabolism. Testosterone metabolities are excreted primarily as c. _____ conjugates.

SECTION 6-2: POST-TEST ANSWERS

1. a. lipo-
   b. hydro-
2. a. cholesterol
   b. pregnenolone
3. a. mitochondrial
   b. microsomal (or smooth endoplasmic reticulum)
4. a. 3
   b. liver
   c. albumin
   d. transcortin
   e. TeBG
5. a. Solubilization of steroids in plasma
   b. Protection of steroids from catabolism
   c. Storage of steroids for later utilization
6. a. TeBG
   b. free
   c. TeBG
   d. increases
   e. increased
   f. free

7. a. dihydrotestosterone
   b. seminal vesicles [other examples possible]
   c. striated muscle
8. a. liver
   b. kidney
   c. glucuronide (sulfate conjugates for androstenedione catabolites)

SECTION 6-3: GONADOTROPINS

OBJECTIVES:

The student should be able to:
   1. Describe the basic structural features, mode of synthesis, storage, release and blood-borne transport of the gonadotropins.
   2. Describe the metabolic clearance and pleomorphism of gonadotropins.
   3. Describe the effects of gonadotropic stimulation on testicular steroidogenesis.
   4. Describe the endocrine control of spermatogenesis.

A. STRUCTURE OF THE GONADOTROPINS

The gonadotropins, luteinizing hormone (LH) [also called interstitial cell stimulating hormone (ICSH)], and follicle stimulating hormone (FSH), are adenohypophyseal glyco-proteins similar structurally to thyroid stimulating hormone (TSH). Like TSH, each of the gonadotropins is composed of two peptide chains, α and β. In humans the 89 amino acids in the α-chains of LH, FSH, and TSH are all in the same sequence. The α-chain of human chorionic gonadotropin (hCG) (a hormone produced by the placenta during pregnancy; see Section 7-4) is also very similar to that of these hormones, differing from them only by the addition of three new amino acids to the N-terminal. Hence, it seems reasonable to conclude that differences in the amino acid sequences of the β-chains of LH, FSH, and TSH must be responsible for the biologic specificity and potency of these double-chained peptide hormones. Nevertheless there is considerable similarity be-tween the β-chains as illustrated by the fact that 41 of the 115 amino acids in β-LH and β-FSH are in the same sequence. The same similarity holds for TSH, clearly suggesting that the evolutionary origins of these three adenohypophyseal hormones are probably very similar. *(Q. 6-11) What effect would you predict this basic structural similarity of LH, FSH, and THS (and hCG) to have on the difficulty of development and specificity of radioimmunoassays for these hormones?* In the laboratory it is possible to separate and recombine (homo- and heterotypically) the α- and β-chains of LH, FSH, and TSH. *(Q. 6-12) Would you predict dimers composed of α-LH/β-FSH to produce physiologic re-sponses similar to dimers composed of α-LH/β-LH? (Q. 6-13) What predominant physio-logic effect would you expect from dimers composed of α-FSH/β-LH, α-FSH/β-TSH, and α-TSH/β-FSH?*

   The adenohypophyseal hormone prolactin (Prl) has also been shown to have tropic actions on the male gonad. Since much more is known about the actions of this hormone in females than in males, discussions of the structural chemistry, synthesis, regulation, and molecular mechanisms of actions are delayed until Chapter 7. However, the potential physiologic actions of Prl in the male are covered briefly here.

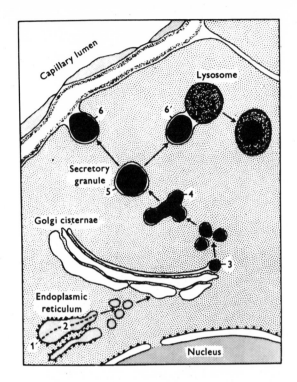

FIGURE 6-4: Synthesis (1 and 2), packaging (3), storage (4–5), lysosomal destruction (6'), and exocytotic release (6) of adenohypophyseal protein hormones; RER designates rough endoplasmic reticulum. (*Source:* Farquhar, 1971.)

B. SYNTHESIS, STORAGE, AND RELEASE OF GONADOTROPINS

The synthesis of the gonadotropins occurs on the rough endoplasmic reticulum of the gonadotropes of the anterior pituitary gland via traditional protein synthetic mechanisms. It is still unclear whether there is only one type of gonadotrope that synthesizes both LH and FSH or whether there is one type of gonadotrope for each hormone. The bulk of the evidence appears to support the former scheme, but the close similarity of the molecular structures of LH and FSH makes the definitive resolution of this problem very difficult. Following their synthesis on the endoplasmic reticulum, LH and FSH are packaged by the Golgi apparatus into microvesicles, which then combine into larger vesicles for storage within the cell, release from the cell via exocytosis, or destruction within the cell by lysosomal enzymes (see Figure 6-4).

C. TRANSPORT, METABOLIC CLEARANCE, AND PLEOMORPHISM

The metabolic clearance rate of gonadotropins in plasma is variable and appears to be at least partially under the control of gonadal steroid hormones. The variability of the MCR is thought to be mediated primarily through changes in the structure of the carbohydrate portions of the glycoproteins before packaging into microvesicles, an alteration referred to as pleomorphism. For example, by means of molecular sieving (a column chromatographic technique that separates molecules based on their size and shape), it was shown that the gonadotropins from female rhesus monkeys behaved as though they were larger than those from males, although the amino acid sequence is the same for both sexes. Gonadectomy increased the apparent size of gonadotropins in both sexes, an effect reversed by administration of exogenous gonadal steroids. Since treatment with the enzyme neuraminidase reduces the apparent size of both LH and FSH from castrated monkeys to the same degree as did treatment with either endogenous or exogenous gonadal steroids, it has been suggested that these gonadal steroids elicit their pleomorphic effects on the gonadotropins by altering the number of sialic acid residues attached to the biologically active protein moiety.

Although TSH also has sialic acid residues susceptible to treatment with neuraminidase, there is no effect on the apparent molecular size of this glycoprotein hormone with castration and/or gonadal hormone replacement. Thus, gonadal hormone-induced pleomorphism appears to be restricted to the gonadotropins. When gonadotropins from male and female rhesus monkeys were injected into rats, it was noted that the hormones from gonadectomized animals (i.e., those with a higher apparent molecular weight) had a longer half-life, and thus biopotency, than those from gonadally intact monkeys. Therefore, pleomorphism may be important to the overall regulation of the biologic actions of gonadotropins. (Q. 6-14) *Would you expect these changes in the MCR and biopotency of gonadotropins to be important in the feedback regulation of testicular steroidogenesis?*

D. ACTIONS OF GONADOTROPINS ON TESTICULAR STEROIDOGENESIS

As described earlier, the controlling step in androgen biosynthesis by the interstitial cells of Leydig is the conversion of cholesterol to pregnenolone (see Figure 6-3). Recent studies have shown that the membranes of Leydig cells contain specific macromolecular protein receptors for LH. The number of these receptors is probaby not a limiting factor for steroidogenesis, since they appear to be nonsaturable within the range of the normal circulating concentrations of LH. Thus regulation of the rate of steroidogenesis does not appear to involve a modulation of the number of LH receptors. In Leydig cells LH stimulates an increase in the activity of the adenylate cyclase enzyme, which is subsequently reflected in increases in both AMP concentration and AMP-dependent protein kinase activity. By a mechanism that is not completely understood, this metabolic sequence culminates in an increase in the synthesis of pregnenolone within 5 minutes. LH also stimulates protein synthesis in the interstitial cells of Leydig, but the time course for this stimulation (approximately 2 hours) is too long for these proteins to be involved in the initial steps of steroidogenesis. However, they may be involved in the maintenance of steroidogenesis. This contention is supported by the observation that inhibitors of RNA and protein synthesis can block the steroidogenic actions of LH in the testis. (Q. 6-15) *How would you expect the phosphodiesterase inhibitors theophylline and caffeine to affect LH-stimulated steroidogenesis?*

Recent studies with rats have shown that FSH can stimulate the aromatization of testosterone to estradiol in the testicular Sertoli cells (see Figures 6-5 and 6-6). The estrogen then appears to diffuse to the adjacent interstitial cells of Leydig, where it can reduce testosterone biosynthesis by a mechanism as yet unknown. Cytoplasmic macromolecular protein receptors for estradiol have been found in Leydig, but not in Sertoli cells. Whether these receptors are involved in the estradiol-testosterone intratesticular negative feedback loop is unknown. Sertoli cells cannot synthesize testosterone from cholesterol because they lack the mitochondrial side-chain cleaving enzymes required for pregnenolone biosynthesis. The presence of testosterone in Sertoli cells occurs as a result of diffusion from the interstitial cells of Leydig.

Research in a variety of species has suggested that Prl may enchance LH-stimulated steroidogenesis by the interstitial cells of Leydig in the testis. The mechanism responsible for this effect appears to involve an increase in either the number or the responsiveness of LH receptors on the Leydig cells. The likelihood that these effects are indirect is supported by the observation that Prl may also enhance secretion of FSH by the

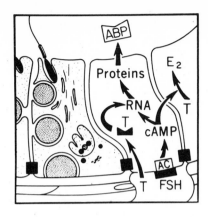

FIGURE 6-5: Actions of testosterone (T) and FSH in the testicular Sertoli cells. ABP = androgen binding protein, AC = adenylate cyclase, E_2 = estradiol. (*Source:* Means et al., 1976.)

anterior pituitary gland. This, in turn, may facilitate steroidogenesis via an effect on the LH receptors of the interstitial cells of Leydig.

E. ENDOCRINE CONTROL OF SPERMATOGENESIS

The process of spermatogenesis within the seminiferous tubules, as well as sperm maturation within the epididymis, involves the interaction of a variety of hormones. The cytologic changes in the sperm cell associated with spermatogenesis are reviewed in Figure 6-6. Although it frequently is stated that the primary action of FSH in males is the stimulation of spermatogenesis, recent studies have shown that the obligatory involvement of FSH is only transitory. It appears to be necessary only for the initial wave of spermatogenesis during pubertal development and not required for the maintenance of spermatogenesis in adulthood. By contrast, testosterone is required throughout life for the continuation of spermatogenesis through the first meiotic division (i.e., primary spermatocyte $\rightarrow$ secondary spermatocyte). Although the actions of androgens are required for spermatogenesis, their effects do not appear to be mediated directly on the developing germ cells (which lack high-affinity cytoplasmic receptors for androgenic steroids); rather, they appear to be mediated in the Sertoli cells (which possess these receptors). (*Q. 6-16*) *Can you think of any reasons for the unlikelihood of finding androgen receptors in haploid spermatids?*

One of the primary effects of both testosterone and FSH on the Sertoli cells is the stimulation of the de novo synthesis of androgen binding protein (ABP) (see Figure 6-5). Although representing only a small fraction of the total chemical composition of the Sertoli-synthesized fluids found in seminiferous tubules, ABP is nevertheless essential for the completion of spermatogenesis. In humans, the chemical composition of ABP appears to be identical to that of TeBG found in blood plasma and synthesized by the liver. As with TeBG and other carrier proteins, the binding of testosterone to ABP has a relatively short half-life (approximately 6 minutes) when compared with its binding to the high-affinity cytoplasmic receptors for testosterone found in Sertoli cells and other target tissues (i.e., $t_{1/2} > 1$ day). Thus ABP acts as a transport protein for testosterone both in the Sertoli cell and following its release into the rete $\rightarrow$ epididymal fluid system (see Figures 6-1 and 6-12). High concentrations of ABP and testosterone are found in the epididymis, where the action of testosterone is required for maturation of sperm. Again testosterone does not act directly on the sperm, but through the high-affinity receptors in the cytoplasm and nucleoplasm of the epididymal cells. These cells are thought to produce nutrients and other factors essential for final maturation of the sperm. The

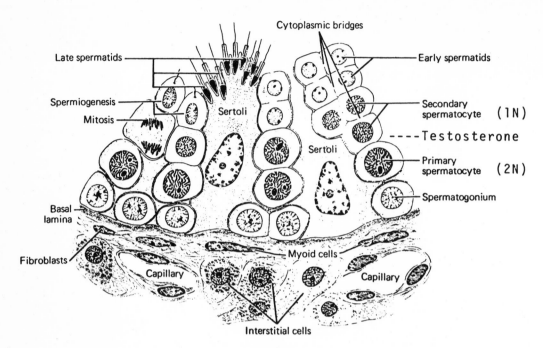

FIGURE 6-6: Diagram of the testis illustrating the cytological changes during spermatogenesis. In man, this process requires approximately 64 days to transform a spermatogonium into a mature spermatid. An additional month may pass before these sperm are ejaculated. (*Adapted from:* Junqueira and Carneiro, 1980.)

genomic actions of testosterone in the epididymal cells are required for the continued production of these nutritive and maturation stimulating factors.

As stated above, de novo biosynthesis of ABP within the Sertoli cells is stimulated by both testosterone and FSH. The action of testosterone in the Sertoli cells is mediated by the classical mobile receptors through genomic mechanisms (see Figure 5-9), whereas the action of FSH is mediated by the classical fixed membrane receptors through the cyclic AMP–protein kinase mechanism (see Figure 6-3). Inhibitors of the synthesis of protein and RNA block the synthesis of ABP stimulated by either testosterone or FSH. The elevation of AMP in response to the action of FSH on Sertoli cells appears to be mediated both by a facilitation of adenylate cyclase and by an inhibition of phospho-diesterase enzymes.

SECTION 6-3: POST-TEST QUESTIONS

1. LH, FSH, and TSH are all a. _____ -proteins, each containing b. _____
_____ peptide chains. The c. _____ chains of these adenohypophyseal hormones all have the same amino acid sequence, while the differences among the d. _____ chains confers the biologic e. _____ to the hormones.

2. Within the gonadotropes of the adenohypophysis, LH and FSH synthesis occurs in the a. _____, packaging into b. _____ occurs in the c. _____, and hormone release at the plasma membrane occurs via d. _____.

3. Steroid hormone-induced changes in the a. _____ acid content of the b. _____ portion of the gonadotropin results in an alteration in their plasma half-life and c. _____ potency. These alterations in molecular composition are referred to as d. _____.

4. Testosterone steroidogenesis in the a. _____ cells of b. _____ is stimulated via the interaction of c. _____ hormone with d. (where or type) _____ receptors resulting in an increase in the activity of the enzyme e. _____, which produces f. (not pregnenolone) _____. This compound is required for the activity of the enzyme g. _____, which phosphorylates proteins whose action is to increase the conversion of cholesterol to h. _____ via the enzyme i. _____.

5. Although both testosterone and FSH have obligatory actions in spermatogenesis, the actions of the a. (former/latter) hormone appears to be required only during the first wave of sperm production during pubertal development. Both these hormones stimulate the de novo synthesis of b. _____ protein within the c. _____ cells. The apparent principal function of this protein is to act as a d. _____ of e. _____ within the f. _____ cells and in the g. _____ fluids.

6. Without testosterone, spermatogenesis is arrested at the a. _____ and sperm already in the b. _____ fail to undergo final maturation.

SECTION 6-3: POST-TEST ANSWERS

1. a. glyco
   b. two
   c. alpha
   d. beta
   e. specificity (or potency)
2. a. rough endoplasmic reticulum
   b. microvesicles
   c. Golgi apparatus
   d. exocytosis
3. a. sialic
   b. carbohydrate
   c. biologic (but not immunologic assay)
   d. pleomorphism
4. a. interstitial
   b. Leydig
   c. luteinizing
   d. membrane (or fixed)
   e. adenylate cyclase
   f. cAMP
   g. protein kinase
   h. pregnenolone
   i. desmolase (cholesterol side-chain cleaving enzyme)
5. a. latter
   b. androgen binding
   c. Sertoli
   d. carrier

     e. testosterone

     f. Sertoli

     g. epididymal (and seminiferous tubule)

6. a. first meiotic division

     b. epididymis

SECTION 6-4: HYPOTHALAMIC HYPOPHYSIOTROPIC HORMONES

OBJECTIVES:

The student should be able to:

1. Describe the chemical composition, biosynthesis, storage, intracellular transport, release, transport in blood, and catabolism of LH-RH (Gn-RH).
2. Describe the actions of LH-RH (Gn-RH) in controlling the secretion of gonadotropins in males.

Luteinizing hormone releasing hormone (LH-RH) is a decapeptide (see Figure 6-7) produced in the hypothalamus of the brain by normal protein synthetic mechanisms. LH-RH synthesis occurs in small (i.e., parvicellular) neurons located primarily in the regions of the arcuate nucleus and median eminence, as well as the preoptic nucleus and organum vasculosum of the lamina terminalis (OVLT). LH-RH-containing neurons have also been detected in septal and retromammillary-rostral mesencephalic brain regions (see Figure 6-8). Following synthesis within the neuronal cell body, LH-RH is packaged into vesicles by the Golgi apparatus, transported by an energy-dependent mechanism down the axon to the synaptic region, where it is stored pending depolarization-induced exocytotic release into the perivascular space (e.g., infundibular "portal" vessels), into the periventricular space (e.g., ventral third ventricle), or into the synaptic cleft adjacent to a postsynaptic receptor of another neuron. LH-RH reaching the gonadotropes in the adenohypophysis via either the direct neural → "portal" vessel → gonadotrope route or the indirect neural → ventricle → tanycyte "portal" vessel → gonadotrope route (see Section 2-2 for further discussion of these systems) can stimulate the synthesis and release of both LH and FSH. The fact that both gonadotropes are released by LH-RH (although release of LH usually exceeds that of FSH), combined with the failure to demonstrate a unique compound capable of stimulating only FSH synthesis and release, has led a number of investigators to question the uniqueness of FSH-RH and to suggest the LH-RH ought to be called gonadotropin releasing hormone (Gn-RH). This suggestion is followed throughout the remainder of this chapter.

    Adenohypophyseal gonadotropes possess high-affinity, plasma membrane-associated receptors for Gn-RH. Binding of Gn-RH to these receptors results in a rapid influx of Ca^{2+} from extracellular fluids (which can be detected using either electrophysiologic or biochemical techniques) leading to an increase in the secretion of preformed gonadotropins via the exocytotic mechanisms described previously (see Section 2-3). The increase in synthesis of LH and FSH following exposure to Gn-RH is thought to involve the

FIGURE 6-7: Primary amino acid sequence of Gn-RH (LH-RH/FSH-RH).

pyroGLU-HIS-TRP-SER-TYR-GLY-LEU-ARG-PRO-GLY-NH$_2$

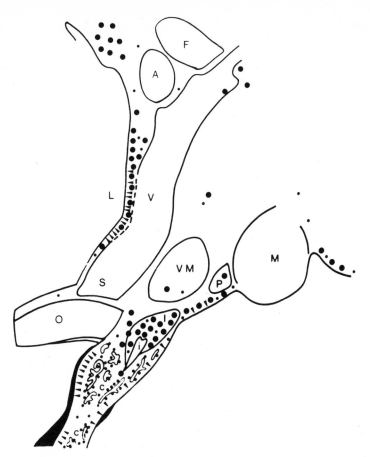

FIGURE 6-8: Sagittal view of the human hypothalamus illustrating the principal Gn-RH containing loci. O = optic chiasm, I = infundibulum, VM = ventromedial nucleus, P = posterior hypothalamus, M = mammillary body, S = septal area, L = lamina termmalis (OVLT), V = third ventricle, A = anterior commissure, F = fornix. (*Adapted from:* Barry, 1977.)

adenylate cyclase → cAMP → protein kinase → phosphorylated protein → protein synthesis mechanism of action discussed previously (see Section 1-3). The receptors for the latter response are probably similar to, or associated with, those involved in the increased mobilization of Ca^{2+}. The calcium ion and cAMP responses to Gn-RH may also relate to the observation that an intravenous infusion of Gn-RH in humans produces a rapid, but biphasic increase in the secretion of LH. The initial response may involve the mobilization of Ca^{2+}, whereas the secondary response may involve an increase in adenylate cyclase activity. The biphasic response to Gn-RH may also reflect the existence of two "pools" of LH within the gonadotropes—a readily releasable pool and a storage or synthesis pool.

Recent research with rodents has revealed hypothalamic enzymes capable of inactivating Gn-RH rapidly. The activity of these enzymes is sensitive to alterations in the concentrations of gonadal hormone in blood, suggesting an involvement of these enzymes in regulating the concentrations of active Gn-RH. Pituitary plasma cell membranes also possess Gn-RH peptidase activity.

Although the details of the mechanisms of action for Gn-RH are still not well understood, it is clear that the physiologic potency of synthetic analogues of Gn-RH correlate with their resistance to destruction by peptidase enzymes and/or with their binding affinity to receptors on the plasma membranes of gonadotropes. Some analogues are extremely potent, whereas others have no action or are capable of blocking the actions of native Gn-RH (*Q. 6-17*) *Does this suggest a possible application for contraception?*

SECTION 6-4: POST-TEST QUESTIONS

1. Gn-RH (LH-RH) contains a. _(how many?)_ amino acids. It is synthetized in neuronal b. (which subcellular region?) _____ in a variety of hypothalamic regions including the c. (give example) _____ .
2. Gn-RH is released via a. _____ from parvicellular nerve terminals into the b. _____ space, c. _____ space, or d. _____ _____ cleft.
3. A single Gn-RH has been suggested because LH-RH stimulates the synthesis and secretion of both a. _____ hormone and b. _____ _____ hormone and no definitive evidence for a unique c. _____ has been reported.
4. Gn-RH binds to a. _____-associated receptors and in doing so apparently stimulates b. _____, which leads to an increase in the secretion of preformed gonadotropins. An increase in the synthesis of gonadotropins following exposure to Gn-RH may require the activation of the c. _____ _____ mechanism.
5. Gn-RH can be inactivated by a. _____ enzymes found in the b. _____ _____ and c. _____.

SECTION 6-4: POST-TEST ANSWERS

1. a. 10
   b. cell bodies (or perikarya)
   c. arcuate-median eminence and preoptic-OVLT
2. a. exocytosis
   b. perivascular
   c. periventricular
   d. interneuronal synaptic
3. a. luteinizing
   b. follicle stimulating
   c. FSH-RH
4. a. membrane
   b. an increase in the influx of extracellular Ca^{2+}
   c. adenylate cyclase → cAMP → protein kinase → phosphorylated protein → protein synthesis
5. a. peptidase
   b. hypothalamus
   c. pituitary membranes

SECTION 6-5: HORMONE SECRETION PATTERNS AND FEEDBACK REGULATION

OBJECTIVES:

The student should be able to:
1. Describe the patterns of secretion of LH, FSH, and testosterone in men.
2. Describe the feedback regulation of secretion of LH, FSH, and testosterone in men.

A. HORMONE SECRETION PATTERNS

In *pubertal* boys there is a sleep-associated increase in the rate of secretion of LH that initiates a subsequent increase in the rate of secretion of testosterone (see Figure 6-9). If the time of onset of sleep is varied, the increases in the rate of secretion of LH and testosterone correlate with the new sleep patterns, not with the time of day. In *adult* males there are pulsatile patterns of secretion for LH and episodic patterns of secretion for testosterone throughout the day. These patterns are not well correlated. However, there are no consistent sleep-associated increases in the secretion of these hormones in *adults,* although there may be slightly more testosterone secreted during nighttime hours than during the day. An appreciation of the fact that the secretions of both LH and testosterone are pulsatile and episodic, respectively, is important both physiologically and clinically. (*Q. 6-18*) *Can basal concentrations of LH and testosterone be assessed using a single analysis of each?* (*Q. 6-19*) *Is the pulsatile secretion of LH reminiscent of another pituitary hormone that you have studied in an earlier chapter?*

B. FEEDBACK REGULATION

Immediately following castration in adulthood there is a rather dramatic and sustained increase in plasma concentrations of LH and FSH. The concentration of Gn-RH in peripheral blood has also been reported to rise after long-term castration, with even

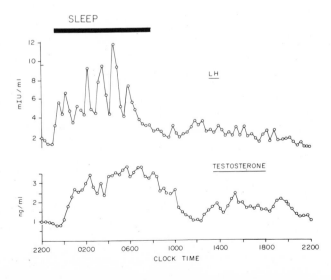

FIGURE 6-9: Plasma LH and testosterone for a 24-hour period in a 12-year-old normal pubertal boy. (*Adapted from:* Weitzman et al., 1975.)

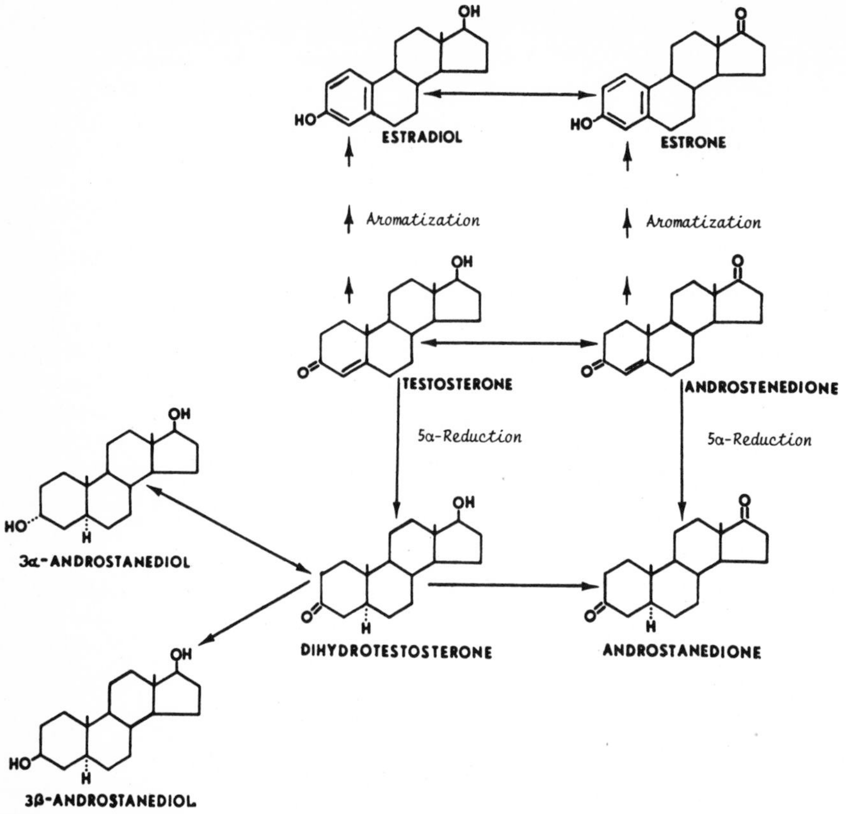

FIGURE 6-10: Schematic representation of androgen metabolism in neural, pituitary, and periph-eral target tissues. Note aromatization and 5α-reduction routes of metabolism. (*Adapted from:* Luttge et al., 1975.)

more dramatic increases occurring if hypophysectomy is also performed. (*Q. 6-20*) Why? Similar, albeit less dramatic, results can be obtained with other conditions that diminish the secretion of testicular hormones (and/or adenohypophyseal hormones in the case of Gn-RH secretion). Since the hypersecretion of LH and Gn-RH can be reversed to varying degrees by replacing the gonadal (and/or adenohypophyseal) hormones, this homeostatic control mechanism appears to represent yet another example of negative feedback similar to that described earlier for thyroid and adrenal cortical hormones. The regulatory effects of gonadal hormones on synthesis, secretion, and/or plasma concen-trations of LH, FSH, and Gn-RH occur by way of the long feedback loop, whereas the regulatory effects of gonadotropins on the synthesis and secretion of Gn-RH occur by way of the short feedback loop.

In adult males, infusion of either testosterone or estradiol at two times their respective endogenous production rates was found to reduce the serum concentration of LH similarly during infusion of the steroid and for several hours after infusion had ended. Since testosterone can be metabolized to an estrogen, the possibility existed that estro-gen was the hormone inhibiting LH secretion even during infusion of testosterone. However, since infusion of the testosterone metabolite dihydrotestosterone, which cannot readily be metabolized (i.e., aromatized) into an estrogen, produced similar overall reductions in serum LH, it is clear that aromatization is not required for testosterone-stimulated inhibition of LH secretion. Other studies in man have shown that circulating dihydrotestosterone probably does not play a major role in the negative feedback regulating gonadotropin secretion. Closer examinations have also revealed that there are subtle differences in the effectiveness of estrogens and androgens in the negative, long feedback loop in human males. For example, infusion of estradiol has been shown to reduce the amplitude, but not the frequency, of the spontaneous LH pulses that normally occur every 2 to 3 hours throughout the day. Infusion of testosterone decreased the frequency but had a slight facilitatory effect on the amplitude of the LH pulses.

In a recent study conducted with adult males rhesus monkeys, the frequency of LH pulses was found to increase from one every 2 to 3 hours in gonadally intact animals to one pulse every hour within 1 day after castration and to one pulse every half-hour by 4 days after castration. This increase in the frequency of LH pulsatile secretion following castration was reversible with exogenous administration of testosterone. In another recent study with adult male rhesus monkeys, the differential effectiveness of testosterone and estradiol on the feedback regulation of gonadotropin secretion following castration was examined in further detail (see Figure 6-11). The concentrations of LH and FSH in serum were maintained at precastration values, when the diurnal episodic secretory pattern and chronic concentrations of testosterone in blood were also maintained at precastration levels. Chronic concentrations of either testosterone or estradiol in blood were accomplished in castrated animals by the subcutaneous implantation of Silastic® rubber capsules containing these steroids. This capsule material allows a constant release of the hormone over relatively long periods of time. Episodic increases in the concentration of testosterone were achieved by bolus injections given systemically each evening. The effects of episodic changes in the concentration of estradiol on the concentrations of LH and FSH were not tested. Removal of the chronic estradiol replacement therapy while continuing the episodic and chronic testosterone therapy did not affect the concentrations of LH and FSH in serum, whereas the removal of both the episodic and chronic testosterone replacement therapy while continuing to administer estradiol via the Silastic® capsule, resulted in a substantial rise in the concentration of gonadotropins in circulation.

Taken together, these various results suggest that whereas physiologic levels of both testosterone and estradiol in blood can affect gonadotropin secretion in the male, they do so by different mechanisms (e.g., differential effects on gonadotropin pulse frequency and amplitude), and of the two hormones, circulating testosterone appears to be much more important than circulating estradiol in negative feedback regulation of gonadotropin secretion. These studies do not preclude the possibility that aromatization of testosterone to an estrogen within the hypothalamus and/or pituitary may also play a role in the negative feedback regulation of gonadotropins in man. This hypothesis is supported by the observation that administration of drugs that block aromatization in adult man greatly reduce, but do not totally block, the ability of exogenous testosterone to suppress the secretion of LH. (Q. 6-21) *In a gonadally intact adult man, what effect should the administration of pharmacologic doses of exogeneous estrogen have on circulating testosterone values? (Q. 6-22) Where is (are) the site(s) of action for this effect of estrogen?*

A wealth of data from laboratory animals suggests that the sites at which testosterone and its metabolites feed back to regulate the secretion of gonadotropins are located in both the hypothalamus and adenohypophysis. These sites contain intracellular macromolecular receptors and enzymes having affinity for testosterone and its metabolites. Additional studies have shown inhibition of secretion of LH, FSH, and/or Gn-RH following the administration of the hormone directly into these areas of brain in situ. Similar results were observed when testosterone was added to the media containing

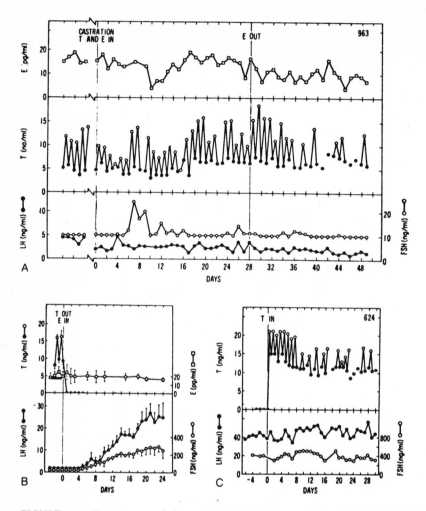

FIGURE 6-11: Time courses of plasma LH, FSH, testosterone (T), and estradiol (E) before and after bilateral castration and exogenous hormone replacement therapy [using chronic release hormone-containing Silastic® capsules supplemented with daily evening systemic bolus injections of testosterone] in an adult male rhesus monkey. a) T and E replacement therapies are initiated immediately after castration. After 28 days the E replacement was withdrawn while T was continued. Note that LH and FSH levels do not increase. b) T replacement was withdrawn while E was continued. In this case LH and FSH values begin to increase within days after loss of T-induced negative feedback. c) T replacement therapy was not initiated until 4.5 years after castration. Note that LH and FSH levels are much higher than in (a) and (b) and that these hyperphysiologic concentrations were not suppressed even though physiologic levels of T were restored. (*Source:* Plant et al., 1978.)

hypothalamic and adenohypophyseal tissues in vitro. In man, the concentration of testosterone in serum must be approximately 150% greater than normal for at least 28 days to reduce markedly the release of LH and FSH in response to the administration of Gn-RH. These findings indicate that testosterone (and/or its locally produced metabolites) can inhibit directly the actions of Gn-RH at the level of the adenohypophysis, but the high doses and prolonged treatment apparently required must be kept in mind when assessing the physiologic significance of these observations for man. It should also be recalled that long-term castration (especially when combined with hypophysectomy) can produce hyperphysiologic concentrations of Gn-RH in peripheral plasma, thus suggesting that reductions in the direct feedback actions of testosterone (and/or LH and FSH) in brain can precipitate a compensatory increase in Gn-RH synthesis and/or secretion. Chronic loss of endogenous androgen stimulation following long-term castration also reduces the responsiveness of the feedback mechanisms affecting secretion of gonadotropin by the hypothalamopituitary axis (i.e., inability to reduce LH and FSH hypersecretion with physiologic levels of testosterone) (see Figure 6-11c).

C. FEEDBACK REGULATION: POTENTIAL ROLE OF INHIBIN

Inhibin is the name given to a hydrophillic, nonsteroidal compound that reduces secretion of FSH, but not LH. Recent work suggests that it is a peptide having a molecular weight of approximately 20,000 daltons that can inhibit both the Gn-RH-stimulated FSH secretion at the level of the adenohypophysis and the FSH-stimulating potency of hypothalamic extracts (i.e., crude FSH-RH) at the level of the hypothalamus. Inhibin appears to be synthesized within the Sertoli cells, from which it can be secreted directly from the basal surface membrane into the lymph and blood supply and/or directly from the luminal surface membrane into the fluid of the rete testis (see Figure 6-12). (*Q. 6-23*) *Can you name another protein synthesized and secreted from the Sertoli*

FIGURE 6-12: The major fluid compartments and flow patterns in the testis. (*Source:* Waites, 1970.)

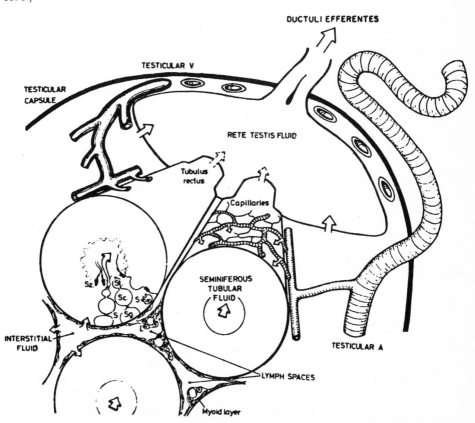

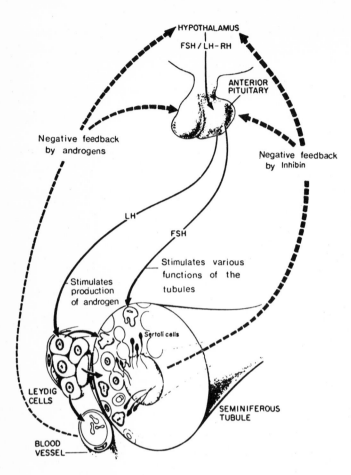

FIGURE 6-13: Summary representation of the interactions between testis, adenohypophysis, and hypothalamus. (*Adapted from:* Setchell et al., 1977; Bloom and Fawcett, 1975.)

cells? Inhibin is thought to be reabsorbed from these fluids in the epididymis by a mechanism similar to that utilized to reabsorb ABP. Presumably the inhibin is then secreted into the local blood supply, where it can be transported to the brain and adenohypophysis. Since active immunization against inhibin in laboratory animals can lead to an increase in FSH secretion without a concomitant increase in LH secretion, the evidence is clearly mounting that this peptide may play a significant role in the feedback regulation of FSH secretion (see Figure 6-13).

SECTION 6-5: POST-TEST QUESTIONS

1. In a. (age?) _____ , but not in b. (age?) _____ human males, there is a sleep-associated increase in c. _____ secretion, which in turn stimulates an increase in d. _____ secretion.
2. Testicular ischemia would probably produce an a. (increase/decrease) in the concentration of LH and FSH in serum, and a(n) b. (increase/decrease) in the concentrations of testosterone and estradiol in plasma. Episodic plus tonic replacement of physiologic levels of c. (steroid) _____ , but not d. (steroid) _____ , is required to maintain normal concentrations of gonadotropins in serum. This homeostatic mechanism is thus an example of a e. (negative/positive) feedback loop. The involvement

of the gonadal hormones indicates that this is a f. ___(long/short)___ feedback loop as contrasted with a g. ___(long/short)___ feedback loop when only the gonadotropins and Gn-RH are involved.

3. Neither LH nor testosterone displays a a. _____ secretory pattern, since plasma analyses reveal b. _____ increases in their concentrations under most standard physiologic conditions.

4. Testosterone and its metabolites influence LH secretion via their direct actions in both the a. _____ and the b. _____.

5. Compared to immediate postcastration replacement therapy, exogenous testosterone treatment following long-term castration is a. (more/less) effective in b. (increasing/decreasing) the concentrations of gonadotropins in serum.

6. A newly discovered peptide synthesized in the a. _____ cells has been shown to inhibit selectively the secretion of b. _____ via its actions in both the c. _____ and the d. _____. This nonsteroidal substance is called e. _____.

SECTION 6-5: POST-TEST ANSWERS

1. a. pubertal
   b. adult
   c. luteinizing hormone
   d. testosterone
2. a. increase
   b. decrease
   c. testosterone
   d. estradiol
   e. negative
   f. long
   g. short
3. a. constant (or nonfluctuating)
   b. pulsatile (or episodic)
4. a. hypothalamus
   b. adenohypophysis (anterior pituitary)
5. a. less
   b. decreasing
6. a. Sertoli
   b. follicle stimulating hormone
   c. hypothalamus
   d. adenohypophysis
   e. inhibin

SELECTED REFERENCES

Bardin, W., 1979, The neuroendocrinology of male reproduction, *Hospital Practice* 14: 65.

Burger, H. and De Krester, D. (Eds.), 1980, *The Testis,* New York: Raven Press.

Conn, P. M., Marian, J., McMillian, M., Stern, J., Rogers, D., Hanby, M., Penna, A., and Grant, E., 1981, Gonadotropin-releasing hormone action in the pituitary: a three step mechanism, *Endocrine Reviews* 2: 174.

Martin, J. B., Reichlin, S., and Brown, B. M., 1977, *Clinical Neuroendocrinology,* Philadelphia: F. A. Davis Co., Ch. 5, p. 93.

Preslock, J. P., 1980, Steroidogenesis in the mammalian testis, *Endocrine Reviews* 1: 132.

7

FEMALE REPRODUCTIVE ENDOCRINOLOGY

SECTION 7-1: ANATOMY OF THE FEMALE REPRODUCTIVE SYSTEM

OBJECTIVES:

The student should be able to:
1. Name the organs supported by the broad ligament.
2. Name the internal (primary) female reproductive organs.
3. Name the accessory (secondary) female reproductive organs.
4. State the functions of the internal (primary) and accessory (secondary) reproductive organs of the female.

The internal (primary) female reproductive organs are located in the pelvis and are supported or anchored by a series of ligaments, chief among which is the broad ligament. This ligament crosses the pelvic region in a coronal plane. Suspended in the midline is the uterus, with the Fallopian (uterine) tubes projecting laterally and attached to the broad ligament via the mesosalpinx. In juxtaposition to the distal end of the tubes are the ovaries, which are anchored via the mesovarium to the broad ligament (see Figure 7-1).

The almond-shaped ovaries are situated near the lateral walls of the pelvis; their exact position varies because of the mobility of their attachment and the effects of pregnancy. Structurally, each ovary consists of a medulla and a cortex surrounded by the dense connective tissue of the tunica albuginea, which is enveloped in turn by the germinal epithelium. Both the cortex and the medulla are contained in the germinal epithelium and tunica albuginea. Follicles are found in the cortex of the ovary, whereas blood vessels, nerves, and lymphatic vessels comprise the medulla. (*Q. 7-1*) *What other endocrine organ has a cortex and a medulla?*

The Fallopian tubes (oviducts) are the site of fertilization of the ovum by sperm cells and serve to transport the fertilized ovum from the ovary to the uterus. Fingerlike projections of the Fallopian tubes, the fimbriae, are in close proximity to the ovaries. Examination of the action of the fimbriae reveals that they sweep across the surface of the ovaries and thus aid in guiding each ovum into the Fallopian tubes. Fimbriae also project from the flared portion of the Fallopian tubes known as the infundibula. Beyond the infundibula, the tube narrows to form an ostium leading to the ampulla, a section that accounts for half the length of the tube. An isthmus forms the final extrauterine portion of the tube.

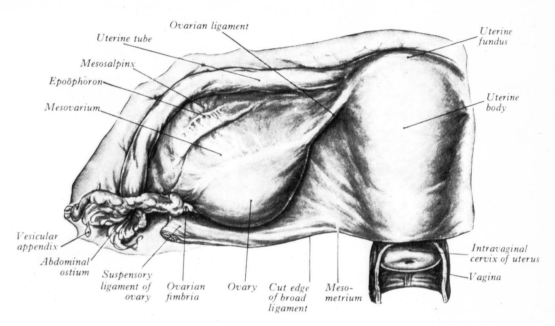

FIGURE 7-1: Various features of the internal organs of reproduction in the human female. (*Source:* Warwick and Williams, 1973).

The uterus is a hollow, thick-walled, muscular organ located in the pelvic midline posterior to the bladder and anterior to the rectum. It is composed of three major portions: fundus, body, and cervix. Superior to the entry point of the Fallopian tubes is the fundus. Inferior to this point the body extends to a slight constriction in the surface of the uterus. Caudal to this constriction is the cervix. The cervix enters the vagina at its upper portion and projects into the vagina for a short distance. The opening into the vagina is the external os. Normally the uterus is positioned at almost a right angle to the anterior surface of the vagina, changing position as the bladder distends or empties. The vagina is a tubular structure situated parallel to the pelvic outlet. Its external orifice is known as the introitus (not shown in Figure 7-1).

The main functions of the internal (primary) reproductive organs include the production of the female sex cells, the ova, and the secretion of estrogenic and progestational hormones that are important to the preparation of the uterus for the reception and development of the fertilized ovum. The internal reproductive organs also play an important role in the process of birth and in the expulsion of the fetus at the end of the gestation period.

The female accessory (secondary) reproductive organs include the mons pubis, the labia minora, the labia majora, the clitoris, the bulbis vestibuli, and the greater vestibular glands, which are located below the urogenital diaphragm and in front of, and below, the pubic arch. The labia form the external covering of the vaginal orifice. In general, the accessory (secondary) reproductive organs function to provide a repository for sperm cells and to aid their movement eventually to the Fallopian tubes, where fertilization of the ovum occurs. Sensory receptors are concentrated in the glans clitoris and serve there as the major source of sensory stimulation during coitus. Lubrication during coitus is provided in large part by the greater vestibular (Barthalin) glands, located beneath the labia minora.

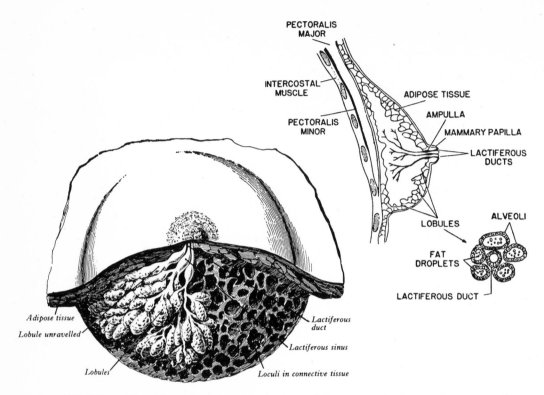

FIGURE 7-2: Frontal and lateral schematic views of the gross and microscopic anatomy of the human breast. (Source: Warwick and Williams, 1973; Jensen, 1980.)

The structure of the breasts is influenced by a variety of hormones, chief among which are estrogens and progesterone. However, the breasts cannot be classified as genital organs in the strictest sense. The breasts are composed of 15 to 20 lobes consisting of glandular, fibrous, and adipose tissue (see Figure 7-2). These components are supported, but not encapsulated, by strengthened subcutaneous tissue. Each lobe is drained by a lactiferous duct. Lobules are formed by the arborizations of the ducts and by the alveolar glands. These glands are the producers of milk, which is drained by the system of ducts to empty at the nipple through 15 to 20 separate openings. Tactile receptors in the breast are located mainly in the end portion of the nipple. The role of the various hormones of the female reproductive system on the development of the breast and the production of milk is discussed in greater detail in Section 7-4.

SECTION 7-1: POST-TEST QUESTIONS

1. Name the three main organs supported by the broad ligament.
   a.
   b.
   c.
2. Structurally each ovary consists of two layers called the a. _____ and b. _____. The layer in which follicles are located is the c. _____.

3. a. Why are the Fallopian tubes important?

   They contain fingerlike projections known as b. _____ .
   What is their function? c.

4. The site of fertilization of the ovum is the uterus. (True/False)
5. The main functions of the internal (primary) reproductive organs are the production
   of a. _____ and the secretion of b. _____ and c. _____
   _____ hormones that are important for d. _____
   _____ .
6. Name six accessory (secondary) reproductive organs in the human female.
   a.
   b.
   c.
   d.
   e.
   f.
7. Describe the three major functions of these accessory (secondary) reproductive
   organs.
   a.
   b.
   c.

SECTION 7-1: POST-TEST ANSWERS

1. a. Ovaries
   b. Uterus
   c. Fallopian tubes
2. a. cortex
   b. medulla
   c. cortex
3. a. They transport of the ovum from the ovary to the uterus.
   b. fimbriae
   c. To sweep the ovum expelled from the ovary into the Fallopian tubes.
4. False
5. a. ova (egg cells)
   b. estrogenic
   c. progestational
   d. the preparation of the uterus for the reception and development of the fertil-
      ized ovum
6. a. Mons pubis
   b. Labia minora
   c. Labia majora
   d. Bulbis vestibuli
   e. Greater vestibular glands
   f. Clitoris
7. a. To provide a repository for sperm cells.
   b. To aid the movement of sperm cells to the Fallopian tubes.
   c. To provide a source of sensory stimulation and lubrication during coitus.

SECTION 7-2: CYCLIC CHANGES IN THE HISTOLOGIC ANATOMY OF THE OVARIES AND UTERUS DURING THE MENSTRUAL CYCLE

OBJECTIVES:

The student should be able to:
1. Describe the development of a primordial germ cell into a mature Graafian follicle.
2. Describe the changes in the ovum occurring just before ovulation.
3. Describe the two phases of the menstrual cycle with respect to the ovaries.
4. Describe the four phases of the menstrual cycle with respect to the uterus.
5. Describe the changes occurring in the endometrium of the uterus that result in menstruation.

Cyclic changes are characteristic of the adult human female reproductive system. To understand their physiologic significance, it is important to describe in general terms the cyclic changes in the histologic anatomy of the ovary and uterus during the normal menstrual cycle.

A. OVARIAN HISTOLOGY DURING THE MENSTRUAL CYCLE

The development of the germ cell in the ovaries of the female (oogenesis) is quite different from spermatogenesis in the testis of the male. In the female, primordial germ cells develop into oogonia early in fetal life. After some mitoses during fetal life, all the oogonia become primary oocytes. They remain in this stage until puberty at 10 to 15 years of age. (*Q. 7-2) Does the production of primary spermatocytes in the male cease long before puberty?* In the fetus at 5 months of development, there are about 6,000,000 potential germ cells. Most of these degenerate, leaving only 700,000 to 2,000,000 potential germ cells at birth, and by puberty only 400,000 remain. Of these, only about 400 germ cells are ovulated during the reproductive life of a woman (i.e., about 0.1%). The remainder of the germ cells never fully mature and degenerate. (*Q. 7-3) Would you predict radiation damage to the gonads to produce a more lasting effect in women or men?*

The ovulatory cycle of the ovary is shown in Figure 7-3. The earliest follicle observed in the ovary is the primordial follicle, located in the periphery of the cortex. It is composed of a primary oocyte surrounded by a single layer of follicular cells. Primordial follicles are the source of the developing follicles.

At the beginning of each menstrual cycle, a number of primordial follicles undergo differentiation into primary follicles. The single layer of follicular cells divides, forming a stratified layer of granulosa cells that surround the primary oocyte. The primary oocyte obtains a thick mucopolysaccharide coat, the zona pellucida, which is secreted by the granulosa cells. Connective tissue surrounding the follicle then differentiates into a highly vascular, secretory theca interna and an outer connective tissue, the theca externa. The cells of the theca interna secrete estrogens in increasing amounts during the course of the maturation of the follicle (see Section 7-3).

As the follicle enlarges, it becomes a secondary or antral follicle. During the course of enlargement, the granulosa cells loosen and secrete a fluid (liquor folliculi), which fills the spaces between the cells. The spaces eventually coalesce to form a single, large fluid-filled cavity (antrum) in the center of the follicle. The fluid displaces the oocyte to the side of the follicle. The granulosa cells surrounding the primary oocyte proliferate and secrete a hyaluronic acid matrix that separates the cells to form a stalk (cumulus oophorus), which supports the primary oocyte and protrudes it into the antrum.

The final result of follicular maturation is a Graafian or mature follicle. As many as 20 follicles may begin to develop synchronously during each ovulatory cycle, but usually

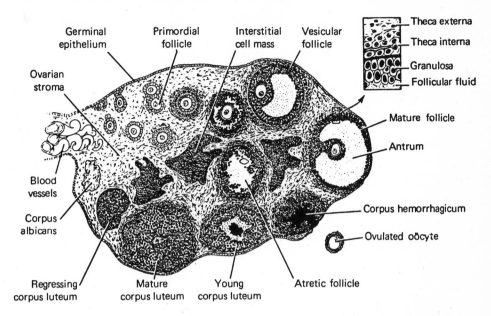

FIGURE 7-3: Diagram of an ovary illustrating the development and regression of the follicles, ovulation, and the development and regression of the corpus luteum. (*Source:* Gorbman and Bern, 1962.)

only a single follicle reaches final maturation. (*Q. 7-4*) *Can you think of an obvious exception to this generalization?* All other developing follicles degenerate, a process known as atresia. This degeneration can take place at any time during the entire developmental process, and atretic follicles are always present in the ovary (see Figure 7-3).

The Graafian follicle is about 10 to 15 mm in diameter and forms a bulge on the outer surface of the ovary. The time required for development from a primordial follicle to a mature Graafian follicle is about 14 days. This period forms the first half of the normal menstrual cycle and is called the follicular phase. (*Q. 7-5*) *How does the time required for oogenesis compare to that required for spermatogenesis?* Rupture of the Graafian follicle and ovulation occur not as a result of increasing pressure within the follicle but most likely as a result of several factors, including the increased production of certain proteolytic enzymes and prostaglandins in the follicle in response to increasing concentrations of FSH and LH in blood (see Section 7-4).

During fetal life, the primary oocyte enters prophase I (a phase of meiosis) and remains suspended in the diploid (i.e., 2N) stage until sometime just preceding ovulation, when the completion of the first meiotic division of the oocyte takes place. The resulting secondary oocyte contains a haploid (i.e., 1N) nucleus and almost all the cytoplasm of the primary oocyte, while the remaining cytoplasm and haploid nucleus are retained in a small polar body (polocyte). The secondary oocyte, surrounded by a layer of "sticky" cumulous cells, is released from the Graafian follicles at ovulation. This oocyte will not enter the second meiotic division unless it is fertilized, an event that usually takes place in the ampulla of the Fallopian tubes (see Figure 7-4). Without fertilization, the ovulated secondary oocyte will degenerate. Upon fertilization, but before fusion of the pronuclei of the two germ cells, the secondary oocyte will divide to form a large ootid and a second small polocyte, both of which have the haploid chromosome number. The first polocyte may also divide to form two more polocytes. All the polocytes eventually degenerate, leaving only one haploid ootid following

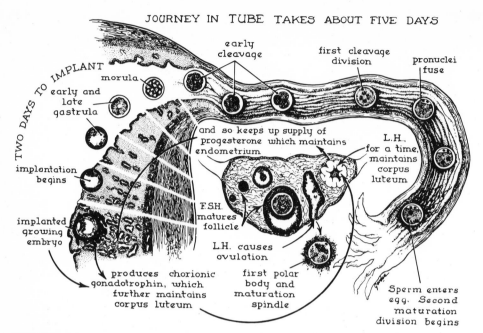

FIGURE 7-4: Hormonal control of follicular maturation, ovulation, development, and function of the corpus luteum, ovum transport, fertilization, meiotic and mitotic divisions, implantation, endometrial preparation, and hCG production and actions. (*Adapted from:* Cormack, 1979; Dickinson, 1933.)

meiosis of the primary oocyte. (*Q. 7-6) In the male, how many spermatids are produced following meiosis of the primary spermatocyte?* Fusion of the haploid pronucleus from the spermatid with the haploid pronucleus from the ootid forms the diploid zygote.

After ovulation, the Graafian follicle undergoes changes to form a corpus luteum (yellow body). The theca interna and granulosa cells of the Graafian follicle accumulate lipid and undergo other changes before transformation into lutein cells. These cells are the source of the second major ovarian hormone, progesterone. Connective tissue, including vascular elements, invade the corpus luteum, making it highly vascular. If pregnancy does not occur, the corpus luteum involutes and ceases to secrete progesterone (and estradiol) about 14 days after ovulation. The resulting connective tissue scar is known as the corpus albicans (white body). The second half of the menstrual cycle is thus referred to as the luteal phase.

B. UTERINE HISTOLOGY AND BLOOD SUPPLY DURING THE MENSTRUAL CYCLE

The uterus also undergoes cyclic changes during the course of the menstrual cycle. As you recall from Section 7-1, the uterus is divided into three portions: fundus, body, and cervix. The body constitutes the major portion of the uterus, and it is in this portion that implantation of the fertilized ovum occurs during pregnancy. When pregnancy does not occur, it is this portion of the uterus that is the source of the menstrual flow.

Histologically, the body of the uterus can be divided into three layers: perimetrium, myometrium, and endometrium. The outermost layer of tissue (perimetrium) is continuous with the rest of the abdominal serosa. Beneath this layer lies a thick muscular coat (myometrium) composed of interlacing smooth muscle bundles surrounded by connective tissue. The mucosa lining the uterus (endometrium) and resting on the myometrium is continuous with the mucosal lining of the Fallopian tubes and vagina. It is the endometrium that undergoes major cyclic changes in response to changes in the concentration of ovarian hormones in blood and is the source of the menstrual discharge. The endometrium also participates in the formation of the placenta during pregnancy (see Section 7-3).

Microscopic examination of the endometrium reveals that it consists of a single layer of columnar epithelium overlying a highly cellular connective tissue stroma and punctuated by many tubelike mucous glands, which are lined with ciliated cuboidal epithelium and are open to the uterine cavity and extend partially into the myometrium. The epithelial lining of the entire endometrium is ciliated before puberty, but after the onset of the periodic destruction of this layer during menstruation, this property of the mucosal lining is apparently lost over large areas of the endometrium. Usually the endometrium is divided into an outer "functional layer" and a deeper "basal layer," which is purported to be "the" source of regenerating endometrium following menstruation. However, recent histologic studies have shown that the human endometrium does not possess a unique epithelial cell population spared from desquamation during menstruation and specialized for the regeneration of the "functional" epithelium. Rather, the stromal and glandular cells remaining after menstruation appear to collapse or shrink to give the erroneous appearance of a separate basal layer. Further details on endometrial regeneration are given later in this section. There is no support for the notion that hyperplasia of stromal cells may participate in the reepithelization of the denuded mucosa.

The principal arterial supply of the uterus originates from the internal iliac arteries. The two uterine arteries that arise from this source anastomose along the surface of the uterus and send branches, called the anterior and posterior arcuate arteries, into the myometrium, where they divide and travel circumferentially around the uterus to anastomose across the midline with similar vessels from the opposite side. The arcuate arteries in turn send numerous radial branches to the deeper regions of the myometrium and adjacent regions of the endometrium. Spiral or helical arteriolar branches from the arcuate arteries nourish the more superficial regions of the endometrium adjacent to the uterine cavity. The spiral arteries proliferate in response to ovarian hormonal stimulation. This hormone-induced vascularization is especially evident during the secretory phase of the menstrual cycle, when the spiral arteries undergo a dramatic increase in length and diameter and become even more tortuous as their linear growth exceeds the rate of endometrial regeneration.

C. UTERINE HISTOLOGY DURING THE MENSTRUAL CYCLE

The menstrual cycle can be divided into four endometrial phases or two ovarian phases. (*Q. 7-7*) *What are the names and approximate lengths of the two ovarian phases?* Each phase is a coordination of the endometrial and ovarian events and is regulated by a complex pattern of endocrine events, discussed in greater detail in later sections of this chapter.

The four endometrial phases are studied most easily starting with the proliferative phase, which actually begins before the cessation of the previous menstrual flow (see Figure 7-5). The superficial areas of the endometrium are largely absent because of the desquamation and expulsion of necrotic tissues during menstrual discharge. The regeneration of the ulcerated mucosa begins within 36 hours after the initiation of menstrual hemmorrhage and may be complete within 140 hours. The mitotic proliferation starts from the edges of the remaining glandular stumps (i.e., the so-called basal layer) and continues until all desquamated portions of the endometrium (including blood clots and any fragments of decidual tissue; see below) are covered by newly regenerated epithelium. During this time the follicular phase within the ovary begins and is charac-

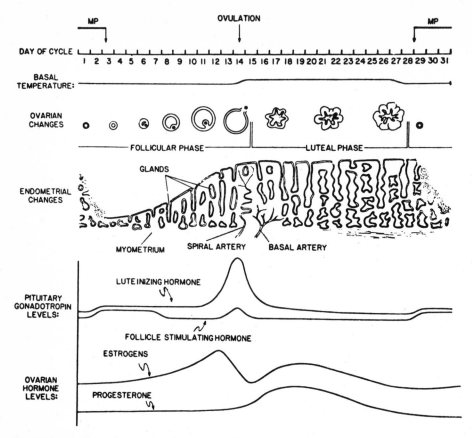

FIGURE 7-5: The endometrial and ovarian cycles and the relative concentrations of estradiol and progesterone in blood. The proliferative phase begins in the repair period and extends through the follicular phase. The secretory period begins after ovulation and extends through the luteal period. The ischemia of the hypertrophied endometrium initiates the onset of the menstrual period (MP). (*Source:* Jensen, 1980.)

terized by the development of numerous follicles and the increased secretion of estrogenic hormones into the follicular fluid and ovarian veins. Like the reepithelization of the endometrium, the development of the follicles also begins during the menstrual phase, but their more observable growth occurs during the last 9 days of the follicular-proliferative phase. This phase of endometrial development ends about 1 day after ovulation.

The secretory phase of the endometrial cycle begins at the same time as the onset of the luteal phase of the ovarian cycle and is characterized by the secretion of copious amounts of mucus from the endometrial glands. The production of mucus reaches a maximum approximately 6 days after ovulation. The comparatively straight tubular glands and spiral arteries that typify the proliferative phase become more tortuous and coiled during the secretory phase. Edema thickens the endometrium during the secretory phase even more than the hyperplasia during the preceding proliferative phase. The purpose of the secretory phase is to ready the uterus for possible implantation of the fertilized ovum. If implantation does not occur, the corpus luteum involutes and ceases its production of progesterone and estradiol (see Figure 7-5).

The loss of hormonal support from the corpus luteum precipitates the regression of the endometrium and the onset of the premenstrual or ischemic phase of the menstrual cycle. The spiral arteries are compressed, blood flow is slowed, and vasodilation is initiated as a consequence of the rapid regression of the endometrium. The spiral arteries then undergo vasoconstriction or spasm, apparently in response to the actions of locally produced prostaglandins, which are known to increase in concentration in the uterine blood during this period of ovarian steroid deprivation. These vascular responses render the superficial endometrium ischemic. The regression of the endometrium involves cellular dehydration, autophagocytosis by the lysosomal enzymes which digest portions of the cell's own cytoplasm, heterophagocytosis by the infiltrating macrophages which ingest cellular debris from the stroma and epithelium, and cellular destruction by powerful lytic enzymes released from lysosomes derived from fragmenting cells and leukocytes released from the ruptured blood vessels. These layers of necrotic cells (mucus epithelium, stromal spongiosum, and in some cases even the outer layers of the myometrium) and ruptured spiral artery fragments desquamate from the uterus.

It is important to note that cellular necrosis and desquamation is not uniform throughout the extent of the endometrium, and the amount of tissue lost appears to correlate with the degree of tortuosity and consequent compression of the spiral arteries (i.e., the more highly developed the arteries, the greater the extent of necrosis and desquamation). The cellular and vascular debris appears to aid in the stimulation of the characteristic menstrual contractions of the myometrium, which facilitate the expulsion of the necrotic material and blood from the uterus. The total fluid loss is variable, but is in the range of 50–70 ml, of which approximately 50% is blood and 50% uterine and cervical secretions. The menstrual fluid typically does not clot because of the presence of a proteolytic enzyme, fibrinolysin, which is released together with the necrotic tissue. After a menstrual phase lasting 3 to 6 days, the secretion of ovarian hormones begins to increase and the endometrial cycle repeats once more.

Cyclic changes in the cellular composition and secretory activity are also apparent in the Fallopian tubes, cervix, vaginal epithelium, and breast tissue. These cyclic changes are all linked to the cyclic changes in secretions of ovarian hormones and they are discussed further in Sections 7-3 and 7-4.

A complete menstrual cycle averages 28 days and ranges from about 22 to 36 days. It may vary considerably between females and from month to month in the same female. The first 5 to 7 years after menarche (i.e., onset of periodic menstruation and ovarian cyclicity at puberty) and the last 6 to 8 years before menopause (i.e., cessation of periodic menstruation and ovarian cyclicity during late middle age) are characterized by wide variability in cycle length as contrasted with the comparative regularity of the length of the menstrual cycle for women 20 to 40 years of age. In addition, there is a clear-cut decrease in the length of the menstrual cycle during these middle years. Although there are exceptions, the greatest variability in the length of the menstrual cycle results from differences in the duration of the follicular phase. It is important to note that day 1 of the cycle commonly is defined as the first day of menstrual flow.

SECTION 7-2: POST-TEST QUESTIONS

1. What part of the ovary contains the primordial germ cells?

2. Many primary oocytes remain in prophase I for 30 years or more. (True/False)
3. The growing follicles develop an antrum because a. _____ is produced by the b. _____ cells.
4. Follicles that are not "selected" to become fully mature or a. _____ follicles undergo b. _____ .
5. Just before ovulation the first a. _____ of the oocyte takes

place. The resulting b. _____ contains a c. ____(2N/1N)____ nucleus and almost all the d. (cytoplasm/nucleoplasm) of the e. _____ oocyte. The remaining cytoplasm and nucleus are found in a small f. _____ _____ .

6. The second meiotic division of the oocyte occurs only if a. _____ takes place. The b. ____(2N/1N)____ pronucleus of the resulting c. _____ fuses with the d. (diploid/haploid) pronucleus of the spermatid to form the e. _____. If fusion of the pronuclei does not occur, the oocyte will f. _____ .

7. After ovulation the Graafian follicle undergoes changes to form a a. _____ _____ , which eventually degenerates to form a b. _____ _____ if pregnancy is not initiated.

8. Where does fertilization usually occur?

9. The hormone secreted predominantly by the developing ovarian follicles is a. _____ , the hormones secreted by the corpus luteum are b. _____ _____ and c. _____ .

10. The uterus can be divided into three portions: a. _____ , b. _____ _____ , and c. _____ . Which of these portions forms the principal source for the material shed during menstruation? d. _____ In which portion does implantation occur? e. _____

11. The body of the uterus can be divided into three layers: a. _____ , b. _____ , and c. _____ . Which of these layers has the thick d. (smooth/striated) muscular coat? e. _____ Which of the layers is highly vascularized, contains many simple glands, and is shed during menstruation? f. _____

12. Follicular phase is to a. (proliferative/secretory) phase as luteal phase is to b. (proliferative/secretory) phase.

13. Day 1 of the menstrual cycle is commonly defined as _____ _____ .

14. Why does the endometrium undergo necrosis just before the initiation of the menstrual flow?

15. When does endometrial reepithelization begin?

16. Why doesn't the blood in the menstrual fluid clot readily?

SECTION 7-2: POST-TEST ANSWERS

1. Cortex
2. True
3. a. fluid
   b. granulosa
4. a. Graafian
   b. atresia (degeneration)
5. a. meiotic division

      b. secondary oocyte
      c. 1N
      d. cytoplasm
      e. primary
      f. polocyte
  6. a. fertilization
      b. 1N
      c. ootid
      d. haploid
      e. zygote
      f. degenerate
  7. a. corpus luteum
      b. corpus albicans
  8. In the ampulla of the Fallopian tubes.
  9. a. estradiol
      b. progesterone
      c. estradiol
10. a. fundus
      b. body
      c. cervix
      d. body
      e. body
11. a. perimetrium
      b. myometrium
      c. endometrium
      d. smooth
      e. myometrium
      f. endometrium
12. a. proliferative
      b. secretory
13. the first day of menstruation
14. The compressed spiral arteries constrict or spasm in response to locally produced prostaglandins. The resulting ischemia leads to tissue hypoxia and eventual necrosis.
15. As early as 36 hours after the onset of menstrual hemorrhaging.
16. It contains a proteolytic enzyme called fibrinolysin, which inhibits the clotting process.

SECTION 7-3: ESTROGENS AND PROGESTINS

OBJECTIVES:

The student should be able to:
1. Describe the basic structural features of the naturally occurring estrogens and progestins.
2. Describe the sites and pathways of biosynthesis of estrogens and progestins.
3. Describe the mechanisms of protein binding and transport of estrogens and progestins in blood.
4. Describe the characteristics of target tissue receptors for estrogens and progestins.
5. Describe several examples of the physiologic actions of estrogens and progestins.
6. Describe the mechanisms for catabolism of estrogens and progestins.

A. STRUCTURE, SITES, AND PATHWAYS OF BIOSYNTHESIS OF PROGESTINS AND ESTROGENS

The naturally occurring *progestins* (e.g., progesterone) are a group of C-21 steroids that are synthesized de novo in all the steroid synthesizing organs. They occupy a central position in the biosynthetic pathways for androgens, glucocorticoids, mineralocorticoids, and estrogens, as well as serving as an end product in themselves. The naturally occurring *estrogens* (estradiol, estrone, and estriol) are a group of C-18 steroids derived from androgens (see Figure 7-6). Although both progestins and estrogens can be synthesized in a variety of tissues, the principal sites of synthesis from acetate and cholesterol are the corpus luteum and the ovarian follicle.

In the ovary, cholesterol (derived from local synthesis, cholesterol ester storage pools, or uptake from the blood) in the theca interna cells (see Figure 7-3) is converted to pregnenolone by a mitochondrial desmolase enzyme. Again, as described in Chapters 5 and 6, this step in steroidogenesis is a critical control point that is subject to modulation by the gonadotropins. Pregnenolone is then converted to androgens by the 4-ene and 5-ene pathways utilizing enzymes localized in the microsomal (or smooth endoplasmic reticular) fraction as described in Section 6-2. In the corpus luteum, progesterone and 17α-OH-progesterone are the principal end products, but considerable amounts of androgen and estrogen are also produced. Recent studies have shown that the testosterone synthesized in the cells of the theca interna (see Figure 7-3) diffuses to the adjacent granulosa cells in which the bulk of the actual aromatization of testosterone to estradiol takes place. As you will recall, a similar separation of biosynthesis and aromatization of

FIGURE 7-6: Overview of estrogen biosynthesis. Note the aromatization of estradiol (E_2) and estrone (E_1) from the 19-hydroxy metabolites of testosterone (T) and androstenedione (AE), respectively. A schematic representation of the synthesis of the catechol estrogens (2-OH-E_2 and 2-OH-E_1) and of the 16-α-hydroxylation pathway yielding estriol (E_3) is also presented. (*Adapted from:* Luttge, 1979.)

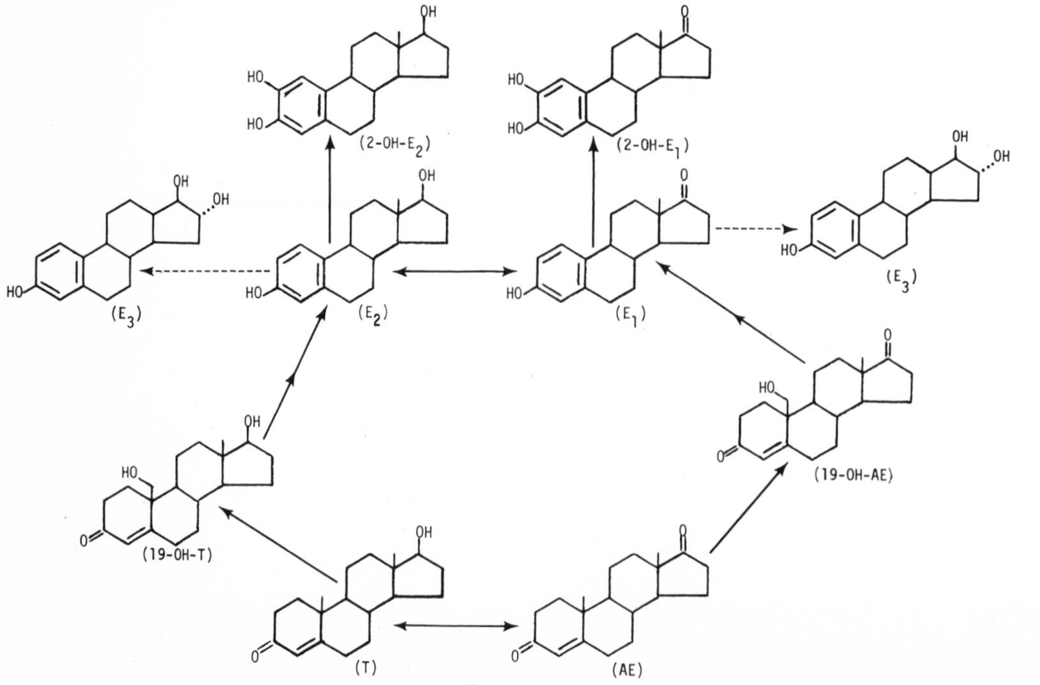

androgens occurs in the testis. (*Q. 7-8*) *What two cell groups in the testis are responsible for these functions?*

The term "aromatization" refers to the conversion of the A-ring of the steroid nucleus from a cyclohexanelike ring to a benzenelike ring. Estrogens frequently are referred to as phenolic steroids because the A-ring has a hydroxyl group located at the C-3 position, thus converting the benzenelike ring to a phenollike ring. The molecular mechanisms underlying the process of aromatization are complex, involving both enzymatic and nonenzymatic steps that have only recently been established. The cellular enzymes involved in this sequence are localized in the microsomal fraction. Although both estradiol and estrone are produced by aromatization of testosterone and androstenedione, respectively, in the ovary and corpus luteum, the synthesis and secretion of estradiol clearly exceeds that of estrone under most circumstances. Estriol is considered to be a product of the catabolism of estradiol and estrone, although it does possess biologic potency as an estrogen and is a major secretory product during pregnancy (see Section 7-4).

B. TRANSPORT AND PROTEIN BINDING OF ESTROGENS AND PROGESTINS IN BLOOD

As described in Chapters 5 and 6, nearly all (> 97%) of the circulating nonconjugated estrogens and progestins are bound to plasma proteins. (*Q. 7-9*) *What is the name of the protein that transports the largest amount of the glucocorticoid hormones* (e.g., cortisol) *in blood?* (*Q. 7-10*) *What performs the same function for androgenic hormones* (e.g., testosterone)? (*Q. 7-11*) *What is the name of the low-affinity, high-capacity protein used for transport of steroids in blood?* Estrogens are bound primarily to testosterone binding globulin (TeBG, also referred to as sex steroid-binding globulin) and albumin, while progestins are bound primarily to transcortin and albumin. In women the total binding capacity of the TeBG in blood normally is in excess of that required to bind all the estrogen in blood. Estrogens bind better than androgens to albumin, but their binding to transcortin is exceedingly low. The high binding affinity of transcortin for progestins forms the basis of a competitive protein binding assay for progestins.

C. CATABOLISM OF ESTROGENS AND PROGESTINS

The catabolism of progesterone and 17α-OH-progesterone by the liver results in the formation of pregnanediol from the former and proganetriol and etiocholanolone from the latter. The catabolism of estradiol and estrone by the liver is a complex and somewhat controversial subject. The liver is responsible for the production of derivatives oxygenated at the C-16 position and hydroxylated at the C-2, C-4, C-6, C-16, and C-18 positions. The 16α-hydroxylation pathway yielding estriol has been regarded commonly as the principal catabolic pathway for estrogens, but several recent studies have indicated that hydroxylation at the C-2 and C-4 positions, yielding the so-called catechol estrogens, may in fact be the major route of catabolism of estrogens by the liver (see Figure 7-6). In humans, estrogens are excreted in urine in the form of conjugates. Estriol, catechol-estradiol, and catechol-estrone are excreted primarily as glucuronide conjugates, whereas estrone is excreted primarily as a sulfate conjugate. (*Q. 7-12*) *In the male, does catabolism of testosterone* (a direct precursor of estradiol in both the male and female) *result in the excretion of glucuronide- or sulfate-conjugated catabolites, and does catabolism of androstenedione* (a direct precursor of estrone in both the male and female) *result in the excretion of glucuronide- or sulfate-conjugated catabolites?* The parallelism between androgen and estrogen catabolism thus represented may be coincidental, but heuristically it is still useful.

D. TARGET TISSUE RECEPTORS AND METABOLISM OF ESTROGENS AND PROGESTINS

Both the estrogens and progestins appear to exert most of their molecular actions through the cytoplasmic macromolecular receptor → nuclear receptor → chromatin acceptor → mRNA synthesis → protein synthesis mechanism discussed in earlier chapters (see Sections 5-6 and 6-2 and Figure 5-11). The intricate and fascinating details of this complex mechanism of action are beyond the scope of this chapter. The number of receptors for progestins in the uterus, breast, and other target tissues has been shown to be dependent on adequate concentrations of estrogen in blood. However, receptors for estrogen are demonstrable even in the ovariectomized animal. In contrast to the situation described in Sections 5-6 and 6-2 for glucocorticoid and androgen receptors, respectively, the activation of both the estrogen and progestin receptors appears to involve a major change in the molecular weight of the steroid-receptor complex. Physicochemical studies of receptors extracted from the nucleoplasm indicate that the activated form of the estrogen- and progestin-receptor complex is probably an aggregate of the nonactivated form of the receptor (normally classified as the cytosolic receptor) with one or more other large proteins. (Q. 7-13) *What is steroid-receptor activation?*

Progesterone can be metabolized to a wide variety of progestins in target tissues, but it is unclear which of these metabolites, if any, is required for progestin-specific actions. By contrast, estradiol does not undergo extensive metabolism in its target tissues, with the possible exception of the little understood formation and function of the catechol-estrogens. Estradiol is thus considered to be the active agent in estrogen target tissues in most situations. For example, it has been found that following the administration of [^{3}H]estrone to gonadectomized experimental animals, virtually all the hormone recovered from the nuclei of uterine endometrial cells is associated with [^{3}H]estradiol. As discussed in Section 7-5, the formation of catechol estrogens in brain may be important in the feedback regulation of prolactin secretion.

E. ACTIONS OF ESTROGENS AND PROGESTINS IN TARGET TISSUES OTHER THAN BRAIN AND PITUITARY

One of the most obvious examples of the actions and interactions of the hormones of the ovary and corpus luteum in the human female consists of the marked changes in the *uterine endometrium* observed during the menstrual cycle (see Section 7-3). The proliferative phase of the cycle is characterized by increasing concentrations of ovarian estrogens in blood which stimulate the rapid hypertrophy and hyperplasia of epithelial cells in the endometrium (see Figure 7-5). The invasion of spiral arteries and the production of both a fibrinolysin and an antifibrinolysin are also stimulated within the endometrium by the actions of estradiol. (Q. 7-14) *What is the eventual function of this fibrinolysin?* (Q. 7-15) *How long does the proliferative phase generally last in a woman 20 to 40 years of age?* The secretory phase of the cycle is characterized by increasing concentrations of corpus luteal progestins and estrogens in blood, which stimulate rapid growth of spiral arteries and increased secretory activity of epithelial glandular cells. At the close of the secretory phase, the concentrations of progesterone and estradiol in blood drop rapidly, precipitating a rapid regression of the endometrium and the onset of menstruation. (Q. 7-16) *How many days after ovulation does menstruation usually begin during the normal menstrual cycle of an adult woman?* (Q. 7-17) *How do you define menarche and menopause?* The sudden drop in the secretion of hormones by the corpus luteum and the consequent onset of menstruation does not occur if fertilization, implantation, and pregnancy are initiated (see Section 7-4).

The actions of estrogens and progestins in the *Fallopian tubes* are analogous in many respects to the actions of these hormones in the uterus. The obvious exception to this generalization is the absence of periodic necrosis and desquamation of the mucous epithelium of the Fallopian tubes. Estrogens increase the number and size of the nonciliated glandular cells in the epithelium, whereas progestins greatly increase their secretory activity. This provides the necessary nutrients (e.g., lactate) for the ovum before fertilization and to the zygote before its release (approximately 5 days after ovulation) into the nutrient-rich uterus (see Figure 7-4). Although estrogens also induce hyperplasia of the ciliated, nonsecretory epithelial cells, the action of these cilia does not appear to play a major role in the intratubal transport of the ovum. These cilia, together with those on the fimbriae, are important in the initial capture and transport of the newly ovulated ovum, together with its surrounding layer of sticky cumulous cells, into the infundibulum and distal portions of the ampulla.

The peristaltic activity of the highly muscular ampulla is thought to be the principal driving force for the intratubal transport of the ovum and zygote. These contractions are regulated by an interaction between the ovarian steroids and sympathetic innervation (and in some cases other hormones such as oxytocin). This interaction is exemplified by the regulation of the ampulloisthmic block. During the follicular phase of the cycle, estrogens facilitate the adrenergic activation of the isthmic musculature, which closes the lumen of each Fallopian tube, thus preventing premature release (i.e., before fertilization and subsequent initial divisions of the zygote) of the ovum/zygote into the uterus. During the luteal phase of the cycle, progestins inhibit this action of estrogen and thus permit the completion of intratubal-uterine transport of the ovum/zygote. A similar interaction between ovarian steroids and sympathetic innervation exists in the uterus. Both tissues exhibit a peak in contractile activity before ovulation and a relative quiescence during the luteal phase. Both tissues also exhibit very active contractile activity during menstruation. (Q. 7-18) *What is the presumed function of this activity in the uterus?*

The glandular cells in the cervix also respond to estrogen and progestin, such that during the early days of the proliferative-follicular phase of the menstrual cycle, the volume of the *endocervical mucus* is low and its viscosity is high. This situation may help prevent sperm penetration into the uterus before ovulation. As the concentration of estrogen in blood increases, the volume of mucus also increases (up to thirty-fold) with a concomitant decrease in viscosity. The elastic property of the mucus also changes such that just before ovulation a drop of endocervical mucus can be stretched into a long fine thread, a characteristic referred to as "*spinnbarkeit*." In addition, a drop of endocervical mucus taken from a preovulatory female can be shown to form a pattern of "*ferning*" or "*palm-leaf arborization*" when spread and dried on a microscopic slide. This pattern occurs as a result of crystallization of sodium chloride contained in the mucus. Both the spinnbarkeit and the ferning are sometimes examined in clinical tests and are characteristic of high concentrations of estrogen in blood. The acellular, alkaline, and watery mucus produced in relatively high quantities by the cervical glandular cells during the late proliferative-follicular phase may also serve to protect sperm from phagocytic destruction, supply additional nutrients for sperm, and act as a reservoir for sperm, thus increasing the probability of fertilization by providing a more continuous release of healthy, motile sperm into the uterus during the periovulatory period. The effects of estrogenic hormones on endocervical mucus are largely reversed with the rising concentrations of progestins in blood during the secretory-luteal phase of the menstrual cycle and during pregnancy.

The number, type, and appearance of cells present in the *vaginal mucosa* also vary in relation to changes in the secretion of ovarian hormones during the menstrual cycle. These hormonally induced cytologic changes are not as striking in the human as they are in lower animals and other primates, yet they form the basis of the important clinical test known as the "*Pap*" smear. This sequence of changes in vaginal epithelial cytology was first described by Stockard and Papanicolaou. Smears of the vaginal mucosa of the human during the latter part of menstruation (i.e, early in the follicular phase when concentrations of estradiol in blood are at their lowest point in the menstrual cycle) contain a few polygonal basophilic cells with vesicular-type nuclei and many polymorphonuclear leukocytes. Similar smears taken during the late follicular phase (i.e., when concentrations of estradiol in blood are nearing the highest point in the menstrual cycle) contain no polymorphonuclear leukocytes and an abundance of polygonal mucosal cells that contain an acidophilic cytoplasm. These are called cornified cells and are characteristic of the effect of high concentrations of estrogenic hormones in blood on the vaginal epithelium. During the early to midluteal phase of the menstrual cycle (i.e., when concentrations of progesterone and estradiol in blood are at their highest point) a greater degree of desquamation of superficial vaginal cells occurs. These cells are angular and have folded edges. The cytoplasm of these cells is basophilic. During the late luteal phase and just before the onset of menstruation (i.e., when concentrations of both progesterone and estradiol in blood are decreasing rapidly), polymorphonuclear leukocytes reappear. Acidophilic staining cells typical of those appearing in smears taken before ovulation again are evident. These precornified cells are present to a lesser extent than the basophilic staining cells. (*Q. 7-19*) *What type of vaginal epithelial cells would you expect to see predominantly in a Pap smear taken from a woman with an estrogen secreting tumor?*

The *breast* is also a major target tissue for ovarian steroids. During the pubertal period, the growth and pigmentation of the nipples and areola and the active proliferation of the ductal systems is believed to be due primarily to the direct actions of estrogen on breast tissue. The completion of mammogenesis is thought to require the actions of progestins and possibly several other hormones including prolactin and cortisol. Estrogens are also important during pregnancy in the proliferation and growth of the ductal epithelium before the initiation of lactation. Progestins appear to have little influence on lactation in humans. The endocrine regulation of lactation is discussed further in Section 7-4. The ductal epithelium of the human breast also undergoes a limited degree of cyclic proliferation and growth during the menstrual cycle. These changes are somewhat similar to those described above for the epithelial linings of the uterus, Fallopian tube, and vagina, and they appear to be the result of the cyclic changes in the secretion of estrogen, progestin, and prolactin during the menstrual cycle.

Estrogens can be demonstrated to have numerous other effects in humans including actions on the *skeleton* (e.g., increased osteoblastic activity, increased retention of calcium and phosphate, early closure of the epiphyses of the long bones, and broadening of the pelvis), *total body protein* (increased with estrogens, but to a much lesser extent than with androgens), *fat deposition* (increases in the breasts, buttocks, and thighs), and *skin* (increased smoothness, thickness, and vascularity). The actions of estrogens and progestins in the feedback regulation of gonadotropin and prolactin secretion are discussed in Sections 7-5 and 7-6. The behavioral actions of these steroids in humans are still understood poorly, but it is clear that the magnitude of the effects is far less dramatic than it is in lower animals and other primates.

The *basal body temperature* of the human female also varies during the menstrual cycle and is thought by some investigators to mirror changes in the concentration of progesterone in blood. When oral or rectal temperatures are measured every morning before arising, a drop of about 0.6°C (1°F) is observed a few days before ovulation. At ovulation there is a sharp rise in body temperature of about 0.6°C followed by a further rise of another several tenths of a degree, after which body temperature remains relatively stable until the close of the luteal phase, when body temperature falls to the premenstrual nadir. Measurement of basal metabolic heat production (as rate of oxygen consumption) under the same conditions has revealed a close parallelism with basal body temperature. This suggests that the changes in body temperature observed during the menstrual cycle reflect changes in metabolic heat production rather than changes in heat dissipation.

As stated above, the increases in basal body temperature and basal metabolic rate have often been claimed to reflect increases in the production of progesterone by the corpus luteum. However, although a correlation between these parameters has been observed in some women, the correlation is relatively poor in others. The possibility that other hormones associated with ovulation may contribute to the change in body temperature remains to be investigated. Even though the mechanisms responsible for the elevation of body temperature associated with ovulation are not understood clearly, this relatively simple measurement has been useful to physicians as well as to women seeking a method to determine the days of their cycle during which pregnancy might occur. (*Q. 7-20*) *How many days during the normal menstrual cycle is a woman at her most fertile condition?*

SECTION 7-3: POST-TEST QUESTIONS

1. Progestins are a. (C-?) _____ steroids that occupy a central position in the biosynthetic pathway of the other four major classes of steroidal hormones: b. _____, c. _____, d. _____, and e. _____.

2. Estrogens are a. (C-?) _____ steroids derived from the b. (C-?) _____ androgens via the process of c. _____, which converts the A-ring of the steroid nucleus from a d. _____-like ring to a e. _____-like ring.

3. Because a hydroxyl group is present in the A-ring, estrogens are also referred to as a. _____ steroids. Estrogens with two hydroxyl groups in the A-ring are referred to as b. _____ estrogens.

4. In the ovary, the biosynthesis of pregnenolone occurs in cells of the a. _____ _____; the actual conversion of androgens to estrogens appears to occur primarily in the b. _____ cells.

5. The liver-synthesized carrier protein transcortin binds the steroids a. _____ _____, b. _____, and c. _____ much better than it binds d. _____.

6. The principal catabolic products of estradiol are a. _____ and the newly emphasized b. _____ estrogens, both of which are secreted primarily as c. _____ conjugates.

7. The principal catabolite of progesterone produced by the liver is _____.

8. The biologic actions of progestins typically require priming the target tissue with estrogen. Why?

9. Describe the synergistic interactions of estradiol and progesterone on the secretory activity of the mucosal epithelium of the uterus and Fallopian tubes.

10. The menstrual cycle of the human female is characterized by a. (increasing/decreasing) concentrations of b. _____ in blood during the proliferative phase, and c. (increasing/decreasing) concentrations of d. _____ and

e. _____ in blood during the secretory phase. Menstruation is precipitated by a rapid f. (increase/decrease) in the concentrations of g. _____ and h. _____ in blood.

11. In the Fallopian tubes, estrogens a. (facilitate/inhibit) the establishment of the ampulloisthmic block. Progestins b. (facilitate/inhibit) this effect. What is the presumed function of the block?

12. How is the ovum/zygote transported from the ovary to the uterus?

13. Estrogen appears to stimulate a(n) a. (increase/decrease) in the viscosity, a(n) b. (increase/decrease) in the elasticity, and a(n) c. (increase/decrease) in the volume of endocervical mucus. What are the presumed functions of these alterations?

14. A Pap smear with an absence of polymorphonuclear leukocytes and an abundance of cornified cells is thought to be a reflection of what type of hormonal environment?

15. In the breast, a. _____ is responsible for the growth and pigmentation of the b. _____ and c. _____ and for the growth and proliferation of the d. _____ system. e. _____ is required for the completion of mammogenesis.

16. Women are usually fertile only during 2 to 3 days of the menstrual cycle. (True/False)

SECTION 7-3: POST-TEST ANSWERS

1. a. C-21
   b. androgens
   c. estrogens
   d. glucocorticoids
   e. mineralocorticoids
2. a. C-18
   b. C-19
   c. aromatization
   d. cyclohexane
   e. benzene
3. a. phenolic

      b. catechol
4. a. theca interna
      b. granulosa
5. a. cortisol
      b. testosterone
      c. progesterone
      d. estradiol
6. a. estriol
      b. catechol
      c. glucuronide
7. pregnanediol
8. The macromolecular mobile intracellular receptors for progesterone are labile. The continued synthesis of these receptors appears to require the actions of estrogen in the target tissue.
9. Estradiol stimulates the hypertrophy and hyperplasia of the glandular cells in the mucosal epithelium of both tissues; progesterone (and its metabolites) stimulates a marked increase in the secretory activity of these cells.
10. a. increasing
      b. estradiol
      c. increasing
      d. progesterone
      e. estradiol
      f. decrease
      g. progesterone
      h. estradiol
11. a. facilitate
      b. inhibit
      It prevents the "premature" release of the ovum/zygote into the uterus. Delaying the ovum in the ampulla enhances the probability of fertilization. Following fertilization, the block provides the necessary time for the early divisions of the zygote before release into the uterus, where implantation in the hypertrophied endometrium should occur.
12. The newly released ovum is swept from the ovary by the fimbriae of the Fallopian tube which, together with the cilia of the infundibular epithelium, rapidly transport the ovum into the ampulla. The layer of sticky cumulous cells that surround the newly ovulated ovum aid in the capture of this cell mass by the cilia of the fimbriae. In the ampulla, peristaltic contractions propel the ovum toward the ampulloisthmic junction. As described in question 11, this junction usually is blocked before the actions of progesterone during the early days of the luteal phase.
13. a. decrease
      b. increase
      c. increase
      They provide a mucous environment that is conducive to sperm survival, maturation, and gradual release into the uterus, thus increasing the probability of fertilization.
14. High blood concentrations of estradiol as might be present during the late follicular phase just before ovulation.
15. a. estradiol
      b. nipple
      c. areola
      d. ductal
      e. Progesterone
16. True. However this period of maximal fertility is highly variable.

OBJECTIVES:

The student should be able to:
1. Describe the basic structural features, mode of synthesis, storage, release, and blood-borne transport of the gonadotropins and prolactin.
2. Describe the metabolic clearance of the gonadotropins and prolactin.
3. Describe the hormonal regulation of steroidogenesis in the ovary and corpus luteum.
4. Describe the hormonal regulation of ovulation, atresia, luteinization, pregnancy, and lactation.

A. STRUCTURE, SYNTHESIS, STORAGE, RELEASE, TRANSPORT, AND CLEARANCE OF THE GONADOTROPINS AND PROLACTIN

Because there are no known sex differences in the structure, synthesis, storage, release, transport, and mechanisms of clearance of LH and FSH, the student should consult Section 6-3 for a discussion of these properties of gonadotropins in males. Although prolactin (Prl) also exists in both sexes, its role in males is not well understood and as a consequence, it was mentioned only briefly in Chapter 6. Prl is a protein with a molecular weight of 22,500 daltons (not a glycoprotein like LH, FSH, and TSH). It contains a single peptide chain of 198 amino acids. (*Q. 7-21*) *How many peptide chains comprise LH, FSH, and TSH and what are they called?* (*Q. 7-22*) *Which of them has the same amino acid sequence for all three hormones?*

Like other protein hormones, Prl is believed to be synthesized on the rough endoplasmic reticulum (RER) via traditional protein synthetic mechanisms and then packaged into microvesicles by the Golgi apparatus. These microvesicles coalesce into larger vesicles before their storage, destruction by lysosomal enzymes, or exocytotic release from the plasma membrane into the perivascular space (see Figure 6-4). Recent studies have indicated that the synthesis of Prl involves the production of a prohormone similar to the well-studied proinsulin system. Preprolactin (Pre-Prl) has 29 additional amino acids joined to the N-terminus. The primary amino acid sequence of this additional peptide segment is very similar to that of the pre- portion of the prohormone for human placental lactogen (hPL), which is discussed later in this section. It is believed that this hydrophobic-rich peptide segment somehow aids in stabilizing the prohormone by facilitating its affinity for membranes. Pre-Prl is converted rapidly to Prl by special proteolytic enzymes within the adenohypophyseal lactotrope (i.e., the cell synthesizing Prl), and it is estimated that in humans only 8–20% of the total Prl in blood is in the form of Pre-Prl. Neither thyrotropin releasing hormone (TRH), which increases the release of Prl (see Section 7-5), nor L-DOPA, which decreases the release of Prl (see Sections 7-5 and 7-6), changes the ratio of Pre-Prl to Prl in blood. Unlike the pleomorphism of the glycoprotein hormones LH and FSH discussed in Section 6-3, the apparent molecular size and consequent metabolic clearance of Prl do not appear to be modified either directly or indirectly by steroid hormones. (*Q. 7-23*) *What are the effects of gonadectomy on the metabolic clearance rate of FSH and, to a lesser extent, LH?*

B. HORMONAL REGULATION OF, AND INTERACTIONS BETWEEN, OVARIAN STEROIDOGENESIS, OVULATION, AND ATRESIA

As discussed in Section 7-2, the primary follicles of the postpubertal women rest in prophase I of meiosis. The transformation from preantral to postantral follicles is stimulated by the actions of FSH and estrogen. The actions of these hormones are believed to be mediated by typical fixed membrane-associated (FSH) or mobile cyto-plasmic and nuclear (estrogen) receptor mechanisms as discussed in earlier chapters. Under the stimulation of FSH and estrogen, the oocyte grows in response to the nutrients it receives from the follicular cells. FSH has been shown recently to stimulate the expansion of the cumulus surrounding the oocyte by facilitating the increased production of an intercellular matrix rich in hyaluronic acid. Although the details of the selection process are still unclear, it is thought that of the 20 or so primary follicles that develop during each ovulatory cycle, the follicle that is, for some as yet unknown reason, secreting the highest amount of estrogen has the highest probability of becoming a fully mature Graafian follicle. The remaining follicles undergo atresia. Recent studies have suggested that 5α-reduced androgens (e.g., dihydrotestosterone and androstane-dione, see Figure 6-10), produced in cells of the theca interna in response to stimulation by LH, can inhibit FSH-stimulated aromatization of testosterone by the granulosa cells. The addition of exogenous FSH can retard the process of atresia, but the continued production of 5α-reduced androgens eventually reduces the production of estrogens in the granulosa cells to such an extent that their necessary supportive actions are inadequate to prevent atresia.

The rupture of the Graafian follicle at ovulation is thought to be the end result of a series of interlocking events. FSH stimulates the production of both follicular fluids and a intercellular cumulous matrix, thereby leading to the expansion of the antrum and a relative thinning of the follicular wall. FSH also stimulates an increased production of a plasminogen activator by the granulosa cells, which in turn catalyze the conversion of plasminogen (synthesized in the kidney and found in relatively high concentrations of ovarian follicular fluids) to the proteolytic enzyme, plasmin. This enzyme may act directly on the follicular wall and/or it may facilitate the production of a collagenase enzyme (from procollagenase precursors) that weakens the intercellular adhesions of the follicular wall. The final stimulant for follicular rupture may, however, result from the action of prostaglandins on the cells of the theca externa, which are rich in microfilaments, actin, and smooth muscle myosin. The intrafollicular production of these prostaglandins is thought to be stimulated by the midcycle surge in LH secretion (see Figure 7-17A). The presumed contraction of these cells, coupled with the thinning and enzymatic weakening of the intercellular adhesions of the follicular wall, may interact to permit the rupture of the Graafian follicle and the release of the ovum. (*Q. 7-24) Is it reasonable to conclude that the rupture of the Graafian follicle results from excessive intrafollicular pressures?*

C. HORMONAL REGULATION OF, AND INTERACTIONS BETWEEN, LUTEINIZATION OF THE GRAAFIAN FOLLICLE AND STEROIDOGENESIS AND ATRESIA OF THE CORPUS LUTEUM

During the later stages in the growth of the Graafian follicle, increasing concentrations of FSH in blood stimulate an *increase* in the number and/or activity of available receptors for LH on the plasma membranes of the cells found in the external layer of the granulosa cells. The increasing concentration of estradiol in follicular fluid further potentiates this *increase* in the number and/or activity of available receptors for LH. Finally, the rapidly increasing blood concentrations of LH stimulate a *decrease* in the number and/or activity of available receptors for FSH. This reciprocal alteration in the number and/or activity of available receptors for the gonadotropins appears to begin just before ovulation and to continue during the remainder of the process of luteinization. The dramatic *preovulatory* increase in the concentration of LH in blood also stimulates a change in steroidogenic pathways in the Graafian follicle such that there is a decrease in the production of estrogen and an increase in the production of progesterone (see Figures 7-17A and 7-17C). Progestrone is, of course, one of the major steroids secreted by the corpus luteum (see Figures 7-5 and 7-17A). (*Q. 7-25*) *What is the other major steroid secreted by the corpus luteum?*

After ovulation the ruptured Graafian follicle involutes and continues to undergo histologic luteinization in response to the actions of LH. The newly formed corpus luteum begins to secrete large quantities of progesterone and, to a lesser extent, estradiol, in response to the continued actions of LH on the luteal cells (see Figures 7-4 and 7-17A). (*Q. 7-26*) *What are the principal physiologic and histologic effects of these steroids on the mucosal epithelium of the uterus and Fallopian tubes during the luteal phase of the menstrual cycle?* FSH does not appear to be involved in these steroidogenic and histologic responses of LH in the corpus luteum.

If fertilization does not occur, LH-stimulated adenylate cyclase activity and steroidogenesis of progesterone and estradiol in cells of the corpus luteum decreases during the second week following ovulation. These decrements in the potency of LH correlate with a decrease during the late luteal phase in the number and/or activity of receptors for LH on membranes of cells of the corpus luteum. This loss in responsiveness to LH by the corpus luteum ultimately culminates in its atresia (see Figure 7-3). (*Q. 7-27*) *What is the name of the tissue scar that remains after the degeneration of the corpus luteum?* The atresia of the corpus luteum can be delayed by giving women substantial quantities of either exogenous LH or human chorionic gonadotropin (hCG). The restorative potency of hCG is analogous to its role in maintaining the corpus luteum following implantation of the fertilized ovum (see Figure 7-4). (*Q. 7-28*) *Where does implantation normally occur?*

D. HORMONAL REGULATION OF FERTILIZATION, IMPLANTATION, PREGNANCY, AND LACTATION

The student should recall that before ovulation the primary oocyte is arrested in prophase I. Both LH and FSH are required to stimulate ovulation and the resumption of meiosis. After ovulation the secondary oocyte proceeds toward the second division of meiosis, but this process is halted at metaphase unless *fertilization* occurs. For this sperm-stimulated completion of meiosis to occur, a "cytoplasmic maturation reaction" must be stimulated in the secondary oocyte. This reaction appears to be produced in the oocyte by the actions of an as yet unknown product or products released from the attached cumulous cells. The production and/or release of this material is in turn stimulated by the actions of estradiol (and possibly 17α-OH-progesterone) in the cumulous cells. After the pronuclei of the germ cells fuse, further mitotic divisions of the zygote are stimulated. During this time period, the actions of estrogen and progestin in the glandular cells of the mucosal epithelium of the Fallopian tubes increase the production of nutrients such as lactate, which is essential for the survival of the dividing zygote.

Generally within 5 days after ovulation, the rapidly increasing concentration of progesterone in blood (secreted by the corpus luteum) stimulates the relaxation of the ampulloisthmic block, thus permitting the release of the embryo (in either the morula or blastula stage of embryogenesis) from the Fallopian tube into the nutrient-rich uterine cavity. Within the next 2 to 3 days, and after further cellular divisions, the blastocyst usually initiates *implantation* in the highly proliferated endometrial mucosa (see Figures 7-4 and 7-5). (*Q. 7-29*) *When does production of mucus by the endometrium reach a maximum?*

Recent investigations have suggested that estrogens (and possibly other steroids) secreted by the blastocyst facilitate the *decidual reaction* (i.e., increased permeability of endometrial capillaries) at the site of implantation. At this stage of embryogenesis, the wall of the hollow, ball-like blastocyst consists of a single layer of cells (the trophoblast) except for the multicellular "embryo," which bulges into the cavity of the blastocyst. Upon contact with the endometrium, the cells of the trophoblast proliferate and apparently secrete lytic enzymes, which aid the implantation of the blastocyst into the endometrial stroma. Epithelial cells surrounding the ulcerated endometrium (which has been healed temporarily with a coagulum formed from fibrin and cellular debris) eventually proliferate to completely enclose the embedded blastocyst (see Figure 7-7).

Following implantation, the cells of the inner layer of the trophoblast (cytotrophoblast) begin to secrete a peptide that has very recently been shown to be immunologically, physicochemically, and functionally very similar, if not identical, to the hypotha-

FIGURE 7-7: Implantation and development of the fertilized ovum and location and development of the decidual lining of the uterus, which make up the maternal portion of the placenta. (*Source:* Ham and Cormack, 1979.)

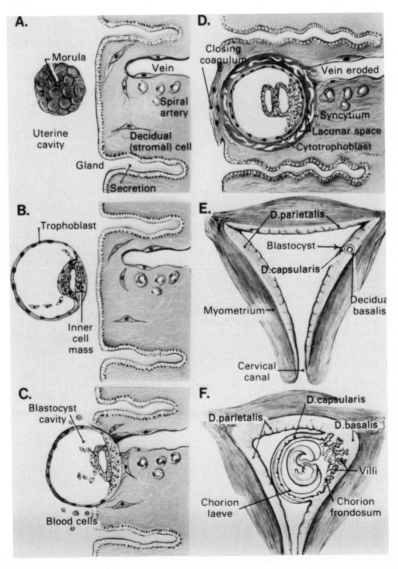

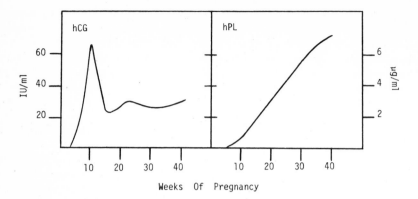

FIGURE 7-8: Patterns of secretion of human chorionic gonadotropin (hCG) and human placental lactogen (hPL) during pregnancy. Placental growth parallels the increase in the secretion of hPL.

lamic hypophysiotropic hormone Gn-RH (or LH-RH). This peptide, originally referred to as placental LH-RH (pLH-RH), stimulates the release of hCG from the cells of the outer layer of the trophoblast (syncytiotrophoblast). pLH-RH can also stimulate the release of LH from the pituitaries of experimental animals. (*Q. 7-30*) *Can you think of another example of a peptide hormone synthesized both in the brain and in a peripheral organ?* Under natural conditions, as the cells of the synctiotrophoblast begin to secrete large amounts of hCG (see Figure 7-8), this glycoprotein (which is composed of two peptide chains similar in amino acid sequence to those of LH) stimulates cells of the corpus luteum to maintain and eventually increase their production of progesterone and estradiol. (*Q. 7-31*) *What other protein hormone will stimulate this response?* The increased concentration of these steroids in blood stimulates further growth and secretory activity of the endometrium (see Figure 7-4). As the placenta begins to form during the next few weeks, it takes over the production of hCG.

Under stimulation by hCG, the corpus luteum grows to approximately twice its maximum size during the nonfertile menstrual cycle. The high rate of secretion of estrogen and progestin by the corpus luteum are required only during the first 11 weeks of *pregnancy*. After this time, the placenta takes over the production of these essential steroids (see Figure 7-9). The placenta also synthesizes and secretes human placental

FIGURE 7-9: Patterns of secretion of progesterone, estrone (E_1), estradiol (E_2), and estriol (E_3) during pregnancy. Note the high levels of estriol secretion.

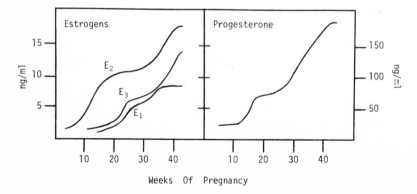

lactogen (hPL) (see Figure 7-8) which, like growth hormone (hGH, see Chapter 8) and Prl, is thought to stimulate breast development in preparation for the production of milk following parturition. It is important to note that very little hPL is transported from the mother to the fetus. (*Q. 7-32*) *Do you know how and why this apparent compartmentalization is affected?* It probably is not coincidental that hGH can stimulate hPL-like actions in breast tissue, since 161 of the 191 amino acids in hPL (a single peptide chain) are in the same sequence as in hGH (also containing a single peptide chain; see Section 8-1).

The actual mechanisms, hormonal and otherwise, that stimulate *parturition* in the female are still unclear. One of the most popular theories, derived from studies with sheep, is illustrated in Figure 7-10. According to this scheme the fetal hypothalamus releases corticotropin releasing hormone(s) (CRH) into the portal blood supply of the adenohypophysis in response to stimuli presently unknown. CRH stimulates the synthesis and secretion of adrenocorticotropic hormone (ACTH) from the corticotropes of the adenohypophysis (see Section 5-7). The increased concentration of ACTH in fetal blood stimulates the adrenal cortex of the fetus to synthesize and secrete glucocorticoids. The increase in the concentration of glucocorticoids has three important effects: a) to increase production of surfactants in the fetal lungs (essential for maintenance of the integrity of the alveoli of the lungs following parturition), b) to increase storage of glycogen in the fetal liver and in skeletal and cardiac muscle (essential for provision of carbohydrates required in the modulation of the concentrations of sugars in blood during early extrauterine life), and c) to increase production of estrogen and prostaglandin $F_{2\alpha}$ by the placenta (essential for the induction of labor). The increase in the local concentration of prostaglandins in placental blood also appears to have three important effects: a) to decrease production of progesterone by the placenta, b) to increase aromatization of androgens to form estrogens in the placenta, and c) to stimulate contractions of myometrial smooth muscle directly. The reciprocal change in the concentrations of progesterone and estradiol in placental blood stimulates an increase in the sensitivity of the myometrium to endogenous contractile agents such as oxytocin and prostaglandins. Thus the release of prostaglandins by the placenta may precipitate the initial uterine

FIGURE 7-10: The pathway by which the fetal lamb may influence the onset of labor in the ewe. Also indicated are the experimental procedures that have been used to modify the activity of the pathway. (*Adapted from: Liggins, 1973.*)

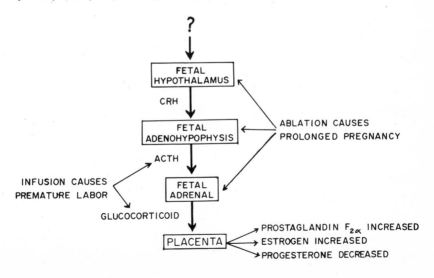

contractions of labor, while oxytocin released from the neurohypophysis in response to cervical stimulation by the fetus may aid in the completion of parturition through its direct actions on the uterine myometrium. (*Q. 7-33*) *What physiologic reaction would you predict in the myoepithelial cells of the breast during labor and delivery?*

Recent findings in humans have suggested that fetal Prl may also participate in the initiation of parturition. In contrast to the findings described above for sheep, the concentrations of ACTH in fetal blood from human beings have been found to decrease during the last few weeks of gestation, even though the concentrations of cortisol in fetal blood continue to increase during this period. This apparent paradox is now attributed tentatively to an increased sensitivity of the fetal adrenal cortex to the stimulatory effects of ACTH. This increase in sensitivity is believed to be the result of a Prl-induced activation of receptors for ACTH in the fetal adrenal. (*Q. 7-34*) *Assuming that this explanation is correct, why do you think the concentration of ACTH in fetal blood decreases during this period?*

The hormonal regulation of *lactation* is exceedingly complex and poorly understood in humans. For example, progesterone, which is known to play an important role in lactation in certain laboratory species, appears to play no significant role in humans. As described earlier, estrogens appear to be essential in the proliferation and growth of the ductal systems of the breast during gestation (see Figure 7-2). These effects, however, as well as the actual development of the secretory alveoli and the production of milk, require the stimulatory actions of either Prl or hPL on the mammary epithelial cells. The exact mechanisms for these diverse effects of Prl and hPL are still unclear, but they appear to involve an interaction with fixed receptors on the plasma membrane of the epithelial cells of the ductal system. Results from laboratory animals suggest that other hormones (e.g., insulin, cortisol, and the thyroid hormones T_4 and T_3) may also be involved in lactation, but the evidence is minimal for a physiologic role of these other hormones in humans.

The concentrations of both hPL and Prl in maternal blood increase dramatically during the latter half of gestation (see Figure 7-8), but these concentrations decrease quickly after parturition (see Figure 7-11). The decrease in the concentration of hPL is,

FIGURE 7-11: Concentrations of Prl in maternal serum during gestation and the immediate postpartum period. Note the change in the scale from weeks to days. (*Adapted from:* Hwang and Friesen, 1971.)

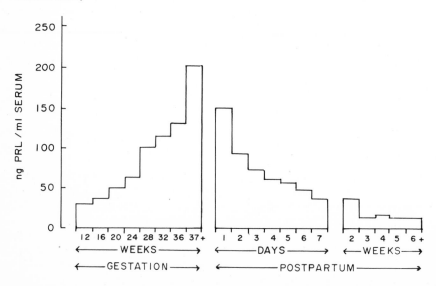

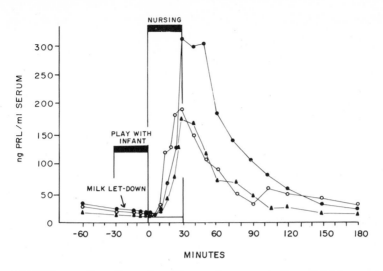

FIGURE 7-12: The effects of suckling on the concentrations of Prl in serum from three different lactating women. Note that although playing with the infant elicits the release of oxytocin as evidenced by the let-down response, this stimulus does not elicit the release of Prl. Suckling, however, is a powerful stimulant for the release of both hormones. (*Adapted from:* Noel et al., 1974.)

of course, due to the loss of the placenta, but the drop in the concentration of Prl may at first seem paradoxical, since it occurs even in nursing women and since this hormone is absolutely required for the maintenance of milk production. Careful monitoring of the concentrations of Prl in blood of nursing women, however, has revealed that the suckling stimulus can elicit a rapid and highly significant increase in the secretion of Prl (see Figure 7-12). The effectiveness of this stimulus (i.e., in bringing about an increase in the secretion of Prl) decreases over a period of weeks following parturition. This decrease is not prevented by frequent bouts of suckling. Although suckling also induces a rapid increase in the secretion of oxytocin, and indirectly the oxytocin-induced let-down reflex essential for milk ejection (see Section 2-3), oxytocin is not the suckling-induced stimulant for the increase in the secretion of Prl. If nursing is terminated, by either the mother or the infant, suckling-induced secretion of Prl and Prl-induced production of milk are also terminated. (*Q. 7-35*) *What physiologic reaction would you predict in the myometrium of the uterus during suckling?*

SECTION 7-4: POST-TEST QUESTIONS

1. LH, FSH, and TSH are all a. _____-proteins, each consisting of b. _____ polypeptide chain(s). Prl is a c. _____-protein consisting of d. _____ polypeptide chain(s).
2. Like LH, a. _____ is a b. _____-protein hormone that stimulates the secretion of c. _____ from the corpus luteum during early pregnancy. Like Prl, d. _____ is thought to be essential for the production of milk during the later stages of pregnancy.
3. Like the pancreatic hormone insulin, the proximate precursor of the adenohypophyseal hormone a. _____ and of the placental hormone b. _____ is a c. _____ hormone.

4. The rupture of the Graafian follicle and the release of the secondary oocyte with its surrounding cumulous layer of the granulosa cells is thought to be facilitated by three principal events in the follicle. Briefly describe each of these follicular events.
   a.
   b.
   c.
   What are the presumed causes for each of these follicular events?
   d.
   e.
   f.
   Which hormones are thought to stimulate each of these presumed causes?
   g.
   h.
   i.

5. Under experimental conditions, the synthesis and secretion of LH, FSH, and hCG can all be stimulated by a decapeptide synthesized in both the hypothalamus and the trophoblast. (True/False)

6. The synthesis of hCG in the a. _____ cells of the trophoblast is stimulated by the release of a b. _____-peptide, which is immunologically, physicochemically, and functionally similar, if not identical, to c. _____ from the d. _____ cells of the trophoblast.

7. The luteinization in the Graafian follicle is stimulated by the actions of the hormone a. _____. This event is facilitated by a b. (increase/decrease) in the number and/or activity of c. (fixed/mobile) receptors for d. _____ found on the plasma membrane of cells in the external layer of the granulosa cells. The change in the number and/or activity of these receptors is thought to be stimulated by the hormones, e. _____ and f. _____.

8. The atresia of the corpus luteum can be delayed by the administration of two protein hormones: a. _____ and b. _____. The atresia of the growing follicle can be delayed by the administration of the protein hormone c. _____. What type of steroid hormone can accelerate the atresia of these follicles? d. _____ Where are these steroids synthesized? e. _____ What protein hormone is thought to stimulate the production of these steroids? f. _____ The same protein hormone is also thought to stimulate a g. (increase/decrease) in the number and/or activity of receptors for the hormone h. _____ found on plasma membrane of granulosa cells. i. What is the proposed mechanism by which the steroids mentioned in (e) accelerate the onset of follicular atresia?

   j. What is the proposed mechanism by which the protein hormone mentioned in (c) delays the onset of follicular atresia?

   Noting that the protein hormones mentioned in (c) and (h) are in fact the same hormone, it is likely that the two proposed mechanisms mentioned in (g) and (i) are either complementary or two different views of the same mechanism.

9. The sperm-stimulated completion of the second division of meiosis by the ovum requires a "cytoplasmic maturation reaction" to occur in the ovum. a. What is the principal hormone involved in stimulating this reaction?

   b. Where is the site of action for this hormone in this situation?

10. Estrogenic hormones secreted by the blastocyst are thought to facilitate the decidual

reaction during (or preceding) implantation of the blastocyst in the endometrium.
(True/False)

11. Although the stimuli eliciting the onset of labor are still unclear in humans, the endogenous biochemicals that stimulate the actual contractions of the myometrium during labor are thought to be a. _____ and b. _____ .

12. What is the proposed role for Prl in the initiation of parturition?

13. The production of milk in the human breast requires the actions of the protein hormone, a. _____ ; the ejection of milk from the human breast requires the actions of the peptide hormone b. _____ .

14. The act of sexual intercourse can produce a rather dramatic effect in the breast of a lactating woman. What is this effect and why does it occur?

SECTION 7-4: POST-TEST ANSWERS

1. a. glyco-
   b. two
   c. nonglyco-
   d. one
2. a. hCG
   b. glyco-
   c. progesterone
   d. hPL
3. a. Prl
   b. hPL
   c. pro-
4. a. Thinning of the follicular wall.
   b. Weakening of the intercellular adhesions in the follicular wall.
   c. Contraction of the cells of the theca externa.
   d. Increased production of the follicular fluids and the intercellular matrix of the cumulus cells surrounding the ovum;
   e. Enzymatic activity of the lytic enzyme plasmin, and/or a collagenase-like enzyme produced by the actions of plasmin on a procollagenase precursor.
   f. Prostaglandin actions on the actin and smooth muscle myosin.
   g. FSH;
   h. FSH (stimulates the production of plasminogen activators that catalyze the conversion of plasminogen into plasmin)
   i. LH
5. True. (A fascinating example of parallel molecular-physiologic evolution.)

6. a. syncytiotrophoblast
    b. deca-
    c. Gn-RH (LH-RH)
    d. cytotrophoblast
7. a. LH
    b. increase
    c. fixed
    d. LH
    e. FSH
    f. estrogen
8. a. LH
    b. hCG
    c. FSH
    d. 5α-reduced androgens (e.g., dihydrotestosterone and androstanedione)
    e. cells of the theca interna
    f. LH
    g. decrease
    h. FSH
    i. inhibition of FSH-stimulated aromatization of androgens to estrogens in the granulosa cells
    j. stimulation of increased aromatization of androgens to estrogens in the granulosa cells
9. a. Estrogen
    b. Granulosa cells of the cumulus surrounding the secondary oocyte
10. True
11. a. oxytocin
    b. prostaglandins
12. Prl is thought to increase the number and/or activity of the receptors for ACTH in the fetal adrenal cortex. This leads to an increase in steroidogenesis of glucocorticoids in spite of the decreasing concentrations of ACTH in fetal blood during this same time period.
13. a. Prl
    b. oxytocin
14. A let-down reaction may occur because of the actions of oxytocin on the myoepithelial cells. The oxytocin is released from the neurohypophysis in response to the activation of magnocellular neurons in the paraventricular nucleus (and possibly the supraoptic nucleus) of the hypothalamus. These hypothalamic neurons are in turn activated by other neurons responding to the tactile stimulation of the vagina during copulation.

SECTION 7-5: HYPOTHALAMIC HYPOPHYSIOTROPIC HORMONES

OBJECTIVES:

The student should be able to:
1. Describe the chemical composition, biosynthesis, storage, intracellular transport, release, blood-borne transport, and catabolism of Gn-RH.
2. Describe some of the same characteristics for the various biochemicals that have been reported to possess PIH or PRH activity.
3. Describe the mechanisms by which the HHHs control the synthesis and secretion of LH, FSH, and Prl in females.

A. GONADOTROPIN RELEASING HORMONE (Gn-RH)

The amino acid sequence, central nervous system localization, life cycle (i.e., synthesis, storage, intracellular transport, release, blood-borne transport, and catabolism) and cellular actions of the hypothalamic hypophysiotropic hormone (HHH) Gn-RH were discussed in Section 6-4. Since there are no significant male-female differences in these aspects of Gn-RH function, no further discussion of them is given here. (*Q. 7-36*) *What are the proposed intracellular and extracellular routes by which Gn-RH is transported from the site of its synthesis (i.e., ribosomes) in neurons of the arcuate nucleus of the hypothalamus to the site of its action (i.e., plasma membranes) in gonadotropes of the adenohypophysis?* (*Q. 7-37*) *Are these the only sites of synthesis and action for Gn-RH?*

B. PROLACTIN INHIBITING HORMONE (PIH)

As discussed in Section 2-2, the tonic secretion of Prl is primarily under the homeostatic control of an inhibitory HHH called prolactin inhibitory hormone (PIH). This unusual form of regulation is illustrated by the dramatic rise in the concentration of Prl in blood following lesions of the basal hypothalamus that destroy the source of the neurons secreting PIH. Either complete transection of the infundibular stalk or hypophysectomy, followed by transplantation of the pituitary to a site other than the sella turcica, also results in dramatic increases in the secretion of Prl. (*Q. 7-38*) *Why would you expect cutting the infundibular stalk to result in an increase in the secretion of Prl?* Further evidence that the secretion of Prl by the pituitary is under tonic inhibitory control includes the observation that pituitaries incubated in vitro release considerable quantities of Prl, while at the same time very little LH, FSH, TSH, ACTH, and GH are released. More than half of all tumors of the adenohypophysis observed in humans (both hormone secreting and nonhormone secreting) are associated with a specific type of endocrine producing cell. (*Q. 7-39*) *From your knowledge of the secretory cells of the adenohypophysis, which type of endocrine producing cell would you expect to find in these tumors and why?* Very recent results obtained with perfusions of dispersed rat pituitary cells in vitro have suggested that the tonic high level of Prl released by these cells is maintained by a steady influx of extracellular calcium, not by the activation of the adenylate cyclase localized in the plasma membranes of these cells. (*Q. 7-40*) *How does this proposed cellular mechanism compare to that proposed for the release of the other adenohypophyseal hormones?*

A large body of evidence supports the hypothesis that dopamine (DA) is a PIH but not necessarily "the" PIH. This biogenic amine was discussed in Section 4-2, and further details on its localization in the brain were presented in Section 2-2. Many studies have shown that the DA synthesized in neurons of the arcuate nucleus of the basal hypothalamus can be released via exocytosis into the perivascular space in the median eminence, where it diffuses into the fenestrated capillaries of the external plexus and is then transported by way of the hypophyseal-portal vessels down the infundibular stalk to the adenohypophysis. The addition of DA to the media used for incubation of pituitary fragments inhibits the spontaneous release of Prl. Exogenous L-DOPA, administered systemically to both humans and laboratory animals, inhibits both the spontaneous and the suckling-induced release of Prl. (*Q. 7-41*) *How is L-DOPA related to dopamine?* Administration of DA agonists (e.g., apomorphine and such ergot alkaloids as bromocryptine) will also inhibit release of Prl, whereas administration of DA antagonists (e.g., pimozide, haloperidol, and perphenazine) will facilitate release of Prl. Detailed analyses of hypothalamic extracts have shown that most of the PIH activity in the extracts can be accounted for by the DA content of the extracts. Thus, though not totally conclusive, these results clearly suggest that DA does not inhibit release of Prl through the release of another PIH, but they fail to rule out the possibility that other endogenous biochemicals may have PIH activity.

Other recent results from the in vitro perfusion of dispersed cells from rat pituitaries described earlier suggest that DA inhibits the spontaneous release of Prl through a reduction in the steady influx of extracellular calcium. For example, the addition of calcium ionophores (chemical agents that facilitate the transmembrane diffusion of calcium) to the perfusion media containing DA was found to stimulate the release of Prl, thus overcoming the inhibition produced by DA. Not yet investigated in this in vitro perfusion system is the potential involvement of the influx of calcium on the DA-induced inhibition of the TRH-stimulated release of Prl. However, earlier studies have suggested that DA may inhibit release of Prl under these conditions through an inhibition of the increase in the activity of adenylate cyclase induced by TRH.

Other putative prolactin inhibitory hormones include the neurotransmitter γ-amino-butyric acid (GABA), and a recently discovered breakdown product of TRH, histidyl-proline-diketopiperazine. In a recent pharmacologic study with rats, evidence was gathered suggesting that DA was not involved in stress-induced release of Prl. Although not excluding the possible involvement of other PIHs, these data were presented as support for the existence of one or more facilitatory HHHs that may also be involved in the regulation of the release of Prl. Further details on these putative facilitatory HHHs are presented below.

C. PROLACTIN RELEASING HORMONE (PRH)

The tripeptide pyroglutamyl-histadyl-proline amide (pyroGlu-His-Pro-NH$_2$) usually is referred to as thyrotropin releasing hormone (TRH) (see Figure 7-13). TRH is also a very potent stimulator of the release of Prl both in vitro and in vivo. Had this property of TRH been observed first, it might have been called Prl releasing hormone (PRH). In humans the facilitation of the secretion of Prl by administration of TRH is clearly more dramatic in women than it is in men (see Figure 7-14). This difference in responsiveness probably is related to the known stimulatory effect of estradiol on the release of Prl (see Section 7-6).

FIGURE 7-13: The primary amino acid sequence for the peptide hypothalamic hypophysiotropic hormones TRH, Gn-RH (LH-RH), and somatostatin (GHIH or SRIH).

$$\text{pyroGLU-HIS-PRO-NH}_2$$

TRH

$$\text{pyroGLU-HIS-TRP-SER-TYR-GLY-LEU-ARG-PRO-GLY-NH}_2$$

GnRH

H-ALA-GLY-CYS-LYS-ASN-PHE-PHE-TRP-LYS-THR-PHE-THR-SER-CYS-OH

SOMATOSTATIN

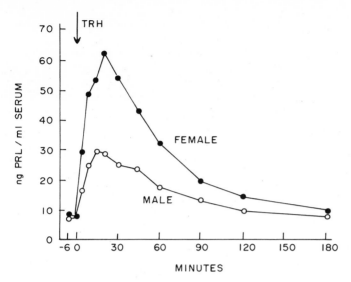

FIGURE 7-14: Concentrations of Prl in serum from men (lower curve) and women (upper curve) following an intravenous injection of thyrotropin releasing hormone (TRH). (*Adapted from:* Jacobs et al., 1973.)

Other hormones have also been shown to modify TRH-induced release of Prl. For example, as described further in Section 3-8 the thyroid hormones thyroxine (T_4) and triiodothyronine (T_3) can inhibit directly the TRH-induced release of TSH from the adenohypophysis. Since recent research with cultured pituitary cells suggests that this mechanism involves a reduction in the number of receptors for TRH found on the cell surface, it should not be too surprising that thyroid hormones can also inhibit the TRH-induced release of Prl from these cells. As mentioned earlier, the administration of L-DOPA can inhibit TRH-induced release of Prl in humans (see Figure 7-15).

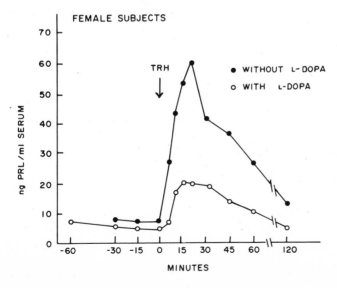

FIGURE 7-15: Concentrations of Prl in serum from women pretreated with or without L-DOPA. An intravenous injection of TRH was given at time zero. (*Adapted from:* Noel et al., 1974.)

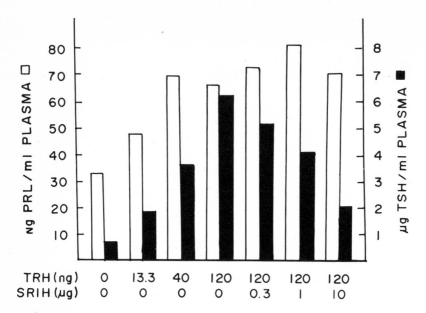

FIGURE 7-16: Dose-response study illustrating TRH-induced secretion of both TSH and Prl, and the inhibition of the secretion of the former, but not the later adenohypophyseal hormone by the administration of the HHH somatostatin (SRIH).

Finally, while the tetradecapeptide somatostatin (GHIH or SRIH) (see Figure 7-13), which originally was named for its ability to inhibit the release of growth hormone (GH) (see Section 8-5), can clearly inhibit TRH-induced release of TSH, it fails to have a similar inhibitory effect on TRH-induced release of Prl (see Figure 7-16). This latter dichotomy is potentially very important to the overall regulation of the release of Prl. For example, although suckling is a powerful stimulant for the release of Prl (see Figure 7-12), it does not stimulate the release of TSH. (Q. 7-42) *If the suckling-induced release of Prl is mediated by the inhibition of the release of PIH, combined with the facilitation of the release of PRH (i.e., TRH release), how can the body prevent the concomitant release of TSH?*

The discussion above clearly supports a role for TRH in the physiologic regulation of the secretion of Prl, but two important questions remain.

1. Although TRH is a sufficient stimulus for increased release of Prl, is it a required stimulant under any particular situation?
2. Although TRH can obviously act as a PRH, is there any reason to believe that it is the only endogenous HHH with PRH activity?

Obtaining a definitive answer to these questions has proved to be a difficult task. (Q. 7-43) *Can you suggest any possible experimental approaches to answering these questions?*

Other putative prolactin releasing hormones include several peptides found in brain tissue, including vasotocin (VIP), neurotensin, substance P, and the endogenous opiates (enkephalins). Since considerable controversy still surrounds some of the findings related to these putative PRHs, the student should use this list as a guide for future reading only.

SECTION 7-5: POST-TEST QUESTIONS

1. Gn-RH is a a. _____-peptide, TRH is a b. _____-peptide, and somatostatin (SRIH) is a c. _____-peptide; the principal candidate for PIH appears to be a d. _____-amine formed by the decarboxylation of e. _____.

2. Although the secretions of LH, FSH, ACTH, GH, and TSH from the adenohypophysis all appear to be regulated by the actions of a. (facilitatory/inhibitory) HHHs, the spontaneous (or tonic) secretion of Prl from the adenohypophysis appears to be regulated by the actions of b. (facilitatory/inhibitory) hormones.

3. Somatostatin a. (facilitates/inhibits) TRH-induced release of b. _____, but not TRH-induced release of c. _____.

4. DA is now thought to a. (facilitate/inhibit) the b. (spontaneous/TRH-induced) secretion of Prl from the lactotrope through c. (facilitation/inhibition) of the d. (influx/efflux) of e. (intracellular/extracellular) calcium. DA may still f. (facilitate/inhibit) the g. (spontaneous/TRH-induced) secretion of Prl from the lactotrope through h. (facilitation/inhibition) in the activity of a membrane-associated enzyme, i. _____.

5. What is the proposed mechanism for triiodothyronine-induced inhibition of TRH-stimulated secretion of Prl (and TSH) from cultured pituitary cells?

6. Both stress and suckling can a. (increase/decrease) the secretion of Prl from the adenohypophysis. DA is now thought to b. (increase/decrease/have no effect on) stress-induced secretion of Prl. It is now thought to c. (increase/decrease/have no effect on) the effects of suckling-induced secretion of Prl.

SECTION 7-5: POST-TEST ANSWERS

1. a. deca-
   b. tri-
   c. tetradeca-
   d. catechol-
   e. L-DOPA
2. a. facilitatory
   b. inhibitory
3. a. inhibits
   b. TSH
   c. Prl
4. a. inhibit
   b. spontaneous
   c. inhibition
   d. influx
   e. extracellular
   f. inhibit
   g. TRH-induced
   h. inhibition
   i. adenylate cyclase

5. Triiodothyronine (T_3) is now thought to reduce the number of receptors for TRH on the plasma membrane of the lactotrope (and the thyrotrope) cells.
6. a. increase
   b. have no effect on
   c. decrease

SECTION 7-6: PATTERNS OF SECRETION AND FEEDBACK REGULATION OF
   · **HORMONES ASSOCIATED WITH THE MENSTRUAL CYCLE OF THE**
      HUMAN FEMALE

OBJECTIVES:

The student should be able to:
   1. Describe the patterns of secretion of LH, FSH, Gn-RH, Prl, estrogen, and progesterone associated with the menstrual cycle of the human female.
   2. Describe the diurnal and/or sleep-associated secretory patterns for these hormones.
   3. Describe the negative and positive feedback regulation of the secretion of LH, FSH, and Prl during the menstrual cycle.
   4. Describe the involvement of neurotransmitters in the regulation of the secretion of LH, FSH, and Prl.

A. SECRETORY PATTERNS OF LH, FSH, Gn-RH, Prl, ESTROGEN, AND PROGESTERONE ASSOCIATED WITH THE MENSTRUAL CYCLE

The rather dramatic fluctuations in secretory patterns of ovarian and gonadotropic hormones that occur during the menstrual cycle were mentioned in Sections 7-3 and 7-4 as part of the discussion of the actions of these hormones on the ovaries and uterus. A more careful examination of grouped data (see Figure 7-17A) reveals clearly the predominant midcycle surge in the secretion of LH and FSH. Although the secretion of FSH is elevated slightly during the follicular phase (relative to the luteal phase), the secretion of LH is low uniformly throughout the cycle except for the peak at midcycle. Grouped data, however, do not reveal that the pattern of secretion of these hormones is actually pulsatile in individual women (see Figure 7-18). Even with these small pulses, the midcycle peak in secretion of gonadotropins is still quite evident in individual women (data not shown).

Examination of the concentration of Gn-RH in blood serum of humans also reveals a midcycle peak, although the variation between individuals is more pronounced and the overall magnitude of the peak less dramatic than that displayed by the gonadotropins (see Figure 7-17B).

The secretion of estradiol shows both a midcycle peak, which generally precedes the surge in the secretion of LH by approximately 1 day, and a more prolonged peak during the luteal phase (see Figure 7-17A). (Q. 7-44) *As described in Section 7-2, what is (are) the sources(s) of estrogen for the two major peaks in the concentration of estradiol in blood during the menstrual cycle?* The secretion of ovarian estrone also shows a small, but significant midcycle peak. In contrast to estradiol, the secretion of progesterone is segregated almost exclusively to the luteal phase of the cycle (see Figure 7-17A). Careful examination of the concentration of progesterone in the blood of women with ovulations certified retrospectively (blood drawn at 8-hour intervals), however, reveals that there is also a small preovulatory peak in the secretion of progesterone that begins to

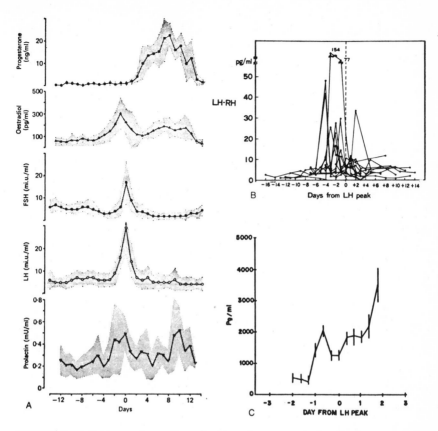

FIGURE 7-17: Patterns of secretion of various hormones during the human ovarian-menstrual cycle. A) Group data on the concentration of progesterone, estradiol, FSH, LH, and Prl. B) Individual data on the concentrations of LH–RH (Gn-RH) in blood and the range of concentrations of LH in the same women. C) Group data on the concentration of progesterone in blood from women in whom ovulation was later established. Note the small preovulatory peak in the secretion of progesterone. (Source: Groom, 1977; Miyake et al., 1980; Laborde et al., 1976.)

increase approximately 22 hours before the surge in the secretion of LH and reaches its acme at approximately 10 hours before the peak in the secretion of LH (see Figure 7-17C). (Q. 7-45) *What is the cellular origin of this progesterone?*

Recent studies have indicated that Prl may also display a menstrual pattern of secretion, typified by peaks in the midcycle and late luteal phases (see Figure 7-17A). It should be noted, however, that the secretion of Prl is much more variable than that displayed by the gonadotropins, although there does seem to be a reasonable relationship between the patterns of secretion of Prl and estrogen. (Q. 7-46) *Based on your knowledge of the various stimuli (both endogenous and exogenous) that may modify the rate of secretion of Prl, can you suggest why the secretion of Prl appears to be much more variable than the secretion of LH during the menstrual cycle?*

Analyses of the concentration of hormones in blood throughout the day have revealed that during the pubertal, but not pre- or postpubertal periods, there are clear sleep-associated peaks in the secretion of LH (see Figure 7-18). A similar sleep-associated peak in the secretion of LH during the pubertal period of the male was described in Section 6-5. The concentration of Prl in blood displays a highly significant increase in

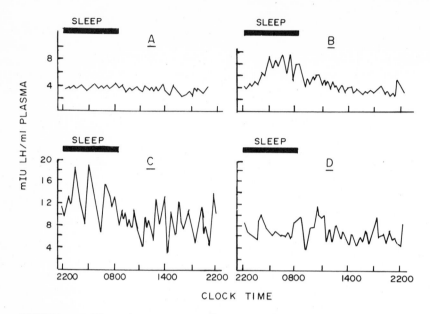

FIGURE 7-18: The 24-hour pattern in the concentration of LH in blood from a representative prepubertal girl (A), an early pubertal girl (B), a later pubertal girl (C), and a young woman (D). Note the pulsatile secretory patterns. (*Adapted from:* Weitzman et al., 1975.)

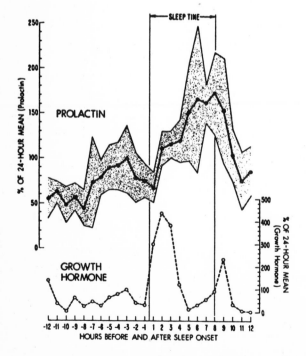

FIGURE 7-19: Concentration of Prl in blood from a group of normal adults during a 24-hour period. Note the sleep-associated peak in Prl and GH secretion. (*Source:* Sassin et al., 1972.)

secretion during the normal nighttime sleeping period (see Figure 7-19). In contrast to LH, the sleep-associated peak in secretion of Prl is observed throughout life, and if the sleeping period is shifted, the peak in the secretion of Prl is likewise shifted regardless of whether there is a similar shift in the light cycle. (*Q. 7-47*) *What would happen to the 24-hour pattern of secretion of ACTH and cortisol under the same two conditions?*

B. FEEDBACK REGULATION OF THE SECRETION OF LH, FSH, AND Gn-RH

As described in Section 6-5, the concentrations of gonadotropins in blood are controlled to a large extent in humans by the negative and positive feedback actions of the gonadal hormones. For example, although the concentration of LH and FSH in plasma from women increases dramatically following ovariectomy, this response can be reversed effectively by the negative feedback actions of exogenously administered estrogen and progesterone. This rather simplistic description of a negative feedback control system cannot, of course, fully explain the relatively consistent, sequentially or concomitantly interrelated *increases and decreases* in the secretion and concentrations in blood of LH, FSH, Prl, estradiol, and progesterone observed during the ovarian-menstrual cycle.

Considerable progress has been made toward an understanding of these negative and positive feedback actions through studies utilizing the female rhesus monkey. The approximately 28-day ovarian-menstrual cycle of secretion of estrogen, progestin, LH, and FSH displayed by these monkeys is strikingly similar to that observed in the human. For example, administration of estrogen to the rhesus monkey during the follicular phase of the menstrual cycle results in a prompt decrease in the concentration of LH and FSH in plasma (i.e., negative feedback) followed by a rather dramatic increase in their concentrations (i.e., positive feedback; see Figure 7-20A). These increases in the concentration of LH and FSH in blood is often equivalent to those displayed during their spontaneous midcycle surges. Pretreatment with relatively high doses of progesterone clearly inhibits the positive, but not the negative feedback actions of estrogen (see Figure 7-20C). The observation that the estrogen-induced surge in the secretion of

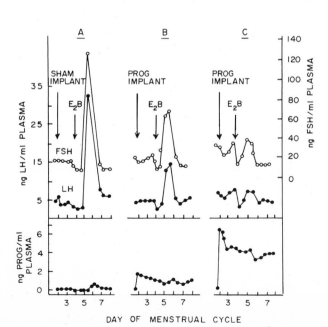

FIGURE 7-20: Plasma concentrations of LH and FSH in female rhesus monkeys receiving subcutaneous implants of Silastic® capsules containing increasing amounts of progesterone (i.e., panels A, B, and C, respectively) followed by acute subcutaneous injections of the powerful synthetic estrogen estradiol benzoate (EB). Plasma concentrations of progesterone are given in the lower portion of each panel. Treatment was initiated during the follicular phase of the ovarian-menstrual cycle. Note the progesterone-induced inhibition of the positive but not the negative feedback effects of EB on plasma concentrations of LH and FSH. (*Adapted from:* Knobil, 1974.)

gonadotropins is inhibited by progesterone forms the basic principle by which the oral contraceptive agents containing estrogen and progesterone protect users against pregnancy. Since very similar results can also be obtained in monkeys subjected to combined ovariectomy and adrenalectomy (to remove the source of all endogenous estrogen and progestin), it is apparent that both the surge in the secretion of LH and FSH during the midcycle phase and the depression in the secretion of these gonadotropins during the luteal phase can be mimicked by recreating an increase in the concentrations of both estrogen and progestin in blood similar to those observed during the last portion of the follicular phase. (*Q. 7-48*) *What effect could this type of treatment paradigm have on the probability of ovulation (and pregnancy) in women with primary (i.e., ovarian origin) hypogonadism?*

The foregoing explanation seems to account for the obvious fluctuations in the secretion of gonadotropin during the ovarian-menstrual cycle, but it fails to provide a role for Gn-RH and for the known differences in the rates of secretion of gonadotropins during different portions of the cycle. For example, although the infusion of Gn-RH in women always results in a biphasic increase in concentrations of gonadotropins in blood similar to that described for men in Section 6-4, the relative magnitude of the amount of LH (and FSH) released both earlier and later during the period of infusion varies at different portions of the cycle (see Figure 7-21). These data have been interpreted as reflecting the differences in the relative sizes of "release" and "synthesis-storage" pools of gonadotropins within the adenohypophyseal gonadotropes. In addition there are differences in the ability of Gn-RH to stimulate the release and the transfer of LH (and FSH) from the synthesis-storage pool to the release pool during various phases of the menstrual cycle (see Figure 7-22).

FIGURE 7-21: Changes in the concentration of LH in serum from women during various portions of the ovarian-menstrual cycle in response to a 4-hour infusion of Gn-RH. The amount of LH released during the first hour of infusion represents the magnitude of the "release" pool of LH, while the amount released during the 3 subsequent hours represents the magnitude of the "synthesis-storage" pool of LH. (*Source:* Hoff et al., 1977.)

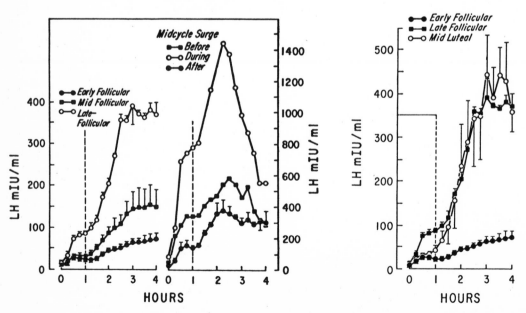

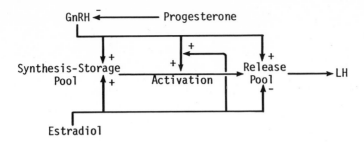

FIGURE 7-22: The effects of estradiol, progesterone, and GnRH on the synthesis, storage, and release of LH in women. Estradiol facilitates the synthesis of LH and the GnRH-activated transfer of LH from the synthesis-storage pool to the release pool, although it retains negative feedback actions on the tonic release of LH and possibly on the synthesis and/or release of GnRH. Progesterone inhibits the synthesis and/or release of GnRH, which in turn facilitates the synthesis of LH and the transfer of LH from the synthesis-storage pool to the release pool. Once in the release pool, Gn-RH facilitates the release of LH. (*Adapted from:* Yen, 1977.)

During the early portion of the follicular phase, when the concentration of estrogen in plasma is low, there is little release of LH during both the first hour of Gn-RH infusion (a reflection of the size of the release pool), and during the subsequent 3 hours (a reflection of the size of the synthesis-storage pool) (see Figure 7-21). As the concentration of estrogen in blood rises during the mid- and late-follicular phase in response to FSH-stimulated ovarian steroidogenesis (see Sections 7-2 and 7-3), the synthesis-storage pool grows much more dramatically than the release pool. However, during midcycle, the magnitude of the amount of LH released during the first hour of infusion of Gn-RH is greater than that released during the last 3 hours of infusion. Thus, at the time of the normal spontaneous surge in the secretion of gonadotropins during midcycle there is comparatively more LH (and FSH) in the release pool of the gonadotrope than during the preceding portions of the cycle. It is important to note that the comparatively large amounts of LH released in response to infusion of Gn-RH during the spontaneous midcycle surge in the secretion of gonadotropins cannot be maintained throughout the entire 4 hours of the infusion. These findings suggest that administration of exogenous Gn-RH increases the rate of release of LH to a level that exceeds the rate of replacement of LH in the synthesis-storage pool. These data also suggest that administration of estrogen stimulates both the synthesis of LH and its transfer from the synthesis-storage pool to the release pool (see Figure 7-22).

During the luteal phase of the cycle, the response to infusion of Gn-RH indicates that the synthesis-storage pool of LH has returned to the level observed during the late follicular phase, while the release pool has decreased to the level observed during the early follicular phase. The last result is especially interesting because the concentration of estrogen in blood during the luteal phase is also elevated considerably (see Figures 7-5 and 7-17A). But why is there no surge in the secretion of LH and FSH at this time, as there is at midcycle? It appears at present that prolonged elevation of the concentration of progesterone in blood inhibits the synthesis and/or the release of Gn-RH from the hypothalamus during the luteal phase of the cycle (see Figures 7-5 and 7-22). (*Q.* 7-49) *Can women ovulate during pregnancy? Why or why not?*

The site(s) of action for the feedback effects of estrogen and progesterone, as well as the regions of the brain controlling the synthesis and release of Gn-RH, have yet to be considered in this discussion. In studies in female rhesus monkeys it has been shown that the patterns of adenohypophyseal secretion of LH and FSH (both pulsatile and surge) continue in a near-normal fashion following lesions that remove all neural input to the hypothalamus. Thus, extrahypothalamic input to the hypothalamus in female rhesus monkeys does not appear to be required for the negative and positive feedback regulation of the secretion of gonadotropins by ovarian hormones. This situation contrasts sharply with that observed in laboratory rodents, in which input to the hypothalamus from preoptic, amygdaloid, and other extrahypothalamic regions of the brain appears to be very important in mediating the positive and, to a much lesser extent, negative feedback actions of ovarian steroids on the secretion of gonadotropins. If the lesions are extended to include the entire hypothalamus, thereby removing the endogenous sources of Gn-RH that normally have access to the adenohypophysis via the portal system, the concentrations of both FSH and LH in blood decrease precipitously and are unresponsive to priming with estrogen in female rhesus monkeys (see Figure 7-23) and in female laboratory rodents (data not shown). (*Q. 7-50*) *Would these lesions destroy all the nuclei in the brain that have been reported to contain Gn-RH?* (*Q. 7-51*) *What should happen to the spontaneous release of Prl in humans with lesions similar to these?*

If monkeys with lesions of the entire hypothalamus are given a chronic intermittent intravenous infusion of Gn-RH, one can observe some rather remarkable effects on the secretion of the gonadotropins. For example, basal concentrations of LH and FSH in the blood of these monkeys begins to rise in a matter of days. Even more surprising, it is then possible to stimulate an unambiguous surge in the secretion of LH and FSH following priming with estrogen (see Figure 7-23). As in the nonlesioned animal (see Figure 7-20), this surge in the secretion of gonadotropins is preceded by a rapid

FIGURE 7-23: Concentrations of LH and FSH in serum from female rhesus monkeys before and after a lesion destroyed all hypothalamic tissue involved in the synthesis and secretion of Gn-RH. The effects of priming with estrogen (upper panel) before, during, and after the chronic intermittent intravenous infusion of Gn-RH (LH-RH) are also shown. Note that in spite of the lesion, the administration of estradiol is still capable of eliciting both a negative and a positive feedback influence on the secretion of gonadotropin, provided replacement therapy with Gn-RH has also been initiated. (*Source:* Nakai et al., 1978.)

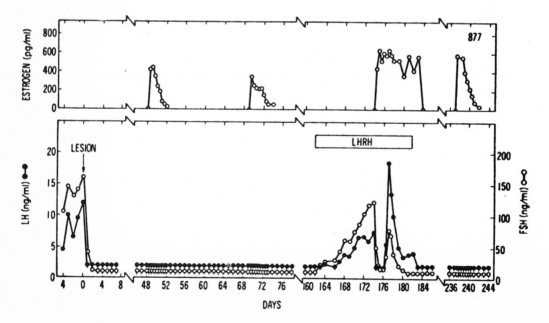

transient decline in the secretion of these hormones (i.e., negative feedback). Attempts to replicate these results by means of a constant infusion of Gn-RH failed. (*Q. 7-52*) *Why do you think this form of replacement therapy was ineffective?* Following the termination of the intermittent intravenous infusion of Gn-RH, priming with estrogen is again ineffective in stimulating a positive feedback-induced surge in the secretion of gonadotropin. It is also interesting to note that the surges in secretion of LH and FSH are apparently self-terminating in that in spite of continued stimulation by Gn-RH and estrogen, the increased secretion of gonadotropins only lasts a few days (see Figure 7-23). (*Q. 7-53*) *Can you think of any reasons for this?* (*Q. 7-54*) *Can you recall any other examples of hormonal secretion that are apparently self-terminating in spite of continued stimulation by the appropriate tropic hormone?*

Thus, it is apparent that the concentration of estrogen in blood can exert both positive and negative feedback actions at the level of the pituitary in the female rhesus monkey. This does not necessarily rule out the possibility that estrogen has additional actions at the level of the hypothalamus. Furthermore, as described earlier, progesterone appears to exert at least some of its negative feedback actions at the level of the hypothalamus as reflected in humans by its inhibition of the synthesis and/or release of Gn-RH. Studies in laboratory rodents, and more recently in bonnet monkeys, have shown that estrogen increases the de novo synthesis of cytoplasmic receptors for progestins within the hypothalamus. Thus, estrogen may act in a similar way in the hypothalamus of humans and thereby regulate the negative feedback actions of progesterone and/or its metabolites.

The exact mechanisms of the positive and negative feedback actions of estrogen in the pituitary are unclear at present. They may involve either an alteration in the number or affinity of receptors for Gn-RH on the gonadotropes and/or an alteration in the postreceptor responsiveness to Gn-RH (e.g., an alteration in the relative efficiency of stimulation of protein kinase). (*Q. 7-55*) *Can you think of any other possibilities?*

C. FEEDBACK REGULATION OF THE SECRETION OF FSH: POTENTIAL ROLE OF FOLLICULOSTATIN

Studies with laboratory rodents have provided increasing evidence for the existence of a nonsteroidal, trypsin- and heat-labile compound that inhibits the secretion of FSH while at the same time having little effect on the secretion of LH. This compound, often referred to as folliculostatin, has a molecular weight of a least 10,000 daltons. It appears to be analogous (and possibly similar chemically) to inhibin, the compound that inhibits the release of FSH and is found in males (see Section 6-5). (*Q. 7-56*) *Where is inhibin synthesized in males?* Folliculostatin appears to be synthesized by the ovarian granulosa cells, found in high concentrations in follicular fluid and effective in inhibiting the release of FSH by a direct action on adenohypophyseal gonadotropes. The concentration of folliculostatin in blood obtained from female rats has recently been shown to be inversely proportional to the concentration of FSH. These and other findings suggest, but clearly do not establish, an apparent causal relation between the increased rate of secretion of folliculostatin and the decreased rate of secretion of FSH. The potential role of folliculostatin in the feedback regulation of the secretion of FSH in the human female remains unexplored.

D. FEEDBACK REGULATION OF THE SECRETION OF Prl

The hormonal regulation of the secretion of Prl appears to involve the actions of a number of hormones including the direct actions of PIHs (e.g., DA) and PRHs (e.g., TRH) on the adenohypophyseal lactotropes, the positive and negative effects of ovarian steroids representing the long feedback loop, and the negative effects of Prl itself, representing the short feedback loop.

As described earlier (see Figure 7-17A), the variations in the concentration of both Prl and estradiol in blood during the ovarian-menstrual cycle seem to be correlated positively. Thus, estradiol exerts a positive feedback influence on the tonic secretion of Prl. This is further evidenced by the fact that ovariectomy results in a decrease in the tonic secretion of Prl, whereas replacement therapy with exogenous estradiol results in a restoration, or even a dose-dependent overshoot, in the tonic rate of secretion of Prl. The administration of exogenous estradiol also increases the magnitude of the Prl released in response to the administration of TRH. Although these findings suggest clearly that estradiol can facilitate the secretion of Prl, they do not delineate the site or sites at which the positive feedback effects are elicited. Research conducted with laboratory animals has established that estradiol has the potential to increase the secretion of Prl through an action both in the brain and in the adenohypophysis.

The evidence that estradiol exerts part of its facilitatory actions on the secretion of Prl at the level of the hypothalamus comes from a variety of sources. There is solid data for the existence of high-affinity, limited-capacity cytosolic and nuclear receptors for estradiol in neurons in the arcuate nucleus, which synthesize and secrete DA into the portal vasculature. Estradiol also binds to intracellular receptors in other neurons in this region of the brain that do not appear to produce catecholamines but may influence the secretion of DA (or other PIHs or PRHs) through their synaptic interactions. Estradiol given systemically can affect the turnover of catecholamines in the hypothalamus.

In a recent study with female rats it was shown that the concentration of DA in blood collected from severed infundibular portal vessels decreased following the systemic administration of estradiol, while the concentration of DA in subsequent blood samples increased after the administration of progesterone. When systemic blood from female rats was treated with a similar regimen of exogenous steroids, but not subjected to collection of portal blood (both groups of rats were subjected to acute ovariectomy during the late follicular phase of the ovarian cycle), it was found that the concentrations of Prl were inversely proportional to the presumed concentrations of DA in portal blood. This suggests clearly that these two estradiol-induced effects (i.e., the decreased rate of release of DA into the portal vasculature and the increased rate of secretion of Prl from the adenohypophysis) are causally related.

The evidence for estradiol exerting part of its facilitatory actions on the secretion of Prl at the level of the pituitary also comes from a variety of sources. High-affinity, limited-capacity intracellular receptors have been found in the lactotropes of female rats. Estradiol given systemically to female rhesus monkeys subjected previously to a transection of the infundibular stalk facilitates the tonic release of Prl (see Figure 7-24). (Q. 7-57) What effect would this operation have on the tonic release of Prl and LH in these monkeys before the administration of estradiol? The magnitude of the TRH-induced release of Prl was also increased following transection of the infundibular stalk (see Figure 7-24). However, since the effect of TRH (at the dose used in this study) appears to be limited to a four-fold increase in the secretion of Prl over the baseline or tonic levels of secretion in females with and without an exogenous source of estradiol, these stimulatory effects may be simply the result of an increase in the amount of Prl available for release in response to TRH.

Recent studies with pituitary primary cell cultures have shown that estradiol can prevent the inhibition of Prl secretion induced by DA and that this steroid can also increase the de novo synthesis of Prl directly through an interaction with the chromatin material in the cultured lactotropes. Since progesterone has been shown to inhibit both of the latter actions of estradiol, it is clear that this steroid can also have direct actions

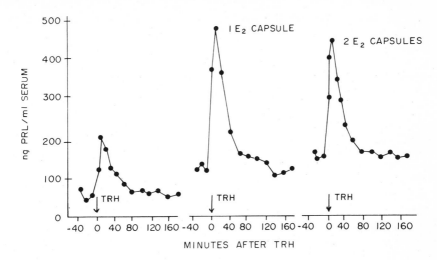

FIGURE 7-24: Changes in concentrations of Prl in blood samples taken from female rhesus monkeys (subjected previously to a transection of the infundibular stalk) following intravenous injection of TRH (at the positions indicated with arrows). Females were also implanted with none, one, or two Silastic® capsules containing estradiol (E_2). Note the change in the baseline or tonic levels of prolactin concentrations in the blood samples after the administration of estradiol. Also note the increase in the magnitude of the effects of TRH on the secretion of Prl. (*Q. 7-58*) *Why are the TRH-induced effects so transient?* (*Adapted from:* Ferin, 1979.)

on the lactotrope that indirectly (i.e., via an inhibition of the actions of estradiol) inhibit the synthesis and secretion of Prl.

A very recent clinical study with young women exhibiting normal menstrual cycles has suggested that 2-OH-estrone, a catechol estrogen produced in the human brain by the 2-hydroxylation of estrone (see Figure 7-6), may play a significant role in the negative feedback suppression of the secretion of Prl. The infusion of this steroid was reported to produce a rapid and profound decrease in the secretion of Prl in most of the volunteer subjects. Although site of mechanism of action for this effect has not been established for the human female, there are several viable possibilities suggested from the literature on studies with female rats and other laboratory species. Catechol estrogens can compete with estradiol for binding to the limited-capacity, intracellular, high-affinity receptors in the hypothalamus and pituitary, they can bind directly to plasma membranes isolated from the hypothalamus and pituitary, and they can compete (n.b., better than any other known endogenous biochemical) with other substrates for the enzyme catechol-O-methyltransferase (COMT). (*Q. 7-59*) *What effect could the latter action have on the local concentrations of endogenous catecholamines such as DA?*

These rather provocative findings suggest that regulation of the secretion of Prl in the human female may be mediated in large part by the positive and negative interactions of two naturally occurring estrogens, estradiol and 2-OH-estrone, by way of the long feedback loop. In light of this possibility, it is relevant to point out that the systemic administration of opiate agonists, which results in an increase in the secretion of Prl, inhibits the activity of estradiol-2-hydroxylase in rat brain, whereas the systematic administration of opiate antagonists, which results in a decrease in the secretion of Prl, facilitates the activity of this enzyme. Since the endogenous opiates (i.e., enkephalins and endorphins) may be involved in the neurotransmitter regulation of the secretion of Prl (see below), these effects on the synthesis of 2-OH-estrone take on added significance. The long-term importance of the catechol estrogens in clinical medicine remains to be clarified, but the student should pay particular attention to these biochemicals in future reading.

The evidence that Prl may regulate its own secretion through a short negative feedback loop on PIH and/or PRH is derived from recent anatomic studies with humans and with nonhuman primates and from recent physiologic studies with laboratory rodents. The anatomic evidence (discussed in detail in Section 2-1) is centered around the following observations:

1. The hypothalamopituitary portal blood flow is bidirectional.
2. There is a recirculation of blood within and between the adenohypophysis and the neurohypophysis.
3. The superior-lateral localization of most Prl secreting microadenomas (i.e., small tumors) suggests that normal lactotropes should release Prl in the region of the pituitary, which appears to be preferentially drained through the superior-proximal neurohypophysis and as such should be preferentially available for transport to the hypothalamus in the portal capillaries.

The physiologic evidence is centered around the following observations:

1. Exogenous Prl applied directly to the basal hypothalamus reduces the tonic secretion of Prl. (Q. 7-60) *Do you think that this effect is due to a lesion in the hypothalamus produced by the cannula?*
2. Prl injected systemically increases DA turnover within the basal hypothalamus.
3. Neurohypophysectomy reduces the concentration of Prl (but not that of LH or TSH) in systemic blood. This effect is thought to be the result of the interruption of the normal routes of exit of Prl (i.e., via the neurohypophysis) from the adenohypophysis to the systemic circulation and to the hypothalamus (see Section 2-1).

The physiologic significance of this putative short feedback loop in the regulation of the secretion of Prl in humans remains to be established.

E. INVOLVEMENT OF NEUROTRANSMITTERS IN THE SECRETION OF LH, FSH, AND Prl

The precise nature of the involvement of neurotransmitters in the regulation of the secretion of the HHHs that control the secretion of the gonadotropins and Prl is still very controversial, especially in humans. Studies in which L-DOPA was administered to humans either orally or through an intravenous infusion have shown that this precursor of the neurotransmitter dopamine can clearly inhibit the secretion of Prl and LH, but not FSH (see Figure 7-25). The inhibition of the secretion of Prl would, of course be expected, since DA appears to be a PIH and as such should be able to inhibit directly the secretion of Prl from the adenohypophysis. DA does not inhibit the increased secretion of LH following the administration of Gn-RH. Thus, it seems likely that the inhibitory actions of L-DOPA were due to inhibition of the synthesis and/or secretion of Gn-RH rather than to inhibition of the action of this HHH at the level of the adenohypophysis.

The fact that the secretion of FSH was not inhibited to the same extent as that for LH raises two obvious questions.

1. Does the administration of L-DOPA inhibit the synthesis and/or secretion of Gn-RH (LH-RH) while at the same time failing to inhibit these properties for an as yet uncharacterized FSH-RH?
2. Is it possible that the secretion of FSH is more sensitive than the secretion of LH to the facilitatory actions of Gn-RH?

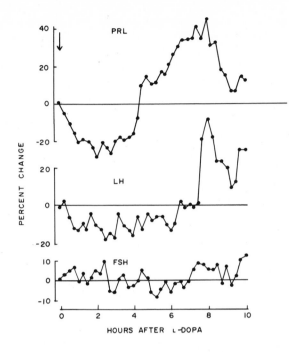

FIGURE   7-25: Mean   percentage changes from the basal concentrations in serum for Prl, LH, and FSH following the oral administration of L-DOPA. The six women represented by these data were normal endocrinologically and were in the early follicular phase of the ovarian-menstrual cycle when L-DOPA was administered. (*Adapted from:* Lachelin, et al., 1977.)

With regard to the second question, a reduction in the amount of Gn-RH reaching the adenohypophysis could potentially have a greater effect on the secretion of LH than on the secretion of FSH because the secretion of FSH may be maintained with lower concentrations of Gn-RH in portal blood than the secretion of LH. Definitive answers to these questions have not been found. (*Q. 7-61*) *How might you examine these questions experimentally?* It is also interesting to note that following the cessation of infusion with L-DOPA (data not shown), or 4 to 8 hours after oral administration of L-DOPA (see Figure 7-25), there is a rebound in the concentrations of LH and Prl in blood to levels greater than those measured before the administration of L-DOPA. (*Q. 7-62*) *What does this period of hypersecretion suggest to you regarding the possible mechanisms by which the administration of L-DOPA inhibits the secretion of LH and Prl in the human female?*

There is a considerable amount of data supporting the contention that serotonin (5-HT) synapses are somehow involved in facilitating the release of a PRH that in turn facilitates the release of Prl. For example, the oral administration of precursors to 5-HT (e.g., L-tryptophan and 5-OH-tryptophan) has been shown to increase the concentration of Prl in blood, whereas the oral administration of drugs that block the action of 5-HT at its receptors on postsynaptic membranes (e.g., methysergide and metergoline) decreases the concentration of Prl in blood. The concentrations of LH and FSH in blood samples from these subjects were not usually altered by these procedures. The demonstration that administration of methysergide to rhesus monkeys can block the increased secretion of Prl induced by the electrical stimulation of the basal hypothalamus but not by the administration of TRH is consistent with the theory that 5-HT synapses facilitate the secretion of a PRH other than TRH. In vitro studies have shown that 5-HT has no direct effect on the tonic secretion of Prl, thus further supporting a neurotransmitter role rather than an HHH role for 5-HT.

Recent studies examining the possible neuroendocrine roles of the endogenous opiates have suggested that the endorphins and enkephalins may be involved in both suckling- and stress-induced increases in the secretion of Prl. Infusions of naloxone, a specific opiate antagonist, inhibited the nocturnal increase in the secretion of Prl in a recent study with six healthy postmenopausal women, suggesting that the endogenous opiates may be involved in regulating the sleep-associated peaks in Prl secretion (see, e.g., Figure 7-19) in humans. Since many of these effects of the endogenous opiates appear to be mediated through a modulation in the synthesis and/or secretion of DA and 5-HT, it is likely that these biochemicals act at synapses other than those that regulate the secretion of PIH and PRH directly. Recent studies have also suggested that GABA may be involved in stimulating the release of PRH and Gn-RH.

It has also been observed recently that electrical stimulation of the amygdala (an extrahypothalamic region of the brain often categorized as belonging to a group of brain structures referred to as the "limbic system") in humans can produce a significant rise in the concentration of Prl in blood, without producing concomitant increases in the concentrations of LH, FSH, GH, and TSH. This result further suggests that one or more of the aforementioned neurotransmitters may be involved in mediating the secretion of PRH and/or PIH in humans.

SECTION 7-6: POST-TEST QUESTIONS

1. In addition to the relative sizes of the midcycle increases in the secretion of LH and FSH [i.e., the peak in the secretion of a. _____ is bigger than that observed normally for b. _____], the secretion of c. _____ during the d. _____ phase of the ovarian-menstrual cycle exceeds that observed during the e. _____ phase, while the secretion of f. _____ is uniformly low during both phases of the cycle.

2. The secretion of estradiol increases to a peak twice during the ovarian-menstrual cycle, the first peak is relatively sharp and a. (precedes/follows) the midcycle peak in the secretion of LH by approximately b. _____ hours. The second peak in the secretion of estradiol is relatively c. _____ and is positioned d. (at the beginning/in the middle/at the end) of the e. _____ phase.

3. Recent studies with humans have revealed that progesterone also has two peaks in its pattern of secretion. The first peak is a. (bigger than/smaller than/the same size as) the second peak. The first peak b. (precedes/follows) the midcycle peak in the secretion of LH by approximately c. _____ hours. The second peak is positioned d. (at the beginning/in the middle/at the end) of the e. _____ phase of the menstrual cycle.

4. The secretion of Prl in women also appears to have two peaks, one during the a. _____ and one during the b. _____. The occurrence of these two peaks in the secretion of Prl correlates roughly with the occurrence of peaks in the secretion of c. _____.

5. During the pubertal period of ontogenesis, the concentrations of both LH and Prl in blood have been shown to increase during a. _____, but only the secretion of b. _____ displays these peaks during adulthood.

6. Experiments with female rhesus monkeys have revealed that pretreatment with relatively high doses of progesterone inhibits the a. (positive/negative), but not the b. (positive/negative) feedback actions of c. _____ on the secretion of the d. _____.

7. Studies with female rats have suggested that progesterone may a. (facilitate/inhibit/have no effect) on the b. (facilitatory/inhibitory) effects of estradiol on the secretion

of Prl. The sites of action for these effects of progesterone appear to be c. _____
_____; the site(s) for the actions of estradiol appear(s) to be
d. _____.

8. Why do the high concentrations of estradiol in blood from women during the luteal
phase of the menstrual cycle fail to elicit a rapid increase in the secretion of LH (i.e.,
similar to the peak in the secretion of LH observed during midcycle)?

9. As the time of the midcycle rapid increase in the secretion of LH approaches, the
size of the hypothetical a. _____ pool of LH b. (increases/decreases)
relatively more rapidly than that of the c. _____ pool of LH.
Estrogen appears to be required for the LH-RH-mediated transfer of LH from the
d. _____ pool to the e. _____ pool.

10. A recent series of studies with female rhesus monkeys has shown that following a
massive lesion of the basal hypothalamus, the positive feedback effects of estrogen
on the secretion of LH are lost unless the animals are pretreated with _____
_____.

11. What is the proposed cellular origin of folliculostatin, and what role has been
proposed for it?

12. Estrogen appears to increase the amount of Prl released from the pituitary in
response to the administration of TRH by increasing the number and/or activity of
the receptors for TRH on the lactotropes. (True/False)

13. Recent studies conducted on humans and laboratory species have suggested that
the positive and negative long feedback actions of estrogen may be mediated by an
alternation in the enzyme a. _____, which converts
estradiol (and estrone) to its b. _____ derivative.

14. In addition to the direct actions of PRH and PIH, and the long feedback loop actions
of estradiol and a. _____ estrone, the secretion of Prl is thought to be
regulated at least in part by the b. _____ feedback actions of
c. _____.

15. Recent clinical studies on the factors regulating the secretion of the gonadotropins
and Prl have suggested that the neurotransmitter a. _____ inhibits the
release of the HHHs b. _____, while the neurotransmitter c. _____
_____ probably facilitates the release of the HHH d. _____.

SECTION 7-6: POST-TEST ANSWERS

1. a. LH
   b. FSH
   c. FSH
   d. follicular
   e. luteal
   f. LH
2. a. precedes
   b. 24 hours

   c. prolonged
   d. in the middle
   e. luteal
3. a. smaller than
   b. precedes
   c. 10 to 22 hours
   d. in the middle
   e. luteal
4. a. midcycle region
   b. luteal phase
   c. estradiol
5. a. sleep
   b. Prl
6. a. positive
   b. negative
   c. estradiol
   d. gonadotropins
7. a. inhibit
   b. facilitatory
   c. both the hypothalamus and the pituitary
   d. also at the level of both the hypothalamus and the pituitary
8. The high concentrations of progesterone in blood are thought to inhibit the release of Gn-RH from the hypothalamus. The actions of this steroid appear to be at the level of the hypothalamus, since it does not inhibit the increased secretion of LH induced by the administration of exogenous Gn-RH.
9. a. release
   b. increases
   c. storage-synthesis
   d. storage-synthesis
   e. release
10. a chronic intermittent intravenous infusion of Gn-RH.
11. Folliculostatin is thought to be synthesized by the ovarian granulosa cells. It is thought to act at the level of the pituitary to inhibit preferentially the secretion of FSH.
12. False. It appears to increase the pool of Prl that is available for TRH-induced release.
13. a. estradiol-2-hydroxylase
    b. catechol (or 2-OH-)
14. a. catechol
    b. negative short
    c. Prl
15. a. DA
    b. Gn-RH
    c. 5-HT
    d. PRH

SELECTED REFERENCES

Buster, J. E., and Marshall, J. R., 1979, Conception, gamete and ovum transport, implantation, fetal-placental hormones, hormonal preparation for parturition, and parturition control, in Endocrinology, L. J. DeGroot, G. F. Cahill, Jr., L. Martini, D. H. Nelsen, W. D. Odell, J. T. Potts, Jr., E. Steinberber and A. I. Winegrad (Eds.), New York: Grune & Stratton, Vol. 3, p. 1595.

Jaffe, R. B. and Monroe, S. E., 1980, Hormone interaction and regulation during the menstrual cycle, in *Frontiers In Neuroendocrinology*, L. Martini and W. F. Ganong (Eds.), New York: Raven Press, p. 219.

Knobil, E., 1980, The neuroendocrine control of the menstrual cycle, *Recent Progress In Hormone Research* 36: 53.

Neill, J. D., 1980, Neuroendocrine regulation of prolactin secretion, in *Frontiers In Neuroendocrinology*, L. Martini and W. F. Ganong (Eds.), New York: Raven Press, p. 129.

Ojeda, S. R., Andrews, W. W., Advis, J. P., and White, S. S., 1980, Recent advances in the endocrinology of puberty, *Endocrine Reviews* 1: 228.

8

GROWTH HORMONE, SOMATOMEDINS, AND SOMATOSTATIN

SECTION 8-1: CHEMICAL CHARACTERISTICS OF GROWTH HORMONE

OBJECTIVES:

The student should be able to:

1. State which tropic hormone is present in the largest amount in the human pituitary gland.
2. State whether the content of growth hormone in the pituitary gland changes with age.
3. Describe some of the chemical characteristics of growth hormone.
4. State whether growth hormone is species specific and describe the consequence of this property for humans.

Removal of the pituitary gland results not only in loss of the tropic hormones controlling the thyroid, adrenals, and gonads, but also in failure to grow. The latter effect can be attributed to the loss of growth hormone or somatotropin. This is the most abundant tropic hormone in the pituitary: 5 to 10 mg of it can be extracted from a single human pituitary gland. This means that from 5% to 8% of the weight of a single pituitary gland is growth hormone. The content does not appear to decline with age.

Human growth hormone is a single chain polypeptide with a molecular weight of 22,000 daltons. It contains 191 amino acids, 2 disulfide bridges, and an α-helical configuration (see Figure 8-1). The disulfide bridges can be reduced without apparent loss of biologic activity. In its chemical structure, growth hormone differs only slightly from pituitary prolactin and human placental lactogen (the latter is secreted by the placenta during pregnancy). Both contain 191 amino acid residues, 2 disulfide bridges, and an α-helical configuration. Both prolactin and placental lactogen have 161 of their amino acids in the same sequence as is found in the growth hormone molecule. The presence of structural similarities between growth hormones and the lactogenic hormones in a number of mammalian species suggests that these hormones may have a common evolutionary origin. (*Q. 8-1*) *How would you expect these structural features to influence the development of a specific radioimmunoassay for growth hormone?*

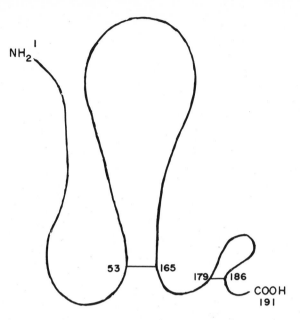

FIGURE   8-1: Two-dimensional representation of the human growth hormone molecule. Disulfide bridges occur between C-53 and C-165 and between C-179 and C-186.

In spite of similarities of structure in the pituitary growth hormones of various mammalian species, there appears to be a species specificity in their biologic action. Only growth hormone extracted from the pituitary glands of primates can stimulate growth in hypopituitary humans, although primate growth hormone can stimulate growth in most subprimate mammalian species. Because of the species specificity of growth hormone, its relatively high concentration in human pituitary glands, and the impracticability at present of synthesizing so large a molecule, pituitaries generally are removed at autopsy and sent to a central processing laboratory where growth hormone is extracted. The human growth hormone available for use in patients is obtained from processed human pituitary glands. Currently some success has been reported in the synthesis of growth hormone by certain bacteria. If this process becomes feasible commercially, it will eliminate the need to collect human pituitary glands. In addition we see in a later section that the somatomedins, which are growth hormone-dependent peptide growth factors, offer the possibility of substituting for growth hormone in stimulating growth in hypopituitary humans.

The reason for the species specificity of growth hormone is not known with certainty, but it is related most likely to the specificity of receptors for growth hormone in primates.

Recent studies have shown that growth hormone as usually isolated from the human pituitary gland is not a single substance but a heterogeneous mixture contaminated with a protease that readily produces hydrolytic products. Two cleaved forms of human growth hormone have been isolated: one has prolactinlike activity and the other has growth promoting activity greater than that of the uncleaved molecule. The importance of these findings lies in the possibility that growth hormone may be converted into more active forms in vivo and that this process of "metabolic activation" could have physiologic significance. This should be kept in mind as you read this chapter. (Q. 8-2) *Do you recall any other examples of hormones that may be converted into more active forms in vivo?*

SECTION 8-1: POST-TEST QUESTIONS

1. Removal of the posterior pituitary gland of an immature mammal results in failure to grow because growth hormone is no longer secreted. (True/False)
2. Growth hormone is a polypeptide containing a. _____ amino acid residues and having a molecular weight of b. _____ daltons. The physiologic activities of two other polypeptide hormones, c. _____ and d. _____ _____, are similar to that of growth hormone because e. _____ _____.
3. Growth hormone content of the pituitary gland of the human decreases with age. (True/False)
4. Why can't bovine growth hormone be used to treat human hypopituitary dwarfs?

5. How is growth hormone obtained for the treatment of human hypopituitary dwarfs?

6. Growth hormone is present in the human pituitary in amounts greater than any other hormone. (True/False)

SECTION 8-1: POST-TEST ANSWERS

1. False
2. a. 191
   b. 22,000
   c. prolactin
   d. placental lactogen
   e. 161 of their amino acid residues are in the same sequence as in the growth hormone molecule.
3. False
4. Growth hormone is species specific with respect to primates.
5. Growth hormone for use in human hypopituitary dwarfs is obtained by removal of pituitary glands at autopsy and extraction of growth hormone from them.
6. True

SECTION 8-2: REGULATION OF THE SECRETION OF GROWTH HORMONE

OBJECTIVES:

The student should be able to:
1. Name the hypophyseal peptidergic hormones that influence the secretion of growth hormone.
2. Describe some of the chemical characteristics of somatostatin.
3. Name the three regions of the brain that influence the secretion of growth hormone.
4. Name the neurotransmitters used by each of these regions of the brain to influence the secretion of growth hormone.
5. Name some stimuli that are known both to stimulate and to inhibit the secretion of growth hormone secretion.
6. Explain why "normal" values for the concentration of growth hormone in plasma have varied widely from laboratory to laboratory.
7. Describe some of the characteristics of growth hormone in blood.

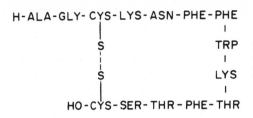

FIGURE 8-2: The amino acid sequence of the tetradecapeptide somatostatin, produced in the hypothalamus.

Much as in the other pituitary trophic hormones studied, the secretion of growth hormone is influenced by hypophysiotrophic hormones secreted at nerve endings in the hypothalamus (see Section 2-2). The HHHs include a hormone to stimulate production of growth hormone, called growth hormone-releasing hormone or factor (GH-RF), and a hormone to inhibit production of growth hormone, called somatostatin. Following secretion at nerve endings, these HHHs are carried by the blood in the hypophyseal portal vessels to the pituitary, where they influence specific acidophilic cells that secrete growth hormone (i.e., somatotropes).

Somatostatin has been isolated and purified from biologic sources and it has been characterized and synthesized in the chemical laboratory (see Figure 8-2). It is a tetradecapeptide (i.e., it has 14 amino acids) that contains a disulfide bridge. The disulfide bridge initially did not seem to be important for biologic activity because the noncyclized form has such activity. The likely explanation for this is that the reduced, noncyclized form is oxidized to the active, cyclized form in the body. Substitution of alanine for cysteine, which prevents cyclization, reduces biologic activity significantly. Somatostatin is discussed in greater detail in Section 8-5. (Q. 8-3) *Can you name another adenohypophyseal hormone whose secretion is strongly influenced by an inhibitory HHH?* (Q. 8-4) *How does the structure of this hormone compare to that for growth hormone?*

GH-RF has been much more difficult to isolate, purify, and characterize than somatostatin. To date its structure is unknown. It is found in the median eminence of the hypothalamus, from which it is released into the hypophyseal portal system (and the third ventricle). Currently it is thought that the secretion of growth hormone may be mediated by any of three regions or "centers" in the brain, the ventromedial and arcuate nuclei of the hypothalamus, and the limbic system. Stimuli that reach the ventromedial nucleus then traverse the arcuate nucleus (see Figure 8-3). Other stimuli may interact with the arcuate nucleus only, to stimulate the secretion of GH-RF. Still other stimuli that reach the limbic system appear to stimulate the release of GH-RF directly. Electrical impulses from the ventromedial nucleus travel via noradrenergic pathways to the arcuate nucleus. From the arcuate nucleus, impulses travel via dopaminergic pathways to the median eminence, where the secretion of GH-RF is stimulated. Electrical impulses from the limbic system travel to the median eminence via nerves that release serotonin at their endings (see Figure 8-3). This also results in the secretion of GH-RF. (Q. 8-5) *Do you recall the effects of serotonin on the secretion of prolactin?* It is possible to divide the stimuli responsible for the release of growth hormone into three categories depending on which of the neurotransmitters mentioned above mediates the response.

Since hypoglycemia is an important stimulus for the release of growth hormone and hyperglycemia is an important inhibitor, it is likely that glucoreceptors in the ventromedial nucleus of the hypothalamus mediate these responses. α-Adrenergic agonists stimulate, while β-adrenergic agonists inhibit, the secretion of growth hormone. It is not surprising then that administration of an α-adrenergic receptor antagonist such as phentolamine before induction of hypoglycemia has been found to prevent the release of growth hormone. These studies suggest that the secretion of growth hormone in response to hypoglycemia is mediated by the ventromedial nucleus and that the neuro-

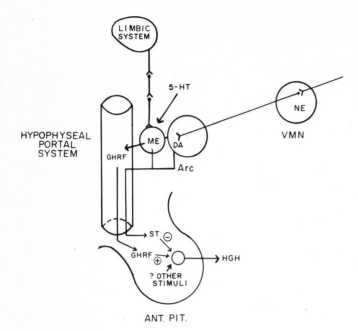

FIGURE 8-3: Three regions of the central nervous system that appear to be important in the control of growth hormone secretion: VMN = ventromedial nucleus, AN = arcuate nucleus, ME = median eminence, GHRF = growth hormone releasing factor, ST = somatostatin, HGH = human growth hormone, DA = dopamine, NE = norepinephrine. Although the major stimuli mediating growth hormone secretion originate in the hypothalamus, it is possible that certain stimuli may act directly on the pituitary gland. (*Adapted from:* Merimee and Rabin, 1973.)

transmitter is norepinephrine. When electrolytic lesions are placed in the ventromedial nucleus of the rat, the release of growth hormone in response to hypoglycemia is suppressed.

Other substances, including glucagon, vasopressin, and L-arginine-HCl, also induce the release of growth hormone from the anterior pituitary in man. Since the release of growth hormone in response to these substances can also be prevented by prior administration of the α-adrenergic antagonist phentolamine, it is believed that these substances act at the level of the ventromedial nucleus, as well.

Administration of L-DOPA also stimulates the release of growth hormone in man. This response is not attenuated if hyperglycemia is induced before administration of L-DOPA. This suggests that L-DOPA acts at a site other than the ventromedial nucleus to stimulate the secretion of growth hormone. L-DOPA is believed to be taken up by nerve terminals in the region of the arcuate nucleus and converted to dopamine by the enzyme DOPA-decarboxylase. The release of dopamine from these nerve endings is followed by release of GH-RF from the median eminence into the hypophyseal portal system. (*Q. 8-6*) *Do you recall the effects of administering L-DOPA on the secretion of LH and prolactin?*

Sleep is a potent stimulator of growth hormone secretion in man (see Figure 8-5). Since the limbic system appears to play an important role in slow wave sleep, it is felt that nerve terminals in the limbic system release serotonin during slow wave sleep. Serotonin may be responsible for mediating the release of GH-RF. (*Q. 8-7*) *Can you name another adenohypophyseal hormone that has a pattern of secretion strongly influenced by sleep?* Fever producing agents (pyrogens) may also induce the release of growth hormone by way of the limbic system, serotonin, and GH-RF (see Table 8-1).

There are also a number of stimuli that induce the release of growth hormone but whose locus of action is unknown; examples include stress, exercise, protein depletion, and estrogenic hormones. Other stimuli are known to inhibit the release of growth hormone; these include obesity, elevation of serum free fatty acid levels, and increases

TABLE 8-1: Classification of Stimuli for Release and Inhibition of Growth Hormone According to the Site at Which They Act

	Ventromedial Nucleus	Arcuate Nucleus	Limbic System	Anterior Pituitary
Transmitter				
Norepinephrine		Dopamine	Serotonin	
Excitation				
Via α-adrenergic receptors by stimuli such as hypoglycemia, vasopressin, L-arginine-HCl		L-DOPA	Deep sleep	GH-RF
Inhibition				
Hyperglycemia; α-adrenergic stimulation		Chloropromazine[a]	Unknown	Somatostatin

[a] Excitation at this level bypasses the ventromedial nucleus. Inhibition at this level can also result in inhibition of excitatory stimuli arising in the ventromedial nucleus.

in blood concentrations of glucocorticoid hormones. The locus of action of these stimuli is also unknown. A current suggestion is that they stimulate the release of somatostatin.

Because of the larger number of stimuli that have the potential both to stimulate and to inhibit the release of growth hormone, it is difficult to state what constitutes the feedback limb from the periphery to the central nervous system to regulate the secretion of growth hormone. Judging from the variety of stimuli, it is likely that there are many feedback limbs. How these are interrelated must await additional experimentation. Section 8-5 introduces the postulate that the somatomedins may act as a feedback limb.

For many years investigators have been aware that values for the "normal" concentration of growth hormone in plasma from various laboratories have differed widely. An explanation for this rather striking variability became available when it was shown that the secretion of growth hormone was episodic and that the concentrations of growth hormone in plasma could vary as much as 16-fold within 3 hours in conscious rats (see Figure 8-4).

A periodicity of about 3.5 hours occurs in the rat. This episodic pattern of secretion of growth hormone was not affected by the light-dark cycle, by feeding, or by the level of activity of the animals. Evidence is lacking that any peripheral stimuli are responsible for initiating the bursts of secretion. Instead, it is more likely that these bursts are initiated by neurons in the central nervous system as part of their inherent "free-running" characteristics.

Some investigators suggest that these episodes of growth hormone secretion may be the critical events that regulate the growth process in the rat. It would then follow that the very low basal concentration of growth hormone would have very little physiologic consequence in spite of the fact that many investigators have designated it the "physiologic concentration."

Although occasional bursts of growth hormone secretion occur in some adult humans when they are awake, a burst of secretion occurs in most humans within about 90 minutes after the onset of slow wave sleep and reaches a peak before the first cycle of rapid eye movement (REM) sleep occurs (see Figure 8-5). The increase in rate of secretion of growth hormone is neither preceded nor accompanied by changes in plasma concentration of glucose, insulin, or cortisol (see Figure 8-5). The factors responsible for initiation of this burst of secretory activity are unknown. It is known, however,

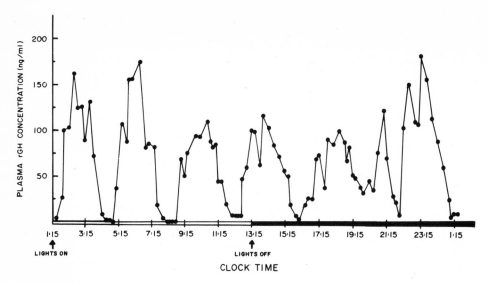

FIGURE 8-4: Mean concentration of growth hormone (rGH) in the plasma of rats during a 24-hour period. The rats were maintained in a room having a 12-hour light-dark cycle. (*Adapted from:* Tannenbaum and Martin, 1976.)

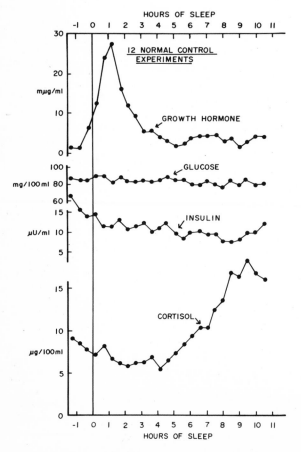

FIGURE 8-5: Plasma concentrations in sleeping human subjects of growth hormone, glucose, insulin, and cortisol. (*Adapted from:* Takahashi et al., 1968.)

that the burst of secretory activity is associated with the period of deep sleep, since it also appears in individuals whose cycle of waking and sleeping is reversed.

Attempts have been made to determine the molecular size of growth hormone in blood. There appear to be primarily two substances with growth hormonelike activity. The one present in the larger amount is about the same size as human growth hormone isolated from the pituitary gland (i.e., about 22,000 daltons). This has been called "little growth hormone." The second is approximately twice as large and has been called "big growth hormone." Procedures such as storage or repeated freezing and thawing of big growth hormone result in the formation of some little growth hormone. It is unknown at present whether big growth hormone is simply a dimer of two little growth hormone molecules or consists of little growth hormone bound to another peptide. The biologic significance of big versus little growth hormone is presently unknown; however, the ratio of little growth hormone to big growth hormone is greater in blood samples taken from patients with acromegaly than in blood samples taken from normal individuals.

SECTION 8-2: POST-TEST QUESTIONS

1. Name two HHHs that affect the secretion of growth hormone.
   a.
   b.
2. These hormones are secreted by nerve terminals within the a. _____ _____ and released into either the b. _____ or the c. _____ _____.
3. When these HHHs reach the anterior pituitary, they either stimulate or inhibit the release of growth hormone from the acidophilic somatotropes. (True/False)
4. Name the three neurotransmitters that are important in the eventual release of growth hormone.
   a.
   b.
   c.
5. a. Which of the neurotransmitters mediates stimuli received by the ventromedial nucleus?

   b. Which mediates stimuli received by the arcuate nucleus?

   c. Which mediates stimuli received by the limbic system?

6. a. Name a stimulus that is believed to act through the ventromedial nucleus to stimulate growth hormone secretion.

   b. What experimental evidence is there for this?

7. Name a stimulus that is believed to act by way of the limbic system.
8. Growth hormone concentration of blood is remarkably constant in mammals. (True/False)
9. Two substances with growth hormonelike activity have been found in blood. They are called a. _____ and b. _____ _____.

SECTION 8-2: POST-TEST ANSWERS

1. a. Growth hormone releasing factor or hormone
   b. Somatostatin
2. a. median eminence (medial basal hypothalamus, etc.)
   b. hypophyseal-portal system (capillary loops of external and/or internal plexus, etc.)
   c. third ventricle (cerebrospinal fluid)
3. True
4. a. Norepinephrine
   b. Dopamine
   c. Serotonin
5. a. Norepinephrine
   b. Dopamine
   c. Serotonin
6. a. Reduction in blood glucose concentration (hypoglycemia).
   b. Lesion of the ventromedial nucleus prevents the release of growth hormone during hypoglycemia. Furthermore, administration of an α-adrenergic antagonist inhibits the release of growth hormone during hypoglycemia.
7. Sleep
8. False
9. a. big growth hormone
   b. little growth hormone

SECTION 8-3: DIRECT PHYSIOLOGIC EFFECTS OF GROWTH HORMONE

OBJECTIVES:

The student should be able to:
1. Name two direct physiologic effects of growth hormone and explain why they are termed "direct effects."
2. State the current information available regarding the mechanisms by which growth hormone stimulates protein metabolism and amino acid transport.
3. State why growth hormone is an anabolic hormone.
4. State the effect of growth hormone on blood glucose and free fatty acid concentrations.
5. State why diabetes mellitus may develop during chronic excess secretion of growth hormone.

It has been known for many years that administration of growth hormone to immature hypophysectomized animals stimulates growth and the synthesis of proteins in skeletal muscles and liver. Synthesis of protein does not begin immediately after administration of growth hormone but becomes apparent approximately one-half hour after treatment. The lag period occurs both in vivo and in vitro and suggests that this amount of time is necessary for stimulation of all cellular processes that culminate eventually in activation of the ribosomes that are important for the process of translation. RNA synthesis occurs only after growth hormone has stimulated ribosomal activity.

It has also been shown that addition of growth hormone to a medium containing the diaphragm of an hypophysectomized rat increases the rate of movement of amino acids from the medium into the muscle cells. A similar effect has been observed in liver and heart. The stimulatory effect of growth hormone on amino acid transport can be prevented by prior administration of inhibitors of protein synthesis. These experiments suggest that growth hormone stimulates the synthesis of a protein that is important in the activation of the amino acid transport mechanism. This mediating protein has never been identified; thus, the effect of growth hormone on amino acid transport has prompted some investigators to label growth hormone as the "insulin for amino acids."

Little information is available regarding the mechanism by which growth hormone stimulates amino acid transport and protein synthesis. Some investigators, using an isolated, perfused rat heart, have shown that addition of growth hormone to the perfusate was accompanied by a decrease in the concentrations of cAMP and cGMP in the tissue. Others have shown that the stimulatory effect of growth hormone on protein synthesis in vitro could be inhibited by substances that increase cAMP levels of tissue such as phosphodiesterase inhibitors. (*Q. 8-8*) *Can you give examples of these inhibitors and explain why they increase the concentration of cAMP?* This has led to the suggestion that growth hormone may act to stimulate protein synthesis by reducing the concentration of cAMP; however, the mechanism for this interaction between cAMP and protein synthesis is not understood clearly.

An important property of the protein synthesis induced by growth hormone is that it does not appear to be a localized effect. The growth induced by growth hormone is proportionate throughout the body. Thus, the individual suffering with an overproduction of growth hormone that originated before puberty may be gigantic (over 8 feet tall), but normally proportioned. (*Q. 8-9*) *What does this suggest to you regarding the target cells and/or receptors for growth hormone?*

Although the syntheses of RNA and protein occur relatively soon after the administration of growth hormone, the rate of DNA synthesis increases only after 24 hours and reaches a maximal rate 48 hours after the start of growth hormone treatment in hypophysectomized rats. The increase in rate of DNA synthesis due to administration of growth hormone may be 10- to 20-fold. This finding is consistent with other evidence that growth hormone promotes cell replication and induces growth by increasing the number, rather than the size, of cells (i.e., hyperplasia rather than hypertrophy).

Because of its effects on protein synthesis, growth hormone is an anabolic hormone. (*Q. 8-10*) *Does this suggest an explanation for the low concentrations of urea in patients receiving injections of growth hormone?* In addition to its effect on amino acid transport and protein synthesis, growth hormone induces an increase in the activity of the enzyme ornithine decarboxylase in the liver. The concentration of the polyamine spermidine has also been shown to increase in the liver within 24 hours after administration of growth hormone. Increases in ornithine decarboxylase activity and the concentration of spermidine are associated with an increased rate of protein synthesis.

It has been known for many years that administration of growth hormone can affect the free fatty acid and glucose concentrations of plasma. There are, however, two distinct effects that depend on the time of measurement of these substrates following administration of growth hormone. Within a half-hour, there is a transient fall in both free fatty acid and glucose concentrations in plasma. This is called the "insulinlike" effect of growth hormone, since it mimics the effect of administration of insulin. However, the effect does not appear to be induced by an increased secretion of insulin. Table 8-2 illustrates the time course of changes in the levels of plasma glucose, free fatty acid, and insulinlike activity of fasted human volunteers after intravenous administration of a large (8 mg) dose of human pituitary extract containing growth hormone. (*Q. 8-11*) *What is the total content of growth hormone in a pituitary gland taken from a normal adult human?*

TABLE 8-2: The Effect of Intravenous Administration of a Growth Hormone Extract (8 mg) on the Concentrations of Glucose and Free Fatty Acids in Blood and on the Insulinlike Activity in Blood of Fasted Humans

	Time (Minutes)						
	0	10	20	30	60	90	240
Blood glucose concentration (mg %)	79 ± 2^a	88 ± 7	70 ± 4	54 ± 2	56 ± 8	74	87 ± 3
Free fatty acid concentration (mEq/liter)	469 ± 55	460 ± 89	356 ± 42	336 ± 51	419 ± 43	793	1476 ± 256
Insulinlike activity in serum (μU/ml)	242 ± 42	—	—	243 ± 73	223 ± 64	—	363 ± 63

Adapted from: Zahnd et al., 1960.

^{a} One standard error of mean.

Insulinlike activity of serum was unchanged throughout the first hour of the study whereas the glucose and free fatty acid concentrations of blood decreased to their lowest values within the first half-hour. By 4 hours after treatment, with growth hormone, the concentration of free fatty acids in plasma had more than tripled but the concentration of glucose was only slightly elevated. The mechanism responsible for the acute reduction in the concentrations of glucose and free fatty acids in blood is not known with certainty. Long-term treatment of laboratory animals with growth hormone leads to depletion of adipose stores in tissues, an increase in the concentration of free fatty acids in serum, and a transfer of lipids to the liver. Generally these effects are accompanied by a decrease in the respiratory quotient (ratio of carbon dioxide produced to oxygen consumed), suggesting that fat was used preferentially as the energy substrate. In some cases of chronic treatment with growth hormone, ketosis has been reported to occur in combination with a reduction in the concentration of bicarbonate in serum. This combination of events induces a change in acid-base balance known as compensated metabolic acidosis. (*Q. 8-12*) *Is this similar to the acidosis seen in diabetes mellitus?*

The increase in the concentration of free fatty acid in plasma observed during chronic treatment with growth hormone is accompanied by an increase in the concentration of glucose in blood. Growth hormone also appears to inhibit the uptake of glucose into cells. It is understandable why the concentration of insulin in plasma would be increased under these conditions. In spite of this increase in the concentration of insulin, growth hormone continues to inhibit the uptake of glucose by cells. This inhibition is the result of a decreased sensitivity of tissues to insulin. Continued administration of excess growth hormone may result in exhaustion of the B-cells of the pancreas and onset of overt diabetes mellitus with an elevated concentration of glucose in blood and a loss of glucose into urine. This effect was first observed by Dr. Bernardo Houssay, the famous Argentine physiologist and Noble Prize laureate. Approximately 20% of patients with elevated concentrations of growth hormone in blood (acromegaly) have frank diabetes and about 25% have abnormal glucose tolerance tests.

SECTION 8-3: POST-TEST QUESTIONS

1. Growth hormone exerts a direct effect on a. _____ and b. _____, where it stimulates c. _____ and d. _____.
2. Why has growth hormone been called the "insulin for amino acids"?

3. Present knowledge suggests that the direct effect of growth hormone on protein synthesis is mediated by activation of the cAMP system. (True/False)
4. Why is the concentration of urea in the blood decreased following treatment with growth hormone?

5. The increase in body size of hypophysectomized rats following treatment with growth hormone is due to an increase in the number, not the size, of somatic cells. This response is accompanied by an increase in the rate of synthesis of DNA. (True/False)
6. Why is growth hormone called an anabolic hormone?

7. What is the "insulinlike" effect of growth hormone?

8. Is the insulinlike effect of growth hormone characteristic of its long-term effects? Explain.

9. Chronc elevation of growth hormone concentration in blood may result in diabetes mellitus. (True/False)
10. Is this effect direct or indirect? Why?

SECTON 8-3: POST-TEST ANSWERS

1. a. skeletal muscle
   b. liver
   c. amino acid transport
   d. protein synthesis
2. Because of its effect in increasing the transport of amino acids into cells for use in protein synthesis.
3. False

4. Amino acids are used for the synthesis of protein and fewer are therefore deaminated.
5. True
6. Because of its effect on protein synthesis.
7. It is the transient reduction in free fatty acid and glucose concentrations of blood that occurs within the first half-hour after administration of growth hormone.
8. No. Chronic administration of growth hormone increases plasma free fatty acid and glucose concentrations.
9. True
10. Indirect. Growth hormone reduces the sensitivity of peripheral tissues to insulin. Continued elevation of the concentration of glucose in blood stimulates pancreatic B-cells to produce insulin. This eventually exhausts the B-cells and results in a deficit of insulin. Diabetes mellitus may then result.

SECTION 8-4: INDIRECT EFFECTS OF GROWTH HORMONE

OBJECTIVES:

The student should be able to:
1. Describe what is meant by the "indirect" effects of growth hormone.
2. Describe the physiologic effects of sulfation factor and its relation to the somatomedins.
3. State where somatomedins are produced.
4. State how somatomedins are transported in the blood.
5. Describe the physiologic actions of somatomedins.
6. Describe the meaning of nonsuppressible insulinlike activity (NSILA) of plasma and its relation to somatomedins.
7. Describe some interactions between somatomedins and other hormones.

Growth hormone increases skeletal growth by stimulating the proliferation of chondrocytes and increasing the synthesis of cartilage matrix of bone. Over two decades ago it was shown that the direct addition of growth hormone to cartilage explants of ribs removed from rats and bathed in an artificial medium failed to stimulate either the incorporation of $[^{35}S]SO_4$ into cartilage glucosoaminoglycans or the incorporation of $[^3H]$thymidine into DNA. Both responses could be elicited if serum from normal rats was added to the artificial medium. Addition of serum from hypophysectomized rats failed to affect the two responses, but pretreatment of the hypophysectomized rat with growth hormone restored the stimulatory effect to the serum. As a result of these studies, it was postulated that growth hormone stimulates the growth of epiphyses of bones indirectly by inducing the production of a factor responsible for increasing the formation of both the protein matrix and the collagen of bone as well as increasing the incorporation of sulfate into cartilage. This factor, designated originally as "sulfation factor," has now come to be known as somatomedin.

Somatomedin activity is present in plasma and to a lesser extent in cerebrospinal fluid, liver, kidney, muscle, and lymph. Most of the available evidence supports the concept that the major site of production is the liver. Among the evidence for this is the release of somatomedin into the perfusate during perfusion of rat liver with an artificial medium. If growth hormone is added to the perfusion fluid, the rate of release of somatomedins is increased. In addition, hepatectomy results in a decrease in the concentration of somatomedins in serum. Somatomedins are released by the liver in association with a high molecular weight protein, but the exact transport mechanism from liver cell to plasma is unknown. In plasma, somatomedins are associated with two types of protein, having molecular weight 120,000 and 70,000 daltons, respectively. A special biologic role for these two carrier proteins has not been established, but it is thought that they increase and/or prolong the activity of somatomedins in plasma. The half-life of somatomedin in the plasma of the rat normally is 3 to 4 hours, but this time can be decreased following hypophysectomy and restored following subsequent replacement therapy with growth hormone. These findings suggest that growth hormone may stimulate the production of carrier proteins for the somatomedins and by doing so increase the half-life and biologic activity of these growth promoting agents. The high molecular weight somatomedin complex secreted by the liver can be converted to smaller molecular weight somatomedins. Three somatomedins have been isolated from serum and are called somatomedins A, B, and C, respectively.

It is now apparent that these three somatomedins have similar actions but differ in their chemical characteristics. All are peptides ranging in molecular weight from approximately 4500 to 7500 daltons. None has yet been characterized. In addition to their ability to stimulate cartilage growth in vitro, they can partially substitute for serum in stimulating the growth and proliferation of a variety of cell types in tissue culture. The cell lines that have been shown to respond to somatomedins include myoblasts, chick embryo fibroblasts, fetal liver cells, ovarian tumor cells, and human glial cells. The growth promoting action of somatomedins is related not only to their effect on chondrogenesis and skeletal growth, but also to their effect on amino acid transport and protein synthesis in skeletal muscles and other tissues. As you learned in Section 8-3, an increase in amino acid transport and protein synthesis in skeletal muscle can also be induced by a direct action of growth hormone.

How much of the normal protein synthesis of muscle and other tissue is related directly to growth hormone, as opposed to somatomedins, remains unknown. However, present opinion favors the possibility that all growth promoting actions of growth hormone occur by way of the somatomedins. An important reason for this is the existence of a number of growth disorders in which the growth rates of children correlate better with serum somatomedin concentration than with growth hormone concentration. For example, Laron dwarfs actually have high concentrations of growth hormone in plasma, but their levels of somatomedins are often below the threshold of detection. Serum somatomedin concentration fails to rise when growth hormone is administered, suggesting that the growth defect is related to a reduced responsiveness of the liver to growth hormone with consequent failure to produce adequate amounts of somatomedins to maintain normal growth (see Table 8-4, Section 8-6). Such examples as these suggest that the growth promoting effects of growth hormone in vivo are indirect and occur by way of the somatomedins (see Figure 8-6).

It is true, however, that growth hormone can stimulate amino acid transport and protein synthesis in vitro. It seems likely at present that the physiologically important, direct effects of growth hormone are related to its antiinsulin actions, which include its ability to induce lipolysis and increase blood sugar (see Figure 8-6).

Students should realize that investigators are still attempting to sort out the direct effects of growth hormone from its indirect effects due to stimulation of secretion of somatomedins. There appear to be some overlaps in their activities as well as some differences. With respect to the latter, growth hormone has an antiinsulin action, whereas the somatomedins appear to possess insulinlike properties. In adipose tissue, somatomedins stimulate lipid synthesis and glucose oxidation. They also inhibit the lipolytic actions of epinephrine. It must be pointed out here that the somatomedins are

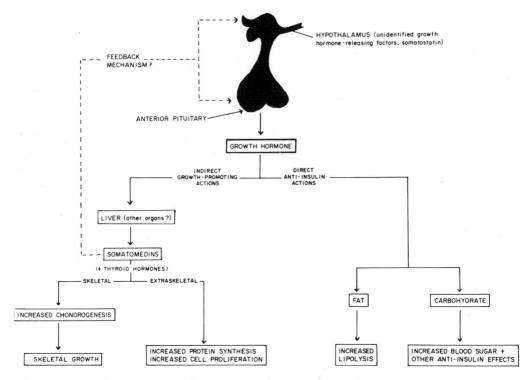

FIGURE 8-6: The multiple actions of growth hormone. The dashed line suggests a feedback mechanism involving somatomedins. (*Adapted from:* Van Wyk and Underwood, 1978.)

considerably more active in their growth promoting activity than in their insulinlike activity.

Of the three somatomedins, A and C appear to have greatest insulinlike activity. This property is related, in part at least, to the fact that they can compete with insulin for insulin receptors on fat cells, chondrocytes, and liver cell membranes. This has raised a question regarding how much of the insulinlike activity of serum is due to insulin. It is surprising to recognize that only 7–10% of the insulinlike activity of serum measured by *biologic assays* can be accounted for by insulin. The remaining insulinlike activity, which cannot be neutralized by specific insulin antibodies, is called nonsuppressible insulinlike activity (NSILA). Recent studies have shown that NSILA is contained in two related peptides that have all the biologic properties of somatomedins A and C and, like them, are more active in growth promoting assays than in assays for insulinlike activity. As mentioned above, it appears that the effects of somatomedins on carbohydrate and fat metabolism in insulin-type bioassays occur only at relatively high doses of somatomedin that may have little physiologic significance. Conversely, the growth promoting effects of insulin, as measured in cartilage and tissue culture assays, occur only with doses of insulin that can be considered unphysiologic. Thus, the important role of somatomedins (and NSILA) is in promotion of growth, and the important role of insulin is in the control of carbohydrate and lipid levels of blood.

Recent measurements of the concentration of somatomedin in the plasma of hypopituitary children, normal adults, and acromegalic adults support its role in growth (see Figure 8-7). Hypopituitary children who have failed to grow have virtually no detectable somatomedin C in their plasma, whereas adults with hypersecretion of growth

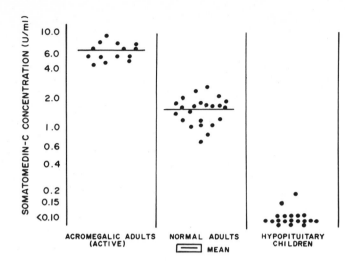

FIGURE 8-7: Concentration of somatomedin C in patients in whom growth hormone is excess (acromegalic), in patients with growth hormone deficiency (hypopituitary), and in normal adults. Somatomedin C was measured by immunoassay. Note that the abscissa is graphed logarithmically. (*Adapted from:* Van Wyk and Underwood, 1978.)

hormone (acromegaly) have levels nearly three times those typical of normal adults. Since the concentrations of somatomedin C are very stable throughout the day and do not respond to stress and provocative testing as does growth hormone, measurement of the concentration of somatomedins in plasma should greatly facilitate the diagnosis of both hypopituitarism and acromegaly.

Critics of the somatomedin hypothesis of growth hormone's action have often pointed out that it has not yet been shown that somatomedins can substitute for growth hormone in restoring the growth rate of hypophysectomized rats to that of normals. One of the difficulties that accounts for this is the lack of availability of purified somatomedins. (*Q. 8-13*) *Why else might the somatomedins be less effective in restoring growth in these hypophysectomized rats than they are in stimulating growth in nonhypophysectomized (i.e., normal) rats?* If purified somatomedins become available and if they can be shown to substitute for growth hormone, it may be possible to treat the hypopituitary growth problems of children with somatomedins instead of growth hormone. At present, human blood appears to be the richest source of somatomedins. Progress will depend on finding a richer source of the somatomedins so that characterizing and synthesizing them will be facilitated.

There are a number of interactions between somatomedins and other hormones. Sustained high concentrations of glucocorticoids, whether induced endogenously or exogenously, inhibit growth. Somatomedin levels of plasma are depressed in such patients while plasma growth hormone concentrations may be unchanged. Chronic administration of glucocorticoid hormones to hypophysectomized rats will inhibit the rise in plasma somatomedin concentration that normally follows administration of growth hormone. Although the primary effect of glucocorticoids is the inhibition of somatomedin production, they may also act peripherally to inhibit the effect of somatomedins on cartilage, fibroblasts, and skeletal muscle (see Figure 8-8).

Large doses of estrogenic hormones inhibit growth in young animals and can actually counteract many of the metabolic effects of growth hormone in acromegalic patients. Estrogens also appear to inhibit the production of somatomedins by the liver. It is less likely that estrogens act to inhibit peripheral responses to somatomedins. Thus, the effect of estrogens on secretion of growth hormone (see Section 8-2) appears to be opposite to their effects on secretion of somatomedins.

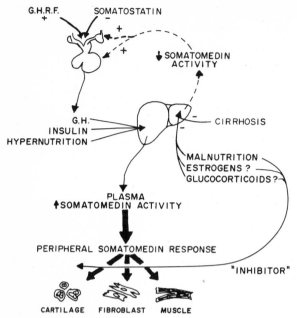

FIGURE 8-8: Factors affecting hepatic production and peripheral response to somatomedins. (*Adapted from:* Daughaday, 1976.)

Malnutrition has also been shown to inhibit the production of somatomedins by the liver. Malnutrition also appears to be associated with the production of a substance that inhibits the peripheral responses to somatomedin (see Figure 8-8). Nutritional status is believed by some investigators to be of primary importance in the production of somatomedins.

In Section 8-2 the feedback limb for the control of growth hormone secretion from the periphery to the hypothalamus and pituitary was said to be unknown. Several investigators have now postulated that the concentration of somatomedins in plasma could act as the feedback limb (see Figure 8-8). A decrease in somatomedin concentration is postulated to increase the secretion of growth hormone. Proof of this, however, must await additional experimentation.

SECTON 8-4: POST-TEST QUESTIONS

1. The experiments that led to the observation of a "sulfation factor" are important to our understanding of the role of growth hormone in the process of growth. Why?

2. Where are somatomedins produced in the largest amount?

3. How many somatomedins are there?

4. Name three of the major physiologic actions of somatomedins.
   a.
   b.
   c.

5. What other actions do somatomedins have at high doses?

6. What is the meaning of "nonsuppressible insulinlike activity of serum"?

7. Nonsuppressible insulinlike activity is contained in two peptides with biologic properties similar to those of somatomedins A and C. (True/False)
8. Insulin has growth promoting properties that are manifest at unphysiologically high levels in blood. (True/False)

SECTION 8-4: POST-TEST ANSWERS

1. They showed for the first time that the sulfation of glucosoaminoglycans in cartilage was not due to growth hormone itself but to a factor in serum. The presence of this factor was dependent on the presence of growth hormone.
2. Liver
3. Three
4. a. Increased chondrogenesis
   b. Increased skeletal growth
   c. Increased protein synthesis
5. Insulinlike effects including decreased lipolysis and decreased blood glucose concentration.
6. Nonsuppressible insulinlike activity of serum is that portion of the total serum insulinlike activity, as measured by a biologic assay, that cannot be neutralized by specific insulin antibodies.
7. True
8. True

SECTION 8-5: PHYSIOLOGIC EFFECTS OF SOMATOSTATIN

OBJECTIVES:

The student should be able to:
1. State where somatostatin can be found in the body.
2. State the half-life of somatostatin in blood.
3. Describe the effect of somatostatin on the secretion of growth hormone.
4. Describe the effect of somatostatin on the release of both glucagon and insulin following the infusion of arginine.
5. State what is currently known about the control of the secretion of somatostatin.
6. Describe the effect of somatostatin on the stomach.
7. Explain how somatostatin is currently believed to act at the level of target cells.
8. Discuss the physiologic role somatostatin may play in regulating the concentration of glucose in blood.

As you learned in Section 8-2, somatostatin is produced in the hypothalamus and is carried by the hypophyseal-portal system to the anterior pituitary gland, where it inhibits the secretion of growth hormone. (*Q. 8-14*) *What type of chemical is the HHH somatostatin?* It had been assumed until recently that somatostatin was produced only in the hypothalamus. It has now been shown that somatostatin can be found in a number of endocrine or endocrinelike cells. It is found in areas of the brain in addition to the hypothalamus, in the pancreas, in the stomach, and in the thyroid gland. Immunohisto-chemical results have suggested that somatostatin may also occur in the prevertebral ganglia, the inferior mesenteric ganglion, and the celiac–superior mesenteric ganglion complex of the guinea pig. A large proportion of all noradrenergic cells in these ganglia also contained somatostatinlike reactivity, which was located in the Golgi complex. These observations are of interest because they represent the first reported example of the concomitant storage of a small biologically active peptide and an amine in the same neuron. This may be the first case of a mammalian neuron producing two putative transmitters. Such a neuron would not conform to the one neuron–one transmitter hypothesis, often referred to as Dale's principle, which was advocated by Sir Henry Dale, the British pharmacologist.

Analysis of various areas of the brain and a large number of peripheral tissues of the rat has shown that the highest concentrations of somatostatin per unit weight of tissue are found the median eminence, arcuate nucleus, and pancreas. It has not been possible to show unequivocally that somatostatin is present in the systemic circulation. How-

FIGURE 8-9: The effect of increasing concentrations of somatostatin in the infusion fluid of the isolated rat pancreas on release of insulin. Glucose (3.0 mg/ml) in the infusion fluid was used to stimulate the release of insulin. (*Adapted from:* Luft et al., 1978.)

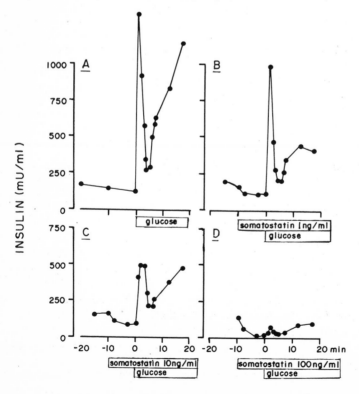

ever, there is a considerable body of evidence for its presence in the hypothalamopituitary circulation and in the hepatic venous effluent. The half-life of somatostatin in blood is approximately one minute. Few data are available on the metabolism of somatostatin, but studies in which exogenous somatostatin was infused into baboons suggest that the kidneys and liver may be major sites of degradation. In view of the very short half-life of somatostatin in the circulation, it is unlikely that it can be considered to be a classic circulating hormone. It is more likely that somatostatin is secreted locally, where it acts either as a regulator of endocrine secretion or a peptidergic neurotransmitter.

In every species tested, administration of somatostatin was found to inhibit the release of growth hormone that normally accompanies such physiologic and pharmacologic stimuli as sleep, exercise, meals, hypoglycemia, administration of arginine and L-DOPA, and direct electrical stimulation of the hypothalamus. In addition, when the circulating concentration of growth hormone was elevated (e.g., in protein-caloric malnutrition, acromegaly, or diabetes mellitus), infusion of somatostatin reduced the elevated level to or toward normal values. Inhibition of growth hormone secretion by somatostatin occurs at the level of the anterior pituitary gland.

During experiments in which the effect of somatostatin on the secretion of growth hormone was studied, several investigators observed by chance that infusion of somatostatin in the proper dose can inhibit completely the release of insulin normally induced by an infusion of glucose (see Figure 8-9). Similarly, infusion of somatostatin can also inhibit the release of both glucagon and insulin normally induced by infusion of arginine (see Figure 8-10). Somatostatin is an effective inhibitor of virtually every known stimulus for the secretion of insulin and glucagon. A given dose of somatostatin

FIGURE 8-10: The effect of somatostatin and an analogue of somatostatin (des-Asn^5-somatostatin) on plasma insulin and glucagon secretions stimulated by infusion of the amino acid arginine. The isolated perfused rat pancreas was used in these studies. (*Adapted from:* Luft et al., 1978.)

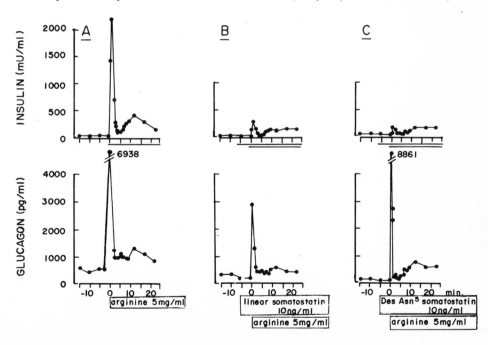

inhibits both to a similar extent. It is now possible, however, to alter the chemical structure of somatostatin, resulting in the production of analogues with relatively greater inhibitory activity for insulin than glucagon, and vice versa. (Q. 8-15) *What does this discovery suggest to you regarding the target cells and receptors for somatostatin in the pancreas?*

In the pancreas, somatostatin is found only in islet tissue. It has been localized by immunohistochemical means to a discrete population of cells known as D-cells. These cells normally constitute approximately 5–15% of the islet cell mass in mammals, whereas glucagon secreting A-cells and the insulin secreting B-cells make up 20–30% and 40–60%, respectively. In man and the guinea pig, D-cells are randomly distributed in islet tissue. As stated earlier, a dose of somatostatin given systemically inhibits A-cells (glucagon) to the same extent as B-cells (insulin). It is possible that somatostatin and glucagon act reciprocally, each to regulate the rate of secretion of the other. Thus, if serum glucagon concentration rises to a certain level, the rate of secretion of somatostatin would increase and inhibit the rate of secretion of glucagon. This could serve the function of limiting the maximal elevation of blood glucose under physiologic conditions (see Section 9-3).

Somatostatin has also been shown to inhibit the release by the stomach of the hormone gastrin, which is important in stimulating the secretion of gastric juice. Other gastrointestinal hormones whose release is impaired by somatostatin include a glucagonlike hormone (gut glucagon), motilin, vasoactive intestinal peptide (VIP), and gastric inhibitory polypeptide (GIP). It is unknown at present whether these effects of somatostatin are direct or indirect. (Q. 8-16) *Can you name two adenohypophyseal hormones whose secretion is inhibited by somatostatin?*

The exact mechanisms by which somatostatin inhibits secretion in pancreas, gastrointestinal tract, thyroid, and pituitary glands are not known with certainty. The picture that appears to be emerging from current research is that somatostatin acts by interfering with some facet of calcium metabolism in target tissues. Thus, somatostatin has been shown to impair the uptake of calcium by pancreatic islet cells. This effect can be reversed by increasing extracellular concentration of calcium. It seems likely that the effect of somatostatin on cellular calcium metabolism may account for its ability to lower the levels of cAMP in the pituitary; to block the elevation of cAMP during glucose-stimulated insulin release in pancreatic islets, and to inhibit hormonal responses to the cAMP analogue dibutyryl cAMP.

By means of synthetic somatostatin, it has become clear that glucagon plays a physiologic role in maintaining blood glucose concentration. Thus, infusion of somatostatin to either normoglycemic or diabetic humans induced a transient fall in the concentration of glucose in blood of 30–50% as a result of a suppression of the release of glucagon, which normally stimulates hepatic production of glucose. These results have suggested to a number of clinical investigators that glucagon may be responsible for the large elevation of blood sugar in insulin-dependent, diabetic patients (see Section 9-5). Infusion of somatostatin during 18 hours after withdrawal of insulin from patients with insulin-dependent diabetes prevented the development of diabetic ketoacidosis by causing sustained suppression of the hyperglycemia and hyperketonemia that would have occurred if somatostatin had not been administered. These studies raise the possibility that somatostatin or analogues of it could prove useful as an adjunct to insulin in the management of patients with diabetes mellitus. In a study testing this, considerably better control of blood sugar was maintained with insulin and somatostatin than with insulin alone (see Figure 8-11). The major limitations in the practical use of somatostatin in the control of diabetes are its very short half-life in the circulation and its effects in inhibiting the secretion of other hormones.

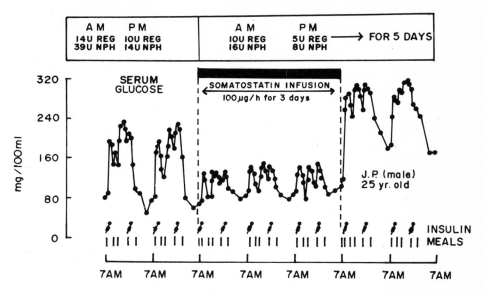

FIGURE 8-11: Effect of a continuous 3-day infusion of somatostatin on serum glucose concentration of a diabetic patient requiring insulin. Note that somatostatin in combination with insulin reduced the variability of serum glucose concentration. Insulin dose is shown at the top of the figure. REG ≡ regular insulin NPH ≡ long-lasting insulin. (*Adapted from:* Gerich, 1976.)

SECTION 8-5: POST-TEST QUESTIONS

1. Somatostatin is an octapeptide. (True/False)
2. Somatostatin has been found in both the central and peripheral nervous systems. (True/False)
3. In addition to being found in neurons, somatostatin can be found in cells of the
   a. _____, b. _____, and c. _____.
4. The half-life of somatostatin in blood is approximately one hour. (True/False)
5. In view of its half-life in the circulation, somatostatin can be considered to be a classic circulatory hormone. (True/False)
6. Administration of L-arginine a. (stimulates/inhibits) the release of growth hormone. Somatostatin b. (stimulates/inhibits) this response. This occurs at the level of the c. (hypothalamus/pituitary).
7. Pancreatic cells that secrete somatostatin are called _____.
8. Somatostatin inhibits the release of glucagon, but not insulin, from pancreatic islet tissue. (True/False)
9. The cells secreting somatostatin in humans occur in the periphery of islet tissue in close association with B-cells. (True/False)
10. Somatostatin is currently believed to act at target tissue by what mechanism?

11. What physiologic role may somatostatin play in the regulation of blood glucose concentration?

12. Name nine hormones whose secretion can be inhibited by what appear to be the direct actions of somatostatin.
    a.
    b.
    c.
    d.
    e.
    f.
    g.
    h.
    i.

SECTION 8-5: POST-TEST ANSWERS

1. False
2. True
3. a. Pancreas
   b. Stomach
   c. Thyroid gland
4. False
5. False
6. a. stimulates
   b. inhibits
   c. pituitary
7. D-cells
8. False
9. False
10. Interfering with some facet of calcium metabolism.
11. It may serve as a mechanism by which the secretion of glucagon is controlled.
12. a. Growth hormone (GH)
    b. Thyroid stimulating hormone (TSH)
    c. Insulin
    d. Pancreatic glucagon
    e. Gut glucagon
    f. Gastrin
    g. Motilin
    h. Vasoactive intestinal peptide (VIP)
    i. Gastric inhibitory polypeptide (GIP)

SECTION 8-6: CLINICAL TESTS USED TO ASSESS THE SECRETION OF GROWTH HORMONE

OBJECTIVES:

The student should be able to:

1. Describe five clinical tests that may be used to assess the secretion of growth hormone.
2. Describe four types of growth disorders.

A. CLINICAL TESTS

It was mentioned in Section 8-2 that the concentration of growth hormone in plasma varies considerably during a 24-hour period in humans and that a burst of secretory activity occurs within an hour of the onset of deep (slow wave) sleep (see Figure 8-5). Measurement of the concentration of growth hormone in serum by radioimmunossay following the onset of deep sleep is a simple method for assessing the secretion of growth hormone under physiologic conditions and may be used as a screening test by awakening the patient one hour after onset of sleep (as determined by an electroenceph-alographic tracing) and obtaining a blood sample. Detection of a normal concentration of growth hormone is evidence that the patient is not deficient in growth hormone. Unfortunately, under these conditions about 30% of normal children will not show an increase in the secretion of growth hormone and other tests must be used.

An additional simple and provocative test for the secretion of growth hormone is strenuous exercise. The standardized test requires that the subject exercise vigorously for 20 minutes. Blood is sampled for measurement of the concentration of growth hormone at the completion of the exercise and 20 minutes later. If an elevation in the concentration of growth hormone in plasma is detected, growth hormone deficiency can be ruled out.

There are a number of pharmacologic agents that can be used to stimulate the secretion of growth hormone. Since hypoglycemia was one of the first stimuli observed to increase the secretion of growth hormone, it is not surprising that small doses of crystalline insulin can provoke the secretion of growth hormone. This test is widely used clinically in the diagnosis of growth hormone deficiency and is believed by some to be of the most reliable of the diagnostic tests.

Other stimuli that can increase the rate of secretion of growth hormone include administration of L-arginine and related amino acids, glucagon, and L-DOPA. Patients are often administered propranolol before receiving arginine, glucagon, or insulin to prevent any interference of the β-adrenergic system with the expected response. Argi-nine, glucagon, and L-DOPA are believed to mediate the release of growth hormone by acting at the level of the hypothalamus to stimulate secretion of GH-RF.

These clinical tests of the secretion of growth hormone are summarized in Table 8-3. Because of the large number of false negative responses (20–30%), possible for any one of the tests, no diagnosis of growth hormone deficiency should be made unless two or more tests have been performed.

B. DISORDERS OF GROWTH

Disorders of growth have been classified into four types (see Table 8-4). These classifications illustrate rather nicely the levels of organization at which an interference with growth may occur. In type I growth hormone deficiency, which is the most common type, the concentration of growth hormone in blood is low. In addition, insulin release after arginine infusion is diminished and there is an extreme responsiveness of glucose concentrations in blood to insulin. In general, these patients exhibit a good therapeutic response to administration of growth hormone. The type I deficiency is in the production of growth hormone by the pituitary gland.

Type II deficiency, which is much less common, is characterized by an exaggerated release of insulin in response to arginine infusion, a decreased responsiveness of glucose concentrations in blood to administration of insulin, and a poor growth re-sponse to administration of growth hormone. Little is known about this category.

Type III deficiency, first described by Laron and colleagues, is characterized by very high concentrations of growth hormone in blood. Release of insulin after arginine

TABLE 8-3: Clinical Tests of the Secretion of Growth Hormone

Test	Test Conditions and Dosages	Time of Growth Hormone Response
Insulin	Regular crystalline insulin	45–75 minutes
Arginine	L-Arginine monohydrochloride	60–120 minutes
Exercise	Magnitude of growth hormone response is related to strenuousness of exercise	20–40 minutes after beginning exercise
Glucagon	Administered intramuscularly or subcutaneously	2–3 hours
Sleep	Growth hormone response occurs with deep sleep	Initial peak within 1 hour after onset of deep sleep
L-DOPA	Growth hormone responses often improved by administering priming doses of L-DOPA for 1 or more days before test dose	30–120 minutes

Adapted from: Van Wyk and Underwood, 1978.

infusion is diminished, and there is an increased responsiveness of glucose concentrations in blood to administration of insulin. The concentration of somatomedin in blood is low or not measurable, even when growth hormone is administered. In this type of deficiency, the liver fails to respond to growth hormone by increasing its production and release of somatomedins. The possibility that receptors for growth hormone in liver are not present in Laron dwarfs has not been established but is a likely explanation for the growth deficiency. (Q. 8-17) *Can you suggest an explanation for the abnormally high concentrations of growth hormone in the blood of the Laron dwarf?*

Type IV deficiency is characteristic of the African pigmy. These individuals have normal concentrations of growth hormone in plasma but the release of insulin is decreased after infusion of arginine. They also exhibit an increase in insulin responsiveness. Their concentrations of somatomedin in blood appear to be normal, but they do

TABLE 8-4: Classification of Disorders of Growth

Type	Concentration of Growth Hormone in Plasma	Arginine-Induced Release of Insulin	Responsivity of the Concentration of Glucose in Blood to Administration of Insulin	Concentration of Somatomedin in Plasma — Basal Level	Concentration of Somatomedin in Plasma — After Administration of Growth Hormone	Response to Exogenous Growth Hormone
I	↓	↓	↑	0	+	Good
II	↓	↑	↓	?	?	Poor
III (Laron)	↑	↓	↑	0	0	Poor
IV (pigmy)	Normal	↓	↑	+	+	Poor

Adapted from: Friesen, 1977.

not increase after administration of growth hormone. (*Q. 8-18*) *On the basis of this information can you theorize why African pigmies are so short?*

Thus types I, III, and IV are examples of growth retardation due, respectively, to a deficiency of growth hormone, a failure of the liver to respond to growth hormone and to produce somatomedins, and a failure of peripheral tissues to respond to somatomedins.

SECTION 8-6: POST-TEST QUESTIONS

1. Administration of either arginine or glucagon will stimulate the release of growth hormone. These substances are believed to act through the ventromedial nucleus to stimulate the secretion of GH-RF. What neurotransmitter mediates this response?

2. Deep sleep also increases the rate of secretion of growth hormone. What area of the brain is believed to mediate this response? a. _____ What is its neurotransmitter? b. _____

3. Administration of L-DOPA increases the rate of secretion of growth hormone. What is the postulated mechanism for this?

4. What effects would you predict on the concentration of growth hormone in blood samples taken from type IV (African pigmy) growth-deficient humans following the administration of insulin?

SECTION 8-6: POST-TEST ANSWERS

1. Norepinephrine
2. a. Limbic system
   b. Serotonin
3. It is thought that L-DOPA is taken up by nerve terminals in the region of the arcuate nucleus and converted to dopamine by the enzyme DOPA-decarboxylase. This, in turn, initiates the release of GH-RF from the median eminence.
4. They should know an increase in the concentration of growth hormone in blood (due to the insulin-induced hypoglycemia) that is similar in magnitude to that displayed by a "normal" individual.

SELECTED REFERENCES

Gerich, J. E. and Patton, G. S., 1978, Somatostatin, physiology and clinical applications, *Medical Clinics Of North America* 62: 375.

Luft, R., Efendic, S., and Hokfelt, T., 1978, Somatostatin—both hormone and neurotransmitter, *Diabetologia* 14: 1.

Phillips, L. S. and Vassilopoulou-Sellin, R., 1980, Somatomedins, *New England Journal Of Medicine* 302: 371.

Van Wyk, J. J. and Underwood, L. E., 1978, Growth hormone, somatomedins and growth failure, *Hospital Practice* 13: 57.

Woods, S. C. and Porte, D., Jr., 1978, The central nervous system, pancreatic hormones, feeding and obesity, *Advances In Metabolic Disorders*, Vol. 9, Levine, R. and Luft, R. (Eds.), New York: *Academic Press*, p. 283.

9

HORMONAL INTERACTIONS IN THE REGULATION OF THE CONCENTRATION OF GLUCOSE IN BLOOD

SECTION 9-1: ANATOMY AND HISTOLOGY OF THE PANCREAS

OBJECTIVES:

The student should be able to:
1. Describe the dual functions of the pancreas.
2. Discuss briefly the innervation of the pancreas.
3. Describe the cell types that make up the islets of Langerhans and the hormones secreted by them.

A. ANATOMY OF THE PANCREAS, AN EXOCRINE AND ENDOCRINE GLAND

The pancreas is an organ located posterior to the liver and stomach and within the curve of the duodenum. It has both an exocrine and an endocrine function. Its exocrine function consists of the secretion of several digestive enzymes, which are released into the gastrointestinal tract by way of the pancreatic ducts. it is estimated that about 99% of the pancreas consists of acinar tissue, which is responsible for the production and secretion of digestive enzymes.

Microscopic examination of the pancreas reveals small areas of endocrine tissue surrounded by acinar cells. These areas have been called islets of Langerhans, and they are known to produce at least six hormones that either act locally or are secreted directly into blood and act at a site distant from the pancreas, or both (*Q. 9-1*) *Could we still call them hormones if they were transported away from the pancreas by a system of ducts?*

B. HISTOLOGY OF THE PANCREAS

At least six different types of endocrinelike cells have been identified within the islets of Langerhans. Those responsible for secretion of glucagon, insulin, and somatostatin have been designated A-, B-, and D-cells, respectively. They account for more than 75% of the cells present in the islets, distributed as follows: A-cells, constitute 20–30%; B-cells, 40–60%; D-cells, 5–15%. In man, A-, B-, and D-cells are scattered randomly throughout the islets. (*Q. 9-2*) *What physiologic role does somatostatin play in the body?* Additional secretory products that have been identified as originating from islet tissue include pancreatic polypeptide (F-cells, 5–15% of islet cells), vasoactive intestinal peptide (D_1-cells, 0–5% of islet cells), and serotonin (EC-cells, 0–5% of islet cells). Of the six hormones secreted by islet tissue, only insulin, glucagon, and somatostatin are discussed in detail in this chapter. Each of these three hormones is known to play a role in the regulation of the concentration of glucose in blood.

C. INNERVATION OF THE PANCREAS

The pancreatic islets are innervated (see Section 4-1). Efferent nerves to the pancreas contain preganglionic parasympathetic fibers (i.e., dorsal trunk of vagus nerve) that originate in the dorsal efferent nucleus of the brain stem and postganglionic sympathetic fibers that originate in the celiac collateral ganglion. The preganglionic sympathetic fibers originate in the intermediolateral portion of the midthoracic spinal cord. Although little solid information is available regarding the afferent nerves from the pancreas, they are believed to reach the spinal cord and central nervous system via the same pathways used by the efferent fibers (i.e., the mixed pancreatic nerve). In spite of our lack of knowledge of afferent pathways, there is experimental evidence for the presence of "receptors" for glucose and insulin in the hypothalamus (see Figure 2-4). These are believed to sense the levels of glucose and insulin, respectively, in blood and to initiate signals to the islet cells of the pancreas. Thus, it has been shown experimentally that electrical stimulation of the ventrolateral portion of the hypothalamus (VLH) induces an increase in the secretion of insulin, whereas lesions placed in this area result in a chronic decrease in the secretion of insulin. When the ventromedial portion of the hypothalamus (VMH) is stimulated electrically, there is an increase in the rate of secretion of glucagon, accompanied by a decrease in the rate of secretion of insulin. Lesioning of this area results in hypersecretion of insulin.

Nervous outflow from the VMH modulates the preganglionic sympathetic splanchnic nerves, which synapse in the celiac ganglion. From there the postganglionic sympa-

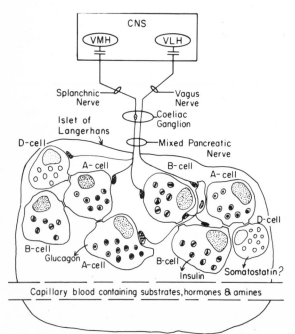

FIGURE 9-1: Innervation of islet tissue of the pancreas: VMH = ventromedial hypothalamus, VLH = ventrolateral hypothalamus. Electrical connections appear as gap junctions on A-, B-, and D-cells. (Source: Woods and Porte, 1978.)

thetic axons enter the pancreas through the mixed pancreatic nerve. Within the islet tissue, the postganglionic sympathetic nerve endings release norepinephrine near both A- and B-cells. Nervous outflow from the VLH modulates the preganglionic parasympathetic nerves, which synapse with ganglion cells in the islets of Langerhans. From there the postganglionic parasympathetic nerve endings release acetylcholine near both A- and B-cells (see Figure 9-1).

There appear to be gaps in the junctions between nerve endings and islet cells. These "gap junctions" readily allow passage into islet cells of both electrical impulses and substances of low molecular weight (<1200 daltons), thus making possible a response of islet cells to both electrical and chemical stimuli. It is also possible that the various cell types in the pancreas may communicate one with the other, since pancreatic cells of all types have been shown to share gap junctions (see Figure 9-1). However, because of the limitation in the size of the chemical molecules that can cross the gap junction, it seems unlikely that a hormone secreted by a particular islet cell could influence the secretory activity of another islet cell by this route. (*Q. 9-3*) *What other mechanisms are there by which the hormones produced by one islet cell could influence another?*

It should be clear from this brief discussion of the innervation of the pancreas that the central nervous system can influence the secretion of the hormones produced by cells of the islets of Langerhans. Section 9-4 also discusses briefly the role of the central nervous system in the control of food intake.

SECTION 9-1: POST-TEST QUESTIONS

1. The pancreas can be classified as both an exocrine and an endocrine gland. (True/False)
2. The pancreas contains small islands of hormone secreting cells called a. _____ _____. These cells are known presently to secrete b. _____ _____ different hormones. Of these, the hormones that are known to play a role in regulation of the concentration of glucose in blood are c. _____, d. _____, and e. _____.
3. Of the three hormones mentioned in (c), (d), and (e) above, _____ is also known for its role in inhibition of the secretion of growth hormone in the anterior pituitary gland.
4. Secretion by cells of the pancreatic islets is influenced by both branches of the autonomic nervous system. (True/False)
5. Cells of the pancreatic islets may communicate one with another by means of a. _____. These allow the passage of b. _____ _____ and c. _____ through the cell membrane and into the cell.
6. Sympathetic nervous stimuli to the pancreas originate in the a. _____ area of the hypothalamus; parasympathetic nervous stimuli originate in the b. _____ area.
7. The "final common" nervous pathway to and from the pancreas, which contains both afferent and efferent sympathetic and parasympathetic fibers, is the _____ _____.

SECTION 9-1: POST-TEST ANSWERS

1. True
2. a. islets of Langerhans
   b. six

      c. insulin
      d. glucagon
      e. somatostatin
3. somatostatin
4. True
5. a. gap junctions
      b. electrical impulses
      c. substances of low molecular weight
6. a. ventromedial
      b. ventrolateral
7. mixed pancreatic nerve

SECTION 9-2: CHEMICAL CHARACTERISTICS, SYNTHESIS, STORAGE, RELEASE, TRANSPORT, AND DEGRADATION OF INSULIN, PROINSULIN, GLUCAGON, AND PROGLUCAGON

OBJECTIVES:

The student should be able to:
1. Describe the chemical characteristics of insulin and proinsulin.
2. Discuss the synthesis, storage, and release of insulin.
3. Discuss the chemical characteristics, synthesis, and release of glucagon.
4. Discuss the degradation of insulin and glucagon.

A. SYNTHESIS, STORAGE, AND RELEASE OF INSULIN

Proinsulin, the precursor of insulin, is produced by standard protein synthetic mechanisms on the rough endoplasmic reticulum of the B-cells of the islets of Langerhans. In humans proinsulin is a single, coiled polypeptide chain containing 86 amino acids (i.e., molecular weight of 9000 daltons) and two disulfide bonds (see Figure 9-2). Proinsulin is also known to be complexed with zinc, but it is not certain whether this occurs before or after packaging in the Golgi apparatus. It is believed that some time is required for the packaged granules to "mature" and for the cleavage of proinsulin to occur. There is evidence that the more mature granules are released from the pancreas first, but some immature granules also can be released. Thus, proinsulin can be detected in plasma by radioimmunoassay. Proinsulin contributes to the estimates of immunoreactive insulin in the blood of humans, but its contribution is less than 20% of the total except in pathologic states such as certain tumors of the islet cells of the pancreas.

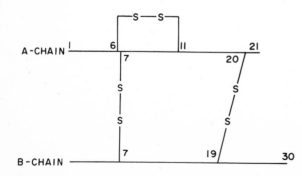

FIGURE 9-2: Highly schematic diagram of the insulin molecule in humans. The numbers indicate specific carbon atoms in each chain.

Within the granules, proinsulin is converted to insulin by a trypsinlike proteolytic enzyme that appears to be unique to the B-cell. Circulating proinsulin does not appear to be converted to insulin peripherally. Proteolytic cleavage reduces the molecular weight from 9000 to 6000 daltons and thus forms insulin and C-peptide, which contains the residue of 3000 daltons. Cleavage occurs at four separate places in the proinsulin molecule (between carbons 30 and 31, 66 and 67, 70 and 71, and 76 and 77) to form a molecule of insulin containing two peptide chains connected by two disulfide bridges. Insulin secreted by the human pancreas contains 51 amino acid residues, 21 of which are in the A-chain and 30 in the B-chain.

Release of insulin occurs by a typical exocytotic process that seems to be initiated by an influx of calcium ions (see Chapter 2 and Figures 2-16 and 9-3). The initial stimulus for this influx is not understood clearly. A current hypothesis is that the influx of calcium ions initiates a contraction or a conformational change in the microtubules of the cell, which are believed to be important in guiding the vesicles or granules to the surface, where they fuse with the cell membranes. The contents are then extruded into the extracellular fluid surrounding the cell. From there insulin diffuses into the blood and is carried to all parts of the body. The C-peptide is released at the same time insulin is released. The released insulin does not appear to be transported in blood by another protein.

Electron microscopic analysis suggests that an endocytotic process follows exocytosis in the pancreas. The endocytotic process represents the movement back into the cell of some of the fused membrane resulting from release of the insulin containing granules. Some of the membrane particles are acted on by lysosomes. Whether they are completely broken down or only fragmented and recycled is not known. It is also believed at present that the Golgi apparatus may be important in processing the membrane fragments. (Q. 9-4) *What would you expect to occur if the vesicular membranes were not retrieved by endocytosis?*

A large quantity of insulin is stored in the pancreas. In man it is about 4 units per gram of tissue or about 200 units for the entire pancreas. There are 24 units per

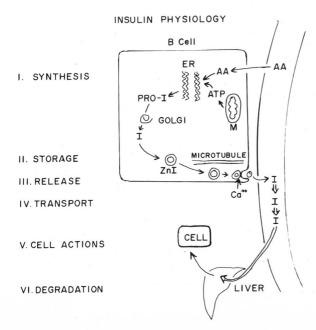

INSULIN PHYSIOLOGY

B Cell

I. SYNTHESIS

II. STORAGE

III. RELEASE

IV. TRANSPORT

V. CELL ACTIONS

VI. DEGRADATION

FIGURE 9-3: Synthesis, storage, release, transport, cellular actions, and degradation of insulin. Amino acids (AA) from blood are used to synthesize proinsulin (PRO-I) by the rough endoplasmic reticulum (ER). Energy for the synthetic process is provided by mitochondria (M) by way of ATP. Newly synthesized proinsulin is transported to the Golgi apparatus, which packages the proinsulin. Either before or after packaging, zinc combines with the proinsulin. During the process of maturing of the granule, proinsulin is converted to insulin. Exocytosis of the granule occurs as a result of an influx of calcium into the cell. Insulin is released into blood, along with C-peptide, and is carried to the liver, where 40–50% of the insulin is degraded; the remainder is available to peripheral cells.

milligram of insulin. From 25 to 50 units or 1 to 2 mg of insulin is secreted daily by adult humans. Thus, if production of insulin by the pancreas were to stop entirely, the insulin stored in the pancreas would be sufficient to supply an adult human for 4 to 8 days. (*Q. 9-5*) *What other endocrine gland has a large storage pool of its hormone?* The concentration of insulin in plasma is about 2 μU/ml and it can increase to levels of 50 to 150 μU/ml after an infusion of glucose. Thus the variation in the concentration of insulin in plasma is from 25- to 75-fold above the minimal concentration.

Fortunately there are very few differences in the insulin molecule among a number of animal species. Pig and man have identical molecules with respect to chain A but have a difference in a single amino acid in chain B (amino acid number 30). It is fortunate that the small differences in the structure of insulin among cattle, pigs, and man do not readily induce production of antibodies when animal hormones are administered to man. (*Q. 9-6*) *What effect would such antibodies have on the biologic effectiveness of insulin?* Currently some success has been reported in the synthesis of insulin by certain bacteria. If the process becomes feasible commercially, it will represent a source of insulin that may be more specific for humans and relatively more simple to produce.

B. CHEMICAL CHARACTERISTICS, SYNTHESIS, AND RELEASE OF GLUCAGON

Glucagon, a product of A-cells of the islets of Langerhans, is a single chain polypeptide containing 29 amino acids and having a molecular weight of 3485 daltons. It is immunologically distinct from insulin. Although the existence of glucagon has been known as long as that of insulin, considerably less is known about its synthesis, storage, and release from A-cells of the pancreatic islets.

It is believed that the synthesis of glucagon proceeds in the same way as that for insulin including the existence of an 18,000 dalton proglucagon molecule. However, zinc is not incorporated into the glucagon molecule. Glucagon is believed to be secreted into extracellular fluid by exocytosis just as is the case for insulin. Details of the synthesis of glucagon are not known with certainty, nor are the details of its cellular release.

About 5 to 10 μg of glucagon can be extracted from each gram of pancreas. (*Q. 9-7*) *How do these figures compare to the number of micrograms of insulin that can be extracted from each gram of pancreas?* Glucagon (like insulin) does not appear to be transported in blood in association with another protein.

C. DEGRADATION OF INSULIN AND GLUCAGON

When insulin is tagged with radioactive iodide and injected into normal humans, less than 15% of the injected dose is present in plasma 1 hour later. Crystalline porcine insulin has been shown to have a half-life of less than 5 minutes in both diabetic and normal humans. Radiolabeled insulin is found to be concentrated mainly by cells in the liver, kidney, and skeletal muscles. The kidney can excrete insulin through its glomeruli, but the insulin is usually completely reabsorbed by the renal tubules and apparently reutilized. Very small amounts of insulin may appear in the urine.

The liver extracts 40–50% of the insulin delivered to it, inactivates it by proteolysis, and excretes it into bile. This accounts for the very short half-life of insulin in blood. Since the vascular supply from the pancreas goes directly to the liver, about 40–50% of the secreted insulin is metabolized before it can exert any effects peripherally. This means that the liver plays an important role in regulating peripheral insulin concentration. (Q. 9-8) *What effects would you predict to occur in an insulin-dependent diabetic following the surgical redirection of the venous drainage of the pancreas to a site other than directly into the liver (i.e., the normal anatomic situation)?*

Glucagon is probably inactivated by the liver just as is the case for insulin, but details of its metabolism are not well known.

SECTION 9-2: POST-TEST QUESTIONS

1. A single, coiled polypeptide chain containing 86 amino acids is the precursor of insulin. It is called a. _____. It is produced by the b. _____ _____ and is transported to the c. _____, where it is packaged. Conversion of the precursor to insulin most likely occurs d. (where?) _____. As a result of this conversion, a residual e. _____ _____ is formed. The packaged granules are released into blood by a process called. f. _____, which is stimulated by an influx of g. _____ ions into the cell.
2. A large quantity of insulin is stored in the pancreas. (True/False)
3. Variations in the concentration of insulin in plasma are very small during the course of a day. (True/False)
4. Glucagon is immunologically distinct from insulin. (True/False) It is secreted by the _____ cells of the islets of Langerhans.
5. The organ largely responsible for the degradation of both insulin and glucagon is the _____.
6. The half-life of insulin in the normal individual is a. _____ _____. It is b. (longer/shorter/the same) for diabetic individuals.

SECTION 9-2: POST-TEST ANSWERS

1. a. proinsulin
   b. rough endoplasmic reticulum
   c. Golgi apparatus
   d. in the packaged granules
   e. C-peptide
   f. exocytosis
   g. calcium
2. True
3. False. The concentration of insulin in plasma can vary from 25- to 75-fold above the minimal concentration.
4. True. A-cells
5. liver
6. a. less than 5 minutes
   b. the same

SECTION 9-3: ACTIONS OF INSULIN AND GLUCAGON AT THE CELLULAR LEVEL

OBJECTIVES:

The student should be able to:
1. State why insulin is called an anabolic hormone.

2. Name the three major tissues in which insulin exerts an anabolic effect.
3. State how insulin stimulates the production and storage of glycogen and trigly-cerides.
4. List some characteristics of the receptors for insulin.
5. State what is known about the second messenger for insulin.

A. INSULIN RECEPTORS AND METABOLIC ACTIONS

Insulin is a hormone of energy storage. For this reason it is called an anabolic hormone. One of its best known actions is to reduce the concentration of glucose in blood. This occurs by four mechanisms: a) an increased uptake of glucose by skeletal muscle and liver, b) a reduction in output of glucose from these tissues, c) an increased uptake of glucose and free fatty acids into adipocytes, and d) an inhibition of the breakdown of triglycerides and release of free fatty acids from them. Insulin also increases the uptake of amino acids and the synthesis of protein and RNA in cells generally. Thus, insulin performs at the cellular level a number of actions that are directed toward the storage of substrates for metabolism.

The mechanism(s) by which insulin facilitates the uptake of glucose, free fatty acids, and amino acids is not known with certainty. Whether a separate mechanism exists for each is also unknown. Uptake of these substrates into cells may be visualized in terms of a direct effect of insulin on cellular membranes (e.g., affecting electrical activity of the cell; inducing conformational changes in the molecules comprising the membrane, and/or other mechanisms affecting their transport across the membrane). However, insulin also affects intracellular enzymes. Thus, in the cases of the liver and skeletal muscle, insulin is known to activate the enzyme glycogen synthetase, which facilitates the production of glycogen from glucose (see Figure 9-4). In adipose tissue, insulin activates acetyl coenzyme A decarboxylase, which facilitates the formation of trigly-

FIGURE 9-4: The major actions of insulin on the intermediary metabolism of certain peripheral cells. Insulin stimulates the formation of glycogen from glucose in hepatic and skeletal muscle cells. It also stimulates the conversion to triglycerides of fatty acids, both those produced endogenously and those taken up from blood. The uptake of amino acids is stimulated in all cells of the body, as is the production of RNA. Insulin is also known to facilitate the movement of potassium intracellularly.

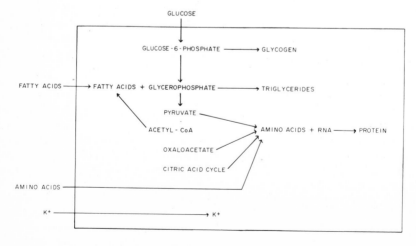

cerides from fatty acids. If insulin could not enter the cell, a second messenger would be necessary to mediate these changes.

Although it is known that the membranes of all cells of the body are permeable to glucose, insulin does not appear to affect the facilitated transport mechanism by which glucose enters most cells. It is only in the insulin-sensitive tissues that transport of glucose into the cell is enhanced, and it is only these cells that are capable of synthesizing glucose into either glycogen or triglycerides for storage in them. Thus, the brain is dependent on glucose as its source of energy, but administration of insulin does not increase the rate of uptake of glucose into its cells or into any of the other insulin-insensitive tissues, such as red blood cells and renal medulla.

When the synthesis of glycogen is stimulated by insulin, potassium enters the cells. The mechanism by which potassium interacts in the synthesis of glycogen is not known with certainty. It is known, however, that the breakdown of glycogen to glucose is accompanied by the release of potassium from the cells (see Figure 9-4).

Insulin manifests its effect at the cellular level by activating receptors located randomly on the surface of the plasma membrane of the cell. This, in turn, triggers the cellular events leading to an increased rate of entry of glucose, free fatty acids, and amino acids, as well as increased rates of synthesis of glycogen, triglycerides, and protein in insulin-sensitive cells. Insulin appears to bind rather loosely to its receptor. The process of binding, however, does not affect the insulin molecule, since dissociated molecules of insulin are still capable of binding to other receptors and activating cellular events. It has been estimated that the surface of one adipocyte may contain as many as 10,000 receptors for insulin. Biologic activity is observed when as few as 10% are activated. The biologic potency of insulin is a function of its binding affinity for its receptor. It has been stated that the receptors for insulin do not differ among mammals and that the differences in biologic activity of insulins from various mammalian species are related to the differences in the chemical characteristics of the insulin molecules.

A great deal of mystery surrounds the fact that only 10% of the receptors for insulin need to be bound to induce a typical response. An interesting, but unexplained, characteristic of the receptor for insulin is negative cooperativity. This occurs when an increase in the number of hormone-receptor complexes reduces the binding affinity for the remaining free receptors. However, other explanations are also possible, such as the existence of two types of receptor, one of high affinity and low capacity and another of low affinity and high capacity. This issue has yet to be resolved.

Biochemical isolation of the receptors for insulin and treatment of the preparation with a phospholipase enzyme increases the binding of insulin as much as four-fold. This eliminates the possibility that the receptor is a phospholipid. (Q. 9-9) Why? However, treatment of the preparation with the enzyme neuramidase, which cleaves and detaches the amino sugar sialic acid from glycoproteins, abolishes both the binding of insulin and the cellular response to it. This suggests that the receptor for insulin may be a glycoprotein.

It might be expected that the insulin would activate cellular mechanisms by way of the cAMP system. (Q. 9-10) Why? In fact, it has been shown that insulin inhibits the enzyme adenylate cyclase, with a resultant decrease in the cellular levels of cAMP. Insulin is the only anabolic hormone that can prevent the catabolic effects of a number of hormones, such as glucagon in liver and epinephrine in adipose tissue, both of which manifest their effects by way of the cAMP system. It is not known at present precisely how insulin prevents these effects, but experimental results show that it can inhibit glucagon-stimulated release of cAMP by hepatic cells of mice in vitro.

As discussed in Chapter 1, it is believed that the hormone-receptor relationship involves two distinct and separable processes: a) recognition and binding and b) activation of cellular mechanisms. In the case of a number of hormones, molecules of similar structure have been synthesized that bind to the receptor but fail to activate cellular mechanisms. This is the mechanism by which many inhibitors of enzymes act. However, no inhibitors are known for insulin. In contrast, there are several known substances that can bind to insulin receptors and activate cellular processes. These include a plant lectin known as concanavalin A, and wheat germ agglutinin. Both are capable of binding to isolated insulin receptors. In addition to these compounds, somatomedins produced endogenously are also known to bind to insulin receptors.

It has become clear that the concentration of insulin in blood in some way influences either the rate of turnover or the availability of binding sites for insulin in the plasma membrane. Thus, a deficiency of insulin per se is accompanied by an increase in available receptor sites. This concept is important to an understanding of the different types of diabetes to be discussed in Section 9-6, in which changes in the adenylate cyclase system would appear to be one of the primary targets of insulin. Whether the intracellular effects of insulin are the result of a reduction in the level of cAMP is unknown. However, there is no evidence for an essential role of cAMP in transport mechanisms influenced by insulin. At present, the "second messenger" for insulin is not known with certainty, although insulin has been shown to increase the concentration of cGMP in certain cells. You may recall from Chapter 1 that this nucleotide often acts opposite to cAMP. (Q. 9-11) *What enzyme is required to increase cellular concentration of cGMP?*

It is not entirely clear, at present, that insulin produces all its cellular effects without entering the cell. Experiments showing that insulin, prevented from entering cells by being bound to large Sepharose® beads, could initiate cellular responses, suggested that the response was initiated at the level of the membrane. It is now known, however, that Sepharose® beads lose insulin and that the freed insulin may have initiated the response. It has also been shown by electron microscopy that small amounts of insulin, or one of its fragment, can enter lymphocytes. However, it does not appear to go beyond 10–15% of the radius of the cell. The insulin, or fragments, that enter lymphocytes appear to localize in lysosomes. Other studies have shown that insulin can bind specifically to isolated cellular nuclei. (Q. 9-12) *What does this suggest?* In summary, although experimental evidence has not yet excluded the possibility that insulin may enter the cell, present consensus is that it exerts its effects by activating membrane receptors that, in turn, activate a second messenger.

As noted above, a great deal of research in the area of receptors for insulin has been carried out on insulin-insensitive tissues such as lymphocytes and red blood cells. At present, the characteristics of the receptors for insulin in the membrane of cells from these tissues appear to be similar to those from insulin-sensitive tissues. (Q. 9-13) *Does this have any physiologic meaning?*

B. GLUCAGON RECEPTORS AND METABOLIC ACTIONS

Glucagon, the hormone secreted by A-cells of the islets of Langerhans, is known to be released only by the following stimuli: hypoglycemia, increased concentration of amino acids in blood, and prolonged or severe exercise.

The physiologic role of glucagon is not known with certainty, but it does act to oppose the effects of insulin. Glucagon increases the concentration of glucose in blood by four mechanisms: a) increasing glycogenolysis, which is mediated by activation of the hepatic phosphorylase enzyme, b) increasing deamination of amino acids, with a resultant increase in urea formation, c) increasing fatty acid oxidation, with the consequent production of hydrogen ions, and d) inhibiting the production of glucose. The production of hydrogen ions is important for the conversion of α-ketoglutarate, oxaloacetate, and pyruvate to glucose, since hydrogen ions are necessary for the conversion of oxaloacetate to phosphoenol pyruvate. Glucagon, in physiologic amounts, is also known to initiate the release of insulin from B-cells. This may be important in preventing an excessive increase in the concentration of glucose in blood, which might otherwise occur if the effects of glucagon were unopposed. Thus, glucagon is a catabolic hormone because of its role in reducing the stores of substrates in liver and adipose tissue. Its effect on carbohydrate metabolism occurs only in liver.

Glucagon is bound by receptors on the membranes of cells of the liver and adipose tissue. Binding does not seem to inactivate the hormone. Analogues of glucagon have been synthesized that bind to receptors but fail to induce cellular activity. The receptors for glucagon, like those for insulin, are most likely glycoproteins.

Glucagon is known to produce its effects by activation of the cAMP system. The release of glucose and free fatty acids occurs as a result of activation of cellular enzymes by cAMP.

SECTION 9-3: POST-TEST QUESTIONS

1. What are the three major target tissues of insulin?
   a.
   b.
   c.
2. What is the effect of insulin on all tissues of the body?

3. What is the definition of an anabolic hormone?

4. In tissues sensitive to its action, insulin performs two important functions. What are they?
   a.
   b.
5. The effects of insulin at the cellular level are mediated by activation of the adenylate cyclase system. (True/False)
6. Receptors for insulin are present only in cell membranes of insulin-sensitive cells. (True/False)
7. Insulin is responsible for maintenance of glucose transport across cellular membranes of all tissues of the body. (True/False)
8. Although there may be as many as 10,000 receptors for insulin on each adipocyte, biologic activity is observed when only 10% are activated. (True/False)
9. The hormone-receptor relationship involves two distinct and separable processes. What are they?
   a.
   b.
10. Analogues of hormones that inhibit cellular activity generally affect which of these two processes?

11. The concentration of insulin in blood affects either the turnover or binding affinity of receptors for insulin. (True/False) This relation is a(n) (direct/inverse) one.
12. Insulin can prevent the catabolic effects of a number of hormones, including glucagon and catecholamines. (True/False) Although the mechanism is not understood, it is known that the effect of insulin on _____ is opposite to that of the catabolic hormones.

13. Only two physiologic stimuli are known to initiate the release of glucagon from A cells of the islets of Langerhans. What are these stimuli?
    a.
    b.
14. Glucagon is known to produce three principal actions in the body. What are they?
    a.
    b.
    c.
15. Glucagon, like insulin, is inactivated during binding to a membrane receptor. (True/False)
16. Glucagon increases plasma concentration of glucose and free fatty acids by activation of the cAMP system. (True/False)

SECTION 9-3: POST-TEST ANSWERS

1. a. Liver
   b. Skeletal muscle
   c. Adipose tissue
2. It increases the transport of amino acids into cells.
3. An anabolic hormone increases the storage of substrates for metabolism, such as glycogen and triglycerides, in cells specialized for these functions.
4. a. Insulin facilitates the transport of glucose and free fatty acids across the membranes of the cells.
   b. Insulin stimulates an activation of enzymes that synthesize glycogen from glucose and triglycerides from free fatty acids.
5. False
6. False
7. False
8. True
9. a. Recognition and binding
   b. Activation of cellular processes
10. Recognition and binding
11. True; inverse
12. True; cAMP
13. a. Hypoglycemia
    b. Increased concentration of amino acids in blood
14. a. Glucagon increases the availability of glucose to peripheral tissue
    b. Glucagon induces the release of insulin from the B-cell
    c. Glucagon stimulates the mobilization of free fatty acids from stored triglycerides of adipose tissue
15. False
16. True

SECTION 9-4: HORMONAL INTERACTIONS IN THE REGULATION OF THE CONCENTRATION OF GLUCOSE IN BLOOD

OBJECTIVES:

The student should be able to:
1. Discuss the extent of the daily variation in the concentration of glucose in blood and the factors that influence it.

2. Discuss the roles of insulin, liver, muscle, and adipose tissue in the storage of glucose.
3. Discuss the hormones that are important in maintaining the concentration of glucose in blood during fasting and their interaction.
4. Discuss gluconeogenesis and the hormones and tissues that play a role in it.

A. STORAGE MECHANISMS FOR EXCESS GLUCOSE

The concentration of glucose in the blood varies in the normal human during the course of a day. Although the subject cannot be discussed in detail here, it should be recognized that hunger and food intake are believed by some investigators to be initiated by the rate of decrease in the concentration of glucose in blood. Glucoreceptors located in the hypothalamus may serve as the sensors and set into motion behavioral mechanisms directed toward an increase in food intake. These may be the same glucoreceptors discussed in Section 9-1, although evidence is not yet clear in this regard. Large increases in the concentration of glucose in blood are associated with eating foods and drinking fluids containing carbohydrates (see Figure 9-5). In fact, the periodic influx of glucose associated with eating and drinking carbohydrates poses a problem to the system, namely, disposal of the glucose. The concentration of glucose in the blood of a normal human rarely exceeds 120 mg/100 ml during the course of a day, although an estimated 10 to 20 times the amount of glucose, and 80 to 90 times the amount of amino acids, present in the entire extracellular fluid, passes through the blood during this time. Thus, it is important for the body to have a mechanism that can be called on to facilitate the storage of excess substrates for energy production. Insulin appears to be the hormone that is important for the storage of these excess substrates.

As the concentration of glucose in blood increases after the ingestion of a meal, the concentration of insulin in blood also increases (see Figure 9-5). The secretion of insulin in response to an increase in the concentration of glucose in blood is very rapid and appears to be adjusted to the extent of the rise and fall in concentration of glucose (see Figure 9-6). Only a barely measurable increase in the concentration of glucose in blood is required to increase the rate of secretion of insulin. The half-time of insulin in blood is only about 8 to 10 minutes (see Figure 9-6). Thus, insulin is both secreted rapidly and metabolized rapidly. (Q. 9-14) *How do these kinetic properties of insulin add to the difficulties faced by the insulin-dependent diabetic?*

The absorption of ingested glucose from the gastrointestinal tract, aided by thyroid hormones, increases the concentration of glucose in blood (see Figure 9-7). The pancreatic B-cells appear to have an advance warning system. Some factor or factors are released by the gastrointestinal tract that appear to be capable of initiating the release of insulin. Two of these have been termed gastric inhibitor polypeptide (GIP) and vasoactive intestinal peptide (VIP). In addition, a glucagonlike hormone may also be responsi-

FIGURE 9-5: Variability of the concentrations of glucose and insulin in a normal human during the course of a day. The times of food ingestion during the day are shown. (*Adapted from:* Cahill, 1977.)

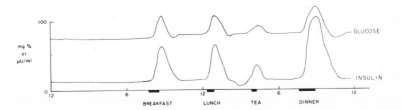

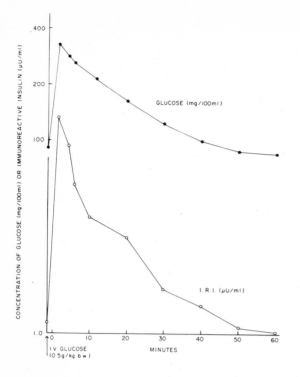

FIGURE 9-6: The response of pancreatic B-cells to the intravenous injection of glucose (0.5 g/kg) into a normal human. Note the rapidity with which the secretion of insulin (I.R.I.) begins. The time required for insulin to decrease half way from its maximal value to its initial value (half-time) is 8 to 10 minutes. (*Adapted from:* Cahill, 1977.)

ble for initiating the release of insulin as glucose is absorbed. This is often referred to as gut glucagon. Thus, both a gastrointestinal hormone and the increase in the concentration of glucose in blood stimulate an increase in the rate of secretion of insulin after a meal. (*Q. 9-15*). *Do you recall the effect(s) of somatostatin on the secretion of insulin, VIP, GIP, and gut glucagon?*

Following the ingestion of a meal, the concentration of amino acids in blood increases. This appears to be an adequate stimulus for the secretion of insulin, which facilitates their entry into cells where they are converted into tissue protein (see Figure 9-7). Somatomedins and growth hormone may also participate. (*Q. 9-16*) *How?* Certain amino acids, particularly the branched chain ones such as valine, leucine, and iso-

FIGURE 9-7: The hormones and organs that are important in regulating the concentration of glucose in blood. The various mechanisms by which rises and falls in the concentration of glucose in blood are corrected are discussed in the text.

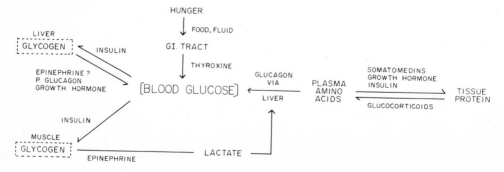

leucine, are also taken up by adipose tissue where they are used as precursors for fat synthesis. Some proteins and amino acids are also converted to fat by the liver. Thus, a high-protein diet can serve as a source of fat.

Some of the glucose that enters the cells of the liver under the influence of insulin is also converted into fat. Since the liver does not store fat normally, it is secreted into blood as a low-density lipoprotein. These are taken up by adipose tissue and used as substrate by the enzyme lipoprotein lipase, to form triglycerides. At present the proportion of a carbohydrate meal that eventually is used by the cells of the liver as substrate for the formation of glycogen, as opposed to fat, is not known with certainty.

B. PRODUCTION OF GLUCOSE DURING FASTING

We have discussed the role of insulin in facilitating the storage of glucose after a meal. It is important at this point to consider the physiologic events that occur between meals and when an individual has fasted for 6 to 12 hours. It has been estimated that the liver spends 18 hours each day putting glucose into blood rather than taking it up. In the periods between meals, the liver is the organ called on primarily to maintain the concentration of glucose in blood so that the organs dependent on it as an energy substrate can maintain their normal function. Thus, the brain appears to require more glucose and oxygen per unit of mass than any other tissue. Since the brain stores no glucose, it depends for its functioning on a proper supply of this substrate. If the supply of glucose is cut off for more than a few minutes, normal cerebration is disrupted. A longer delay in supplying glucose may result in irreversible damage and possibly death. This suggests the necessity for close regulation of the concentration of glucose in blood.

As the concentration of glucose in blood decreases, the concentration of insulin in blood also decreases, while the concentration of glucagon increases. Glucagon stimulates glycogenolysis from the liver to supply the needed glucose. Recent evidence indicates that the rise in the concentration of glucagon in blood is not due to an increase in its rate of secretion but rather it is due to a reduction in its rate of catabolism. Glucagon initiates glycogenolysis by activation of the cAMP system.

Recent studies in dogs have shown that the response to infusion of glucagon in physiologic amounts, and in the absence of antecedent hyperinsulinemia, is to double the output of glucose from the liver within 5 to 7 minutes after initiation of the infusion. Surprisingly, the stimulatory effect of the infused glucagon lasts only about 30 minutes in spite of continued infusion. This refractoriness is not due to depletion of glycogen from the liver. If epinephrine is now added to the infusion fluid containing glucagon, the output of glucose from the liver increases again. If the order of infusion of the hormones is reversed, the same effects occur. These results suggest that the production of glucose from glycogen by the liver is evanescent when stimulated by either glucagon or epinephrine alone (see Table 9-1). The hepatic refractoriness appears to be selective for the hormone whose concentration is greater when glucagon and epinephrine are administered simultaneously.

Recent studies suggest that an increase in glucagon concentration in plasma induces a "down" regulation of receptors for glucagon in the liver. Although reasons for this have not yet emerged, it appears that an increase in the concentration of cortisol in blood, as discussed below, transforms the evanescent action of glucagon and epinephrine to a persistent stimulatory effect on glucose production (see Table 9-1). This suggests the need for several catabolic hormones to maintain the concentration of glucose in blood during fasting.

The catabolic hormones glucagon and epinephrine appear to affect the concentration of glucose in blood not only by stimulating the release of glucose from the liver but also by affecting the utilization of glucose by peripheral cells. Thus, epinephrine plays a role

TABLE 9-1: Interactions of Glucagon, Epinephrine, and Cortisol in the Regulation of the Concentration of Glucose in Blood

Physiologic Effect	Response to			
	Glucagon	Epinephrine	Glucagon + Epinephrine	Cortisol + Glucagon + Epinephrine
Glucose production				
Magnitude	↑↑	↑	↑↑↑	↑↑↑↑
Duration	Transient	Transient	Transient	Persistent
Glucose utilization	↑	↓↓	↓↓	↓↓

Adapted from: Felig et al., 1979.

in glycogenolysis in liver and muscle. The latter tissue is unable to break down glycogen directly to glucose because it does not contain the enzyme glucose-6-phosphatase. The lactate produced when glycogen from muscle is broken down is transported to the liver, where it is converted to glucose by the process of gluconeogenesis (see Figure 9-7). At the same time epinephrine appears to inhibit utilization of glucose by peripheral tissue while stimulating the release of free fatty acids from adipocytes for use as a metabolic substrate by these tissues. Glucagon plays a role in glycogenolysis in the liver, but it also appears to increase the utilization of glucose by peripheral tissues.

After 12 hours of fasting, the glycogen content of the liver is almost depleted. The liver then begins to convert from glycogenolysis to the process of gluconeogenesis. The muscle, by way of an increase in blood concentration of the glucocorticoid cortisol, from the adrenal cortex, begins breaking down its protein to amino acids. These amino acids are transported to the liver, where they are deaminated to form glucose (see Figure 9-7). The liver derives the energy it needs for the process of gluconeogenesis to occur from fat and free fatty acids released from adipocytes by glucagon and epinephrine. Other tissues of the body using fatty acids as substrates under these conditions are able to metabolize the fatty acids to two carbon (acetate) fragments. These condense, two at a time, to form acetoacetate and β-hydroxybutyrate. The concentration of these "ketones" in blood is roughly directly proportional to the gluconeogenic activity of the liver and inversely proportional to the concentration of insulin in blood. (*Q. 9-17*) Why?

The release of amino acids by glucocorticoid hormones during fasting and starvation does not appear to be a random event. It appears to be primarily a release of the so-called glucogenic amino acids, glutamine and alanine. It is not understood clearly how this comes about, but it has been suggested that during the process of breakdown of protein from muscle, serine and methionine are converted to alanine. Isoleucine, leucine, and valine are converted to carbon dioxide and ammonium ions, which are used in the formation of glutamine, while arginine, histidine, lysine, proline, and glycine are released into the circulation. It should be emphasized that gluconeogenesis by liver can be stimulated not only by glucagon but by an increase in the concentration of amino acids in blood as well.

It is important to recognize that the role of cortisol in maintenance of the concentration of glucose in blood is its initiation of the breakdown of muscle protein to amino acids and its retardation of the down-regulation (or evanescent action) of glucagon and epinephrine (see Table 9-1). Cortisol does not appear to initiate the process of gluconeogenesis in the liver; glucagon and amino acids are probably responsible for this.

C. THE ROLE OF THE PERIPHERAL NERVOUS SYSTEM IN THE SECRETION OF INSULIN

It has often been observed that stimuli initiating an increase in the rate of secretion of insulin produce an initial "spike" increase that declines rapidly and is followed by a more gradual increase in the rate of secretion. The spike increase is associated with an immediately releasable pool of insulin, while the more gradual increase is associated with a pool that is dependent on newly synthesized insulin. (*Q. 9-18*) *Can you name any other hormones that have a similar pattern of secretory activity?*

A number of factors affect the rate of secretion of insulin. The most powerful physiologic stimulus is an increase in the concentration of glucose in blood. In addition, an increase in the concentration of amino acids in blood also increases the rate of secretion of insulin. Administration of a β-adrenergic agonist, such as isoproterenol, or a parasympathetic agent, such as metacholine, will increase the rate of secretion of insulin. Glucagon, both pancreatic and gut, as well as certain other hormones of gastrointestinal origin, such as gastrin, can also increase the rate of secretion of insulin. Even growth hormone has also been reported to increase the rate of secretion of insulin under certain conditions in vitro.

β-Adrenergic receptors on both the A- and B-cells of the islets of Langerhans can initiate secretion of glucagon and insulin, respectively, when stimulated by appropriate agonists. On the other hand, the α-adrenergic receptors on both cells inhibit secretion. It is of interest that administration of epinephrine to man is accompanied by an increase in the rate of secretion of glucagon and a reduction in the rate of secretion of insulin. This suggests that the same dose of epinephrine is seen as a β-adrenergic agonist by the A-cell and as an α-adrenergic agonist by the B-cell. An adequate explanation for this observation is not yet available. Isoproterenol, a relatively pure β-adrenergic agonist, stimulates the release of insulin and glucagon, both of which can be blocked by prior administration of the β-adrenergic antagonist, propranolol.

It is accepted generally that an augmentation in the release of insulin and glucagon following stimulation of β-adrenergic receptors is due to activation of the cAMP system. However, there is still considerable doubt regarding the mechanism by which α-adrenergic receptors mediate an inhibition of the release of insulin and glucagon, even though stimulation of α-adrenergic receptors has been shown to reduce the levels of cAMP in islet cells. The mechanism by which inhibition occurs may be related to alterations in intracellular concentrations of calcium, since a calcium ionophore has been used to reverse the inhibition of the secretion of insulin induced by epinephrine. (*Q. 9-19*) *Can you recall the name of another hormone that appears to display a similar mechanism of action (i.e., inhibition of extracellular calcium influx)?*

Acetylcholine, the neurotransmitter of the parasympathetic system, augments the release of both insulin and glucagon in vitro. This response is mediated by muscarinic receptors, since it is blockable with atropine. It is interesting that chronic vagotomy failed to affect the normal fasting concentrations of insulin and glucagon in blood in a number of species. However, in patients with truncal vagotomy, the increase in the rate of secretion of insulin following an oral load of glucose was less than that in individuals with an intact vagus.

Electrical stimulaton of the vagus nerve in the dog and baboon increases the concentration of insulin in blood. This response can be prevented by the prior administration of atropine. Electrical stimulation of the mixed pancreatic nerve in the dog stimulates the release of both insulin and glucagon. Administration of atropine under these conditions blocks the secretion of insulin but not glucagon. This suggests that the increase in the rate of release of insulin following stimulation of the mixed pancreatic nerve is mediated by parasympathetic, cholinergic fibers, whereas the increased rate of release of glucagon is mediated by sympathetic fibers.

D. SOMATOSTATIN

Somatostatin is a tetradecapeptide that was first isolated from brain, where it plays the role of a hypophysiotropic hormone inhibiting the secretion of growth hormone from the anterior pituitary gland (see Sections 2-2 and 8-2). Somatostatin has also been found in large quantities in the pancreas. It is an effective inhibitor of virtually every known stimulus for the secretion of both insulin and glucagon (see Figures 8-9 and 8-10). (Q. 9-20) *Does a given dose of somatostatin inhibit the secretion of insulin and glucagon to the same extent, or is it more effective against one or the other hormone?*

The release of somatostatin from pancreatic tissue is stimulated by an increase in the concentration of glucose, arginine, leucine, glucagon, and the β-adrenergic agonist isoproterenol, in blood. Substances that elevate the concentration of cAMP in islet tissue, such as theophylline and cAMP analogues, also stimulate the release of somatostatin. In contrast, epinephrine, acetylcholine, and inhibitors of cellular metabolism inhibit the release of somatostatin. This indicates that D-cells, which produce somatostatin, are under metabolic, hormonal, and neural control. Most agents that increase the secretion of somatostatin also increase the secretion of insulin. The present state of knowledge suggests that somatostatin is more likely to control the secretion of glucagon rather than its synthesis. This suggests that somatostatin may play a role in inhibiting the release of glucagon when an increase in the concentration of insulin in blood is required for storage of excess glucose (see Section 8-5).

E. HORMONAL INTERACTIONS IN REGULATION OF THE CONCENTRATION OF GLUCOSE IN BLOOD

It is often difficult to integrate into a meaningful scheme the many factors that can affect the secretion of hormones concerned with the regulation of the concentration of glucose in blood. Furthermore, to sort out the factors that are important physiologically from those that may be seen only in the laboratory under experimental conditions presents an additional challenge.

Some investigators feel that the regulation of the concentration of glucose in blood can be accounted for most simply by a knowledge of the concentration of insulin and glucagon in blood. For example, the data shown in Table 9-2 reveal that the concentration of insulin in plasma is graded to the net influx of carbohydrate into blood, whereas

TABLE 9-2: Effect of Varying Metabolic and Nutritional Conditions on the Concentrations of Insulin and Glucagon in Human Plasma

Metabolic or Nutritional Condition	Net Influx of Carbohydrate into Blood (g/min)	Hormones	
		Insulin (mU/ml)	Glucagon (pg/ml)
Large carbohydrate meal	>0.5	200	50
Small carbohydrate meal	0.3	75	50
Intravenous infusion of glucose	0.1	25	50
Fasting	0	10	150
Diabetes	−0.1	5	300

Adapted from: Cahill, C. F., Jr., 1977.

the concentration of glucagon is unchanged under these conditions. In contrast, the concentration of insulin in plasma is reduced during fasting while that of glucagon is tripled. In uncomplicated diabetes in which the secretory function of the B-cells of the pancreas is reduced but not abolished, the concentration of insulin in plasma is reduced even further while the concentration of glucagon is very high. The potential role of this excessive secretion of glucagon in exacerbating diabetes is further discussed in Section 8-5 and 9-6.

SECTION 9-4: POST-TEST QUESTIONS

1. The most potent physiologic stimulus for the secretion of insulin is hyperglycemia. (True/False)
2. Insulin is the hormone that is primarily important for storage of excess substrates. (True/False)
3. A fairly large increase in the concentration of glucose in blood is required to increase the rate of secretion of insulin. (True/False)
4. A hormone(s) released by the gastrointestinal tract is capable of initiating the release of insulin. What physiologic significance could this have?

5. How does insulin aid in maintaining the concentration of glucose in blood after ingestion of a meal that is high in carbohydrates?

6. An increase in the concentration of amino acids in blood is an important stimulus for the secretion of insulin. (True/False)
7. Name three hormones that are important in maintaining the concentration of glucose in blood during fasting.
   a.
   b.
   c.
8. What role does each hormone in question 7 play?
   a.

   b.

c.

9. How do the hormones discussed in questions 7 and 8 interact?

10. Approximately how long will the glycogen stores in liver last during fasting?

11. What happens to maintain blood concentration of glucose after the stores of glycogen are depleted?

12. What happens to the secretion of insulin during fasting?

13. How does the liver differ from other tissues in its metabolism of fatty acids?

14. What is gluconeogenesis? What role does cortisol play in it?

15. One of the physiologic events accompanying administration of glucagon is the release of free fatty acids from adipocytes. (True/False)
16. Substances that elevate cAMP levels in islet cells also stimulate the release of somatostatin. (True/False)

SECTION 9-4: POST-TEST ANSWERS

1. True
2. True
3. False. Experimental evidence indicates that a barely detectable increase in the concentration of glucose in blood will increase the rate of secretion of insulin.
4. It could serve as an advance warning signal to the B-cells of the pancreatic islets that the concentration of glucose in blood is soon to be increased by the food in the gastrointestinal tract.
5. Insulin concentration in blood increases as the concentration of glucose increases. Insulin stimulates the transport of glucose into liver, muscle, and adipose tissue and facilitates the conversion of glucose to glycogen and triglycerides for storage.
6. True

7. a. Glucagon
    b. Epinephrine
    c. Cortisol
8. a. *Glucagon* stimulates the release of glucose from glycogen in the liver as well as initiating the release of free fatty acids from adipocytes.
    b. *Epinephrine* also stimulates the release of glucose from glycogen in the liver and in addition can stimulate the breakdown of glycogen to lactate in muscle. The lactate must be transported to the liver to be converted to glucose. Epinephrine also initiates the release of free fatty acids from adipocytes.
    c. *Cortisol* stimulates the breakdown of protein in muscle to amino acids, which are transported to the liver, where they are transformed into glucose by the process of gluconeogenesis.
9. The effect on glucagon or epinephrine or both combined on the conversion of hepatic glycogen to glucose is evanescent. If cortisol is present in an elevated concentration in blood, the effects of glucagon and epinephrine on glycogenolysis are persistent. Thus, the three hormones interact to facilitate glycogenolysis.
10. Approximately 12 hours.
11. Gluconeogenesis occurs and fatty acids are released from storage.
12. Insulin secretion decreases and its concentration in blood becomes very low.
13. The liver is unable to metabolize fatty acids to carbon dioxide and water as is the case for other tissues. Instead it metabolizes fatty acids to two carbon fragments that condense to form acetoacetate and β-hydroxybutyrate.
14. Gluconeogenesis is the formation of glucose from amino acids or lactate by the liver. Cortisol stimulates the breakdown of muscle protein to amino acids and makes available the substrate for gluconeogenesis to the liver.
15. True
16. True

SECTION 9-5: CLINICAL TESTS OF PANCREATIC ISLET FUNCTION

OBJECTIVES:

The student should be able to:
  1. Describe a test of B-cell function used clinically to assess adequacy of the secretion of insulin.
  2. Describe a test of A-cell function used clinically to assess adequacy of the secretion of glucagon.

A. GLUCOSE TOLERANCE TEST

Administration of an oral load of glucose (100 g) to a normal human after an overnight fast results in an increase in the concentration of insulin in blood within half an hour to levels of approximately 150 μU/ml from initial levels of 70 to 80 μU/ml. Within 2 hours, the concentrations of both insulin and glucose in blood have returned to their initial levels. The increase in the concentration of glucose in blood is accompanied by an increase in the concentration of insulin, which is responsible for the reduction in the concentration of glucose (see Figure 9-8). Obesity can affect the concentration of insulin in blood in that more insulin appears to be secreted, although the concentration of glucose in blood goes no higher than that in a nonobese individual.

A diabetic individual has a higher initial concentration of glucose in blood and a

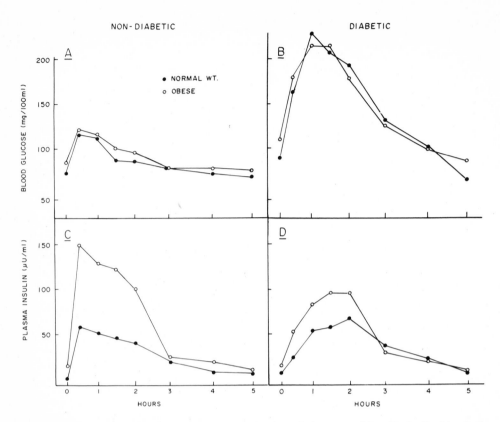

FIGURE 9-8: Time course of increase in concentration of glucose and insulin in the blood of nondiabetic (left) and diabetic (right) subjects after oral ingestion of a load of glucose. The responses of both obese subjects and subjects of normal weight are compared in both nondiabetic and diabetic groups. (*Adapted from:* Perley and Kipnis, 1966.)

higher and more prolonged elevation of the concentration of glucose following the oral load of glucose than is the case for a nondiabetic individual (see Figure 9-8C). Between 80% and 90% of diabetic patients (i.e., those with type 2 or noninsulin-dependent diabetes) have an increase in the concentration of insulin that may be even greater than that of the normal, nonobese individual. Obesity, in combination with this form of diabetes, again exaggerates the secretory response of insulin to an oral load of glucose, but the concentration of insulin in plasma does not reach that of the nondiabetic obese individual.

In a second subdivision of diabetes (i.e. type 1 or insulin-dependent diabetes) representing 10–20% of all diabetics, the secretion of insulin is impaired because of destruction of B-cells in the pancreas. These individuals have the same abnormal glucose tolerance as those with type 2 diabetes but have virtually no increase in the concentration of insulin following the oral load of glucose. The measurement of insulin used in the glucose tolerance test is made by means of a radioimmunoassay.

B. TEST OF ADEQUACY OF RESPONSIVENESS TO GLUCAGON

An increase in the concentration of most amino acids in blood will increase the rate of secretion of glucagon in humans. For example, within 5 minutes after initiation of an infusion of arginine at a rate of 11.7 mg per kilogram of body weight per minute, the

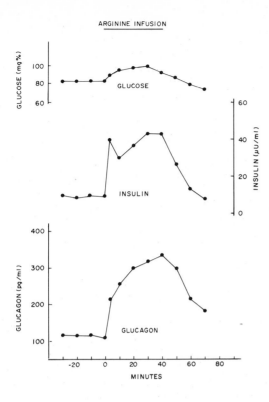

FIGURE 9-9: Concentrations of glucose, insulin, and glucagon in plasma accompanying an intravenous infusion of the amino acid arginine for 40 minutes at a rate of 11.7 mg/kg/min in man. (*Adapted from:* Unger, 1974.)

concentration of glucagon in plasma may have nearly doubled, and by 20 minutes, it may have tripled (see Figure 9-9). Maximal concentrations of glucagon may be attained by the end of a 40-minute infusion. A failure to obtain an increase in the concentration of glucagon by at least 75 pg/ml during the 40-minute infusion is regarded as evidence of a reduced responsiveness of A-cells.

Figure 9-9 also illustrates the increase in the concentraton of insulin in plasma that normally follows an infusion of arginine. Whether the increase is mediated by glucagon acting at the level of the B-cell of the pancreatic islet to stimulate the release of insulin or by the small rise in the concentration of glucose in plasma accompanying the infusion is not known with certainty. The mechanism by which infusion of a variety of amino acids stimulates the secretion of glucagon is also unknown.

SECTION 9-5: POST-TEST QUESTIONS

1. A diabetic human generally has a   (higher/lower)   concentration of glucose in blood after an overnight fast.
2. Describe the abnormal glucose tolerance curve that results from administration of a standard oral load of glucose to a diabetic human.

3. Following an oral load of glucose, the concentration of insulin in plasma in the majority of diabetic patients, measured by radioimmunoassay, is   (greater/less)   than that of nondiabetic individuals.

4. What effect has obesity on the glucose tolerance curve of nondiabetic and diabetic individuals?

5. Infusion of amino acids such as arginine into humans is accompanied by an a. (increase/decrease) in the concentration of glucagon in plasma. Maximal levels are reached within b. _____ minutes after initiation of the standard infusion of arginine. The concentration of insulin c. (increases/decreases) under these same conditions. What is this response related to?
   d.

SECTION 9-5: POST-TEST ANSWERS

1. higher
2. There is an exaggerated rise in the concentration of glucose and a prolonged length of time required for the return of the concentration of glucose to the pretest value.
3. greater
4. Following ingestion of a glucose load, obese individuals have a greater rise in the concentration of insulin in their blood than nonobese individuals. This occurs regardless of whether they are diabetic.
5. a. increase
   b. 40
   c. increases
   d. An increase in the concentration of glucagon in plasma acting directly on the B-cell of pancreatic islet tissue or to the rise in the concentration of glucose in plasma accompanying the infusion of arginine.

SECTION 9-6: DIABETES MELLITUS

OBJECTIVES:

The student should be able to:
1. Describe two types of diabetes and the predominant problem contributing to the disease in each case.
2. Name the types of diabetes into which the majority of patients fall.
3. Describe some effects of either or both lack of insulin and failure of receptors to respond on carbohydrate, fat, and protein metabolism.
4. State why polydipsia, polyuria, and polyphagia occur in untreated diabetics.
5. Describe the Somogyi effect on control of glucose concentration in blood.

A. TYPES OF DIABETES

Diabetes mellitus is a disease characterized by an inability to control the concentration of glucose in blood. In this disease both insulin and its receptors on the surface of cells play a role. The specific role of each depends on the types of diabetes under consideration.

By tradition, diabetes has usually been classified according to the age of onset of the disease as either "juvenile" or "maturity onset." It has become apparent as more is learned about the secretory activity of the pancreatic islets and the status of the receptors for insulin that diabetes mellitus can be divided into two general types.

In type 1 ("insulin-dependent") diabetes, insulin is absent, or nearly absent, although the receptors for insulin are unaffected. Between 10% and 20% of all known diabetics are in this category. The lack of insulin in this type of diabetes results from total or near-total destruction of the B-cells of the pancreatic islets. Hence, these patients must depend on an exogenous supply of insulin. A major objective in their therapy is to try to mimic the daily secretion of insulin as it would occur physiologically. This is very difficult to do by injections of insulin, even though two types of insulin, a long-lasting and a short-lasting one, have been developed. (Q. 9-21) *When would you inject each of these to try to mimic the secretion of insulin under normal circumstances? (See Figure 9-5 for a hint.)* Because of the difficulty in mimicking the physiologic secretion of insulin by exogenous injection, this type of diabetes is often called "brittle." The control of type 1 diabetes requires the maintenance of a delicate balance between food intake, exercise, and dosage of insulin. A new method for treating this type of diabetes is an infusion pump, which is programmed electronically to deliver extra insulin at times paralleling the peaks shown in Figure 9-5.

Type 2 diabetes is characterized by normal or near-normal concentrations of insulin in blood. Often the concentration of insulin is even above normal. This suggests that the problem may be either at the level of the receptors for insulin on cell surfaces or in the activation of cellular processes by the receptor. This type of diabetes is present in 80–90% of all known diabetics.

It is interesting that a majority (75% or more) of type 2 diabetics consists of obese patients. They have an elevated basal level of secretion of insulin, although the level of secretion measured after either meals or a glucose ·challenge may be the same as, or slightly higher than, that of normals. The basal concentration of insulin in blood shows an excellent inverse correlation with the number of receptors for insulin. That is, the higher the level of the basal concentration of insulin in blood, the lower the number of receptors. With appropriate therapy, the numbers of receptors increase, blood concentration of glucose decreases, and insulin concentration in serum returns to normal basal levels.

Although there appears to be a close relation between obesity and diabetes, the mechanism is not well understood. It is believed that obesity, resulting from overeating, occurs first and is followed some years later by diabetes.

Type 2 diabetes also includes a relatively rare group of patients who are thin and have elevated levels of insulin in their blood but have receptors for insulin that bind the hormone poorly. The receptors, present in normal numbers, are almost completely inactivated by antibodies directed against them. The severity of their disease correlates directly with the titer of the antibody in their blood.

Type 2 diabetes also includes several small groups of patients who have high levels of insulin in their blood, and a normal number of insulin receptors with normal affinity. Although the exact mechanism contributing to this type of diabetes is unknown, it is likely that the receptors are unable to transmit their message to the cellular processes that govern the activities of the cell.

B. EFFECT OF LACK OF INSULIN AND/OR FAILURE OF RECEPTORS TO RESPOND

The "poly" triad, often cited as characteristic of untreated diabetics, consists of polydipsia (excessive drinking), polyuria (excessive urine output), and polyphagia (excessive eating). The physiologic effects of diabetes have also been described as "starvation

in the midst of plenty." This is also an appropriate description also because the physiologic response observed when insulin is either absent or severely lacking are those
characteristic of the catabolic hormones epinephrine, growth hormone, and cortisol.

Withdrawal of insulin from a severely diabetic human results in an interconnected
series of events that can end in death if uncorrected. Either lack of insulin or the
response to it has effects on carbohydrate, fat, and protein metabolism. In addition,
effects on fluid and electrolyte balance are observed.

1. Effects of Diabetes on Carbohydrate Metabolism. The physiologic responses of the
untreated diabetic are similar to those that occur during starvation. Thus, the concentration of glucose in blood rises because of reduced peripheral utilization of glucose,
increased mobilization of glycogen from storage, and gluconeogenesis initiated by
catabolic hormones. The concentration of glucose in blood may rise to such high levels
that the renal tubules can no longer reabsorb all the glucose brought to them by way of
glomerular filtration. Glucose then appears in urine. The large amounts of glucose
filtered through the glomeruli of the kidneys act as an osmotic diuretic and increase
both urinary flow (polyuria) and urinary loss of electrolytes (sodium, chloride, and
bicarbonate) as well. These effects result in dehydration and hemoconcentration which,
in extreme cases, can lead to peripheral circulatory failure, hypotension, and death.

In the absence of insulin, as much as 400 g of glucose may be lost in urine daily. This
amounts to 2200 milliosmols of glucose. Assuming a maximal concentrating ability of
the kidneys to be 1100 milliosmols/liter, 2 liters of urine would be required to excrete
the glucose alone. Since urea is also formed as a result of the gluconeogenic process that
occurs in these patients, it also requires water for excretion. It is not uncommon,
therefore, for such diabetic patients to excrete 3 to 4 liters of urine daily. Because of the
excessive urine output, large amounts of water must be ingested. This illustrates the
polyuria and polydipsia that occur in untreated diabetes.

Polyphagia (excessive eating) is also associated with the excessive loss of glucose into
urine. If as much as 400 g of glucose is lost into urine daily and the caloric value for
glucose is 4.0 kcal/g, then 1600 kcal is lost per day—sufficient to supply the total daily
caloric needs of a sedentary student. This large loss of a source of energy is one factor
stimulating polyphagia when insulin is lacking.

2. Effect of Diabetes on Metabolism of Fat. Glucose is unable to enter liver, muscle,
and adipose tissue cells in the diabetic patient. Under these conditions, fat is mobilized
from storage in adipose tissue. (*Q. 9-22*) *What hormones are responsible for this?* The
liver becomes flooded with fatty acids, most of which can be oxidized only to the two-
carbon fragment, acetyl-coenzyme A. The fragments aggregate into acetoacetic and β-
hydroxybutyric acids. These acids and their related ketones produce a number of
effects. The first is a metabolic acidosis. The deep and rapid breathing that is characteristic of diabetic ketoacidosis (called Kussmaul breathing) occurs next. This is a continuing attempt by the body to compensate for the acidosis. (*Q. 9-23*) *Why does this type of
breathing tend to raise the pH of the blood?* The excessive concentration of ketones in
blood, and ultimately in the glomerular filtrate of the kidneys, exceeds the ability of the
renal tubules to reabsorb them and they appear in urine. In the process of being
excreted, fixed base (e.g., bicarbonate) is also lost. This contributes to a net loss of
sodium from the body. Some measurements of the constituents of the blood of severely
ketoacidotic patients are shown in Table 9-3. These measurements illustrate the elevated concentrations of glucose and urea in blood, the elevated osmolarity of plasma, as
well as the reductions in the concentrations of bicarbonate, chloride, and sodium in
plasma.

TABLE 9-3: Excretion of Glucose, Nitrogen, and Minerals in Diabetes Mellitus

Case[a]	Urine Volume (ml)	Glucose (g)	Ketones (g)	Nitrogen Total (g)	Minerals		
					Na (mEq)	K (mEq)	C (mEq)
Controlled with insulin (average 12 days)	1209 (1536)	0 (0)	0.1 (0.1)	11.8 (14.4)	89 (85)	58 (67)	83 (88)
Without insulin (severe acidosis, 4 days)	2621 (2004)	150 (125)	17.7 (0.5)	18.7 (18.3)	174 (121)	152 (81)	131 (108)
Recovery with insulin (5 days)	1020 (1010)	0 (0)	0.3 (0.2)	11.4 (13.5)	66 (35)	8 (46)	89 (32)

[a] Data from case 2 in parentheses.

3. *Effect of Diabetes on Metabolism of Protein.* In untreated diabetes the glucocorticoid hormones are secreted in excess and body proteins are broken down to amino acids, initiating the process of gluconeogenesis. This results in an excessive concentration of amino acids and urea in blood. The excretion of the excessive amounts of urea requires additional water, which contributes to the dehydration of the patients observed under these conditions.

It is not clear why the adrenal cortex should secrete excessive amounts of cortisol to elevate the concentration of glucose in blood when concentrations are already high. It is clear, however, that whatever signals the adrenal cortex to activity, it is not the concentration of glucose in blood but probably is a factor associated with the concentration of intracellular glucose. The Argentine physiologist Bernardo Houssay was the first to show that removal of the anterior pituitary gland from a dog was accompanied by a reduced concentration of glucose in blood. He wondered what would happen if he removed the pituitary from a pancreatectomized, diabetic dog. When he performed this experiment, which gained him a Nobel prize, he observed a return to normal of the concentration of glucose in blood. Some years later, C. N. H. Long, an American physiologist, showed that similar effects occurred if the diabetic dog was adrenalectomized. It is now clear that increased secretion of glucocorticoid hormones under these conditions contributes to an elevation of the concentration of glucose in blood. (Q. 9-24) *Why do you suppose the elevation in the concentration of glucocorticoids in blood does not lead to a suppression in the secretion of ACTH sufficient to reduce the secretion of glucocorticoids to near-normal levels? (Q. 9-25) Would you recommend that the adrenal glands be removed as one aspect of treatment of diabetes? Why or why not?*

C. SOMOGYI EFFECT

Diabetics who are being treated with insulin to control their disease often have episodes of uncontrolled hyperglycemia. Many, on finding glucose in their urine, administer additional insulin to themselves and a vicious cycle begins. This is called the Somogyi effect. It illustrates that the responses of the body to lowering of the concentration of glucose in blood are powerful.

When excess insulin is injected initially and the concentration of glucose in blood is lowered, epinephrine, growth hormone, and glucocorticoid hormone are secreted to return the concentration of glucose in blood to normal. However, the increase in the concentration of glucose in blood initiated by these catabolic hormones overshoots normal concentration. Since insulin is unavailable to reduce the concentration of glucose, this substance appears in urine. If the patient becomes alarmed and administers more insulin, more glucose appears in the urine. This illustrates the importance of a normal check-and-balance system between insulin and the catabolic hormones in the regulation of the concentration of glucose in blood. (*Q. 9-26*) *Can you think of a relatively simple treatment for this problem?*

It is beyond the scope of this chapter to discuss the treatment of diabetes and the pathologic consequences of long-term lack of treatment. It is clear, however, that an understanding of the physiologic effects of diabetes requires a thorough understanding of both physiology and biochemistry, for there are virtually no systems of the body that remain untouched by this disease.

SECTION 9-6: POST-TEST QUESTIONS

1. Diabetes is a disease whose hallmark is an inability of the pancreas to produce insulin. (True/False)
2. In type 1 diabetes, the predominant problem is a. _____ _____. It is the result of b. _____ _____ .
3. Type 1 diabetes constitutes about _____ to _____ (%) of all known diabetics.
4. What is the standard therapy for patients with type 1 diabetes?

5. The concentration of insulin in the blood of type 2 diabetics is a. (normal/abnormal). This type of diabetes is seen in b. _____ to _____ (%) of all known diabetics. The major portion of type 2 diabetics consists of c. _____ _____ patients.
6. The basal concentration of insulin in the blood of type 2 diabetics shows an excellent a. (direct/inverse) correlation with the number of receptors for insulin. What does this suggest about the predominant problem in this type of diabetes?
   b.

7. What is the "poly" triad observed in untreated diabetic patients?
   a.
   b.
   c.
8. Why does glucose appear in the urine of the untreated diabetic?

9. The increased amount of glucose in urine results in an osmotic diuresis and a large loss of substrate for production of energy. (True/False)
10. What is the net result of these two effects?
    a.
    b.

11. An abnormality of fat metabolism manifested by untreated diabetics is an increase in the concentrations of a. _____ and b. _____ acids in blood.

12. The deep and rapid breathing characteristic of diabetic ketoacidosis is called a. _____ breathing. This occurs as a continuing attempt by the body to compensate for what abnormal conditions?
    b.

13. Removal of the anterior pituitary of a diabetic dog returned the concentration of glucose in blood toward normal levels. Why?

14. Administration of insulin in excessive amounts to an insulin-dependent diabetic can result in the appearance of large amounts of glucose in urine. Why does this occur?

SECTION 9-6: POST-TEST ANSWERS

1. False
2. a. an absence, or near absence, of insulin
   b. destruction of the B-cells of the islets of Langerhans
3. 10–20
4. Administration of exogenous insulin.
5. a. normal
   b. 80–90
   c. obese
6. a. inverse
   b. Either the responsiveness of the receptors to insulin or the activation of cellular mechanisms beyond the receptor is affected.
7. a. Polydipsia
   b. Polyuria
   c. Polyphagia
8. The large amounts of glucose filtered through the glomeruli of the kidneys exceed the ability of the renal tubules to reabsorb it. Under normal circumstances, all glucose filtered by the glomeruli is reabsorbed by the renal tubules and the urine contains no glucose.

9. True
10. a. Dehydration
    b. Polyphagia
11. a. β-hydroxybutyric
    b. acetoacetic
12. a. Kussmaul
    b. The metabolic acidosis resulting from the inability to metabolize the large amounts of fatty acids mobilized as a result of the absence of insulin.
13. The glucocorticoid hormone cortisol is responsible for the initiation of gluconeogenesis in the absence of insulin. This results in a further elevation of the concentration of glucose in blood in the diabetic dog. Removal of the anterior pituitary gland removes the source of the tropic hormone that stimulates the adrenal cortex to secrete cortisol. The net result is a reduction in concentration of glucose.
14. This is the Somogyi effect. It is produced as a result of an increased secretion of catabolic, counterregulatory hormones that increase the concentration of glucose in blood after they have been reduced by administration of insulin. Since the amount of insulin that can be produced endogenously is insufficient to prevent an overshoot in the concentration of glucose, the renal threshold to reabsorb glucose is exceeded and it appears in urine.

SELECTED REFERENCES

Cahill, G. F., Jr., 1978, Metabolic effects of insulin, in *Clinical Endocrinology: A Survey of Current Practice*, C. Ezrin, J. O. Godden, and P. G. Walfish (Eds.), New York: Appleton-Century-Crofts, p. 19.

Felig, P., Sherwin, R. S., Somen, V., Wahren, J., Hendler, R., Sacca, L., Eigler, N., Goldberg, D., and Walesky, M., 1979, Hormonal interactions in the regulation of blood glucose, *Recent Progress in Hormone Research* 35: 501.

Gerich, J. E. and Lorenzi, M., 1978, The role of the autonomic nervous system and somatostatin in the control of insulin and glucagon secretion, in *Frontiers in Neuroendocrinology*, W. F. Ganong, and L. Martini (Eds.), New York: Raven Press, p. 265

Roth, J., 1980, Insulin receptors in diabetes, *Hospital Practice* 15, 98.

Unger, R. H. and Orci, L., 1977, the role of glucagon in the endogenous hyperglycemia of diabetes mellitus, *Annual Review of Medicine* 28: 119.

10

CALCIUM HOMEOSTASIS: PARATHYROID HORMONE, CALCITONIN, AND VITAMIN D

SECTION 10-1: ANATOMY OF THE PARATHYROID GLAND; HORMONES CONCERNED WITH CALCIUM HOMEOSTASIS

OBJECTIVES:

The student should be able to:
1. Describe the number and location of the parathyroid glands in man.
2. Discuss the importance of parathyroid hormone in maintenance of the concentration of calcium in plasma and the physiologic consequence of a reduction in the secretion of parathyroid hormone.
3. Describe the mechanisms involved in the synthesis and secretion of parathyroid hormone as well as its chemical characteristics.
4. Describe the secretion, chemical characteristics, and physiologic role of calcitonin.

A. ANATOMY OF THE PARATHYROID GLAND

The parathyroid glands of man are located on the posterior surfaces of the lateral lobes of the thyroid gland. Man has four glands; two are located superiorly and two inferiorly in the thyroid gland. They are rather small glands in adult man, about the size of a pea, and average from 3 to 6 mm in length, 2 to 4 mm in breadth, and 0.5 to 2 mm in thickness. The total weight of the four glands is about 120 mg. As was the case with thyroid tissue, parathyroid tissue may often be found throughout the neck and in the mediastinum. Both the location and the number of the parathyroid glands vary considerably among the various species of mammals. The blood supply to the parathyroid glands comes chiefly from the inferior thyroid arteries. The nerve supply appears to be mainly vasomotor; it originates from the superior and recurrent laryngeal nerves.

Microscopic examination of parathyroid tissue from an adult human reveals two general types of cell: chief cells and oxyphil cells. The chief cells are more numerous and appear to be the source of parathyroid hormone. The oxyphil cells have pycnotic nuclei, and it has been assumed that they are senescent chief cells. These cells have an affinity for acid dyes.

The parathyroid glands are ectodermal in their developmental origin. Embryologically, they originate from the posterior halves of the third and fourth pairs of pharyngeal pouches. Portions of the third pair of pharyngeal pouches form the inferior pair of parathyroid glands, while portions of the fourth pair of pharyngeal pouches form the superior pair of parathyroid glands.

B. HISTORICAL ASPECTS OF THE PHYSIOLOGY OF THE PARATHYROID GLANDS

It was assumed until the end of the nineteenth century that removal of the thyroid gland was fatal. This mistaken assumption occurred because the animals from which the thyroid gland was removed also lost their parathyroid glands, since these are embedded in thyroid tissue. The breakthrough came when it was noted that thyroidectomy in rabbits was compatible with life. Further experimentation revealed that the rabbit has a pair of accessory parathyroid glands located near but not in the thyroid gland. When these were removed, the animal died.

Removal of the parathyroid glands, and loss of the source of production of parathyroid hormone, is accompanied by tetany. This is characterized by a decrease in the concentration of calcium and an increase in the concentration of phosphate in plasma, carpal and laryngeal spasms, epileptiform convulsions, and elevation of body temperature. Death often results from asphyxiation due to spasticity of respiratory muscles. The convulsions can be prevented either by an intravenous infusion of a solution containing calcium or by administration of parathyroid hormone. Hence, parathyroid hormone is important in the maintenance of a constant concentration of calcium in plasma.

C. SECRETION OF PARATHYROID HORMONE

Parathyroid hormone (PTH) has been isolated and characterized. It is a peptide containing 84 amino acids arranged in a linear sequence. It has a molecular weight of 9500 daltons. All the known biologic effects of parathyroid hormone are contained in the first 34 amino acids. This chain has been synthesized and is available commercially.

PTH is synthesized by the same assembly, production, and packaging system used for all peptide hormones (see Section 1-2). In addition, it appears to be assembled on the rough endoplasmic reticulum as a pre-pro-parathyroid hormone of 115 amino acids with a molecular weight of about 13,000 daltons. This is cleaved to pro-parathyroid hormone containing 90 amino acids (about 10,200 daltons) before leaving the area of its synthesis. Either before or during transport of pro-PTH to the Golgi apparatus, six amino acids are cleaved from it to form PTH (1–84). PTH is then packaged in the Golgi zone and stored in membrane-bound secretory granules. Release of PTH from the storage granules occurs when plasma concentration of ionized calcium decreases. (Q. 10-1). *How does PTH get from the secretory granules in the parathyroid gland to the blood draining the gland?* If the concentration of ionized calcium in plasma does not decrease for long periods of time, the granules containing PTH appear to be broken down, the PTH cleaved, and the amino acids recycled. The half-life of PTH in blood is 15 to 20 minutes. The kidney is an important site for metabolism of the hormone. (Q. 10-2) *How much, if any, of the pro-PTH and PTH fragments would you predict to be released from the parathyroid gland?*

A reduction in the concentration of ionized calcium in plasma not only stimulates the release of packaged PTH from the cytoplasm of parathyroid cells, it also stimulates the synthesis of PTH. The intracellular signals that couple hormone release with hormone secretion are unknown. It is clear, however, that increased secretion is necessary, since there is only enough hormone stored in secretory granules to maintain basal secretion of PTH for 5 to 6 hours. At maximal stimulation, stored hormone would last only 60 to 90 minutes. (Q. 10-3) *How do these times compare to those for the thyroid and steroid hormones?* On the other hand, an increase in the concentration of ionized calcium in plasma decreases the synthesis of PTH. However, even a very marked elevation in the concentration of calcium in plasma does not seem to turn off completely the secretion of PTH. Profound, chronic decreases in the concentration of magnesium in plasma inhibit secretion of PTH, although acute decreases may actually stimulate secretion. The mechanism by which these changes occur is not well understood. Several other factors have been shown to stimulate the secretion of PTH in addition to a reduction in the ionized concentration of calcium and magnesium (acutely) in plasma. These include cAMP, β-adrenergic agonists, and prostaglandin E. Secretion of PTH can be inhibited by both β-adrenergic antagonists and α-adrenergic agonists in addition to elevated levels of ionized calcium and reduced levels of magnesium (chronically) in plasma.

It should be apparent that parathyroid hormone is very important in the maintenance of a relatively constant concentration of calcium in blood. It does this by three mechanisms (see Section 10-4): a) by acting at the level of bone to stimulate the breakdown of its mineral components with the consequent release of calcium and phosphate into blood; b) by acting indirectly by way of stimulation of production of physiologically active vitamin D to facilitate the reabsorption of calcium from the gastrointestinal tract, as well as c) to stimulate reabsorption of calcium from urine. It should also be apparent that a reduction in the concentration of ionized calcium in plasma can result in tetany and death. We see later that there is an elaborate mechanism to maintain the constancy of the concentration of calcium in plasma and that the dominant controller in this mechanism is the concentration of PTH in blood.

D. SECRETION OF CALCITONIN

Calcitonin is a hormone that is synthesized and secreted in mammals by specialized cells located in the thyroid gland called parafollicular or clear ("C") cells. These cells are derived from the embryonic neural crest and, similar to the cells of the adrenal medulla, they must migrate to their final destination in the thyroid gland. The physiologic function of calcitonin in man is not known with certainty. This hormone appears to be released when plasma concentration of calcium exceeds approximately 10 mg/100 ml, and it may play a role in lowering plasma concentration of calcium under these conditions. Since the concentration of calcium in plasma rarely exceeds this level in normal man, its requirement for the maintenance of the concentration of calcium in plasma seems minimal. However, certain experiments suggest that secretion of calcitonin may be associated with the transient hypercalcemia that accompanies the absorption of calcium from the gastrointestinal tract following ingestion of a meal. In this way, it may protect against a more prolonged hypercalcemia. In support of this is the fact that certain gastrointestinal hormones, including gastrin, cholecystokinin-pancreozymin, glucagon, and secretin, have been shown to stimulate the secretion of calcitonin. Of these, gastrin appears to be the most potent. The concentrations of these hormones in plasma increase after a meal, and this phenomenon could play an important role in the timing of the increased secretion of calcitonin to coincide with the increase in concentration of calcium in blood. Interestingly, the relationship appears to be reciprocal in that calcitonin can inhibit the secretion of both gastrin and hydrochloric acid by the stomach. This has led some investigators to hypothesize the existence of a "gastroenterothyroid axis," which may control the secretion of both gastrin and calcitonin.

Other substances are known to stimulate the secretion of calcitonin both in vivo and in vitro. These include β-adrenergic agonists dopamine, acetylcholine, and thyroxine.

The mechanism of synthesis of calcitonin by parafollicular cells appears to be similar to other peptide hormones (see Section 1-2). Cell-free translation of human C-cell mRNA produces a calcitoninlike peptide of 15,000 daltons. This "pre-pro form" of calcitonin is thought to contain the typical leader sequence, which is cleaved to yield a prohormone of approximately 12,000 daltons and a final secretory product of 3500 daltons. The calcitonin monomer contains 32 amino acids arranged in a linear chain.

The sequence of the amino acids is known for pig, beef, sheep, and human calcitonin. Attempts to shorten the molecule and maintain biologic activity have been unsuccessful. Calcitonin is not a fragment of the parathyroid hormone molecule.

Thyroidectomized humans, whose presumed source of calcitonin has been removed, have no difficulty in maintaining a normal concentration of calcium in plasma if excessive ingestion of calcium is prevented. When thyroidectomized rats are given diets high in calcium, hypercalcemia develops. This does not occur in intact rats, which suggests that a function of calcitonin may be to prevent an excessive rise in the concentration of calcium in plasma that may occur following ingestion of meals or fluids high in calcium.

Pharmacologic doses of calcitonin can be shown to inhibit dramatically the resorption of bone and the efflux of calcium from bone. It appears to do this by a direct inhibitory effect on the cells that are responsible for bone resorption (osteoclasts). Calcitonin does not appear to affect absorption of calcium from the gastrointestinal tract. However, it does appear to increase renal excretion of calcium and phosphate into urine. Calcitonin appears to produce its cellular effects by way of the cAMP system, as is also the case for parathyroid hormone. Data on the effects of the administration of "physiologic doses" of calcitonin, especially on bone cells, are needed to clarify the physiologic role of this hormone.

The relationship between the concentration of calcium in plasma, on the one hand, and the concentrations of parathyroid hormone and calcitonin in plasma, on the other hand, are shown in Figure 10-1.

FIGURE 10-1: Relationship among the concentrations of parathyroid hormone (PTH), calcium, and calcitonin (CT) in plasma. Calcitonin is undetectable when the concentrations of calcium are below about 10 mg/100 ml; whereas the concentration of PTH is undetectable when the concentrations of calcium are above about 10 mg/100 ml.

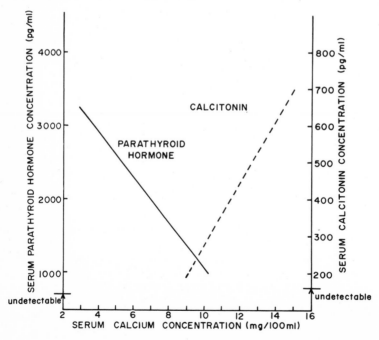

SECTION 10-1: POST-TEST QUESTIONS

1. There are three pairs of parathyroid glands in man. Two pairs are located in the thyroid gland with one pair adjacent to it. (True/False)

2. Each parathyroid gland is about the size of a a. _____. Embryologically these glands originate from the b. _____.

3. The cells of the parathyroid tissue that secrete parathyroid hormone are called the chief cells. (True/False)

4. Removal of the parathyroid glands is accompanied by a condition known as

   _____.

5. List five factors which characterize the tetany accompanying hypoparathyroidism.
   a.
   b.
   c.
   d.
   e.

6. Why does death often result after removal of the parathyroid glands?

7. How can this condition be treated?

8. Parathyroid hormone is produced as a pre-pro-hormone in the rough endoplasmic reticulum and is then converted to proparathyroid hormone before leaving its area of synthesis. (True/False)

9. Parathyroid hormone is packaged into granules by the Golgi apparatus. (True/False)

10. Release of the contents of the granules into blood occurs as a result of a reduction in the concentration of ionized calcium in plasma. (True/False)

11. Is the mechanism triggering the release of insulin from the cytoplasmic granules of B-cells in the islets of Langerhans different from that for the release of PTH from granules in the parathyroid gland? Why?

12. Name the three organs on which parathyroid hormone acts to maintain the constancy of the concentration of calcium in blood.
   a.
   b.
   c.

13. Calcitonin is secreted by the parafollicular cells of the parathyroid gland. (True/False)

14. The physiologic functions of calcitonin in normal man are not known with certainty. (True/False)

15. Calcitonin concentration in plasma increases linearly with increases in the concentration of calcium in plasma beyond 10 mg/100 ml. (True/False)

16. Pharamacologic doses of calcitonin prevent resorption of both bone and calcium efflux from it. (True/False)

17. This treatment also increases the rate of absorption of calcium from the gastrointestinal tract. (True/False)

SECTION 10-1: POST-TEST ANSWERS

1. False
2. a. pea
   b. third and fourth pairs of pharyngeal pouches
3. True
4. tetany
5. a. Decrease in the concentration of calcium in plasma
   b. Increase in the concentration of phosphate in plasma
   c. Carpal and laryngeal spasms
   d. Epileptiform convulsions
   e. Elevation of body temperature
6. The tetany produces a paralysis of the respiratory muscles resulting in asphyxiation and death.
7. It can be prevented or relieved by infusion of solutions containing calcium.
8. True
9. True
10. True
11. Yes. An influx of calcium into the B-cell is believed to initiate the secretion of insulin. A similar mechanism could induce the secretion of parathyroid hormone only if the reduction in concentration of calcium in plasma induced, in some fashion, a release of bound calcium endogenously.
12. a. Bone
    b. Gastrointestinal tract
    c. Kidney
13. False
14. True
15. True
16. True
17. False

SECTION 10-2: FACTORS AFFECTING CALCIUM AND PHOSPHATE HOMEOSTASIS

OBJECTIVES:

The student should be able to:
1. Discuss the role of the gastrointestinal tract in calcium homeostasis.
2. Discuss the role of bone in calcium homeostasis.
3. Discuss the role of the kidneys in calcium homeostasis.
4. Discuss the significance of an increased excretion of hydroxyproline into urine.
5. Describe the physiologic importance of ionized calcium as opposed to bound calcium in plasma.
6. Discuss the factors influencing the concentration of phosphate in plasma.

A. CALCIUM HOMEOSTASIS

The concentration of calcium in plasma has been called "one of nature's physiologic constants." It requires gross metabolic aberrations of long duration to produce a hypocalcemia of more than a minimal degree in animals with intact, functioning parathyroid glands. The intricate mechanisms maintaining the constancy of the concentration of calcium in plasma are discussed in this and subsequent sections.

1. *The Gastrointestinal Tract as a Source of Calcium.* Calcium enters the body by way of the gastrointestinal tract with food and water. Not all the ingested calcium is absorbed by the gut. The daily absorption of calcium from these sources is about 200 mg, or about 20% of the amount ingested daily. Absorption appears to take place most readily in the upper portion of the small intestine (duodenum) where the environment is more acid as a result of contact with the gastric juice. The importance of this acidification has been shown in the gastrectomized dog. Such animals develop bowed front legs and a swayed back as a result of deficient calcium absorption and a consequently weakened skeleton. The absorption of calcium also takes place in the other portions of the small intestine (ileum and jejunum), but the rate of absorption is slower. However, the total amount of calcium absorbed in the ileum and jejunum is actually greater than in the duodenum, since these are much longer, hence provide a longer transit time during which the calcium may be absorbed. The amount of calcium absorbed from the gastrointestinal tract is actually greater than the approximately 200 mg extracted from the daily intakes of food and fluid. Intestinal secretions release into the intestinal tract an additional approximately 400 mg/day. All but 60 to 150 mg of the calcium contained in these secretions is reabsorbed. The remainder is excreted into feces and has been termed endogenous fecal calcium.

There are two major components to the absorption of calcium in the intestines. The first and most important is an active transport process, which is saturable and requires both metabolic energy and vitamin D. There is also a passive diffusion of calcium out of the intestine. This requires neither metabolic energy nor vitamin D and is not saturable. It becomes important only when high levels of calcium are present in the intestine. The active transport of calcium out of the small intestine is aided by a specific calcium binding protein, the synthesis of which requires a vitamin D derivative, probably 1,25-dihydroxy vitamin D (see Figure 10-2, in Section 10-3-A). The precise intracellular mechanism that is important for the transport of calcium up its concentration gradient is not known clearly. It is known, however, that active transport is promoted by chronic ingestion of a low-calcium diet. The converse occurs when calcium intake is high. The mechanism by which vitamin D interacts in this process is unclear.

2. *The Skeleton as a Source of Calcium.* Calcium is the most abundant cation in the body. About 99% of the body's calcium (about 1000 g) is contained in the skeleton, which serves a major mechanical function for the body, namely, to bear weight and to act as a point of attachment for muscles. The remaining 1% of the body's calcium is located in plasma, extracellular fluid, and soft tissues. The concentration of calcium in plasma is 10 mg/100 ml. Of this, 3 mg/100 ml is bound to protein (albumin) and another 1 to 2 mg/100 ml is complexed with citrate, lactate, and other ions. The remainder, 5 to 6 mg/100 ml, is ionized or diffusable calcium and constitutes about 50% of the total concentration of calcium in plasma. It should be emphasized that it is the ionized calcium that appears to be important physiologically. (*Q. 10-4*) *How is this reminiscent of the steroid hormones you have studied in earlier chapters?*

The concentration of calcium in plasma is in equilibrium with a portion of bone known as the exchangeable stores. This amounts to about 5 to 6 g of calcium. In the absence of the parathyroid glands, this equilibrium will maintain the concentration of calcium in plasma at 5 to 6 mg/100 ml. The remainder of the calcium in bone, referred to as the nonexchangeable stores, constitutes the remaining 99% of skeletal calcium. It is the nonexchangeable calcium that is acted on by parathyroid hormone. Under its influence, osteocytes (osteoclasts) release calcium and phosphate from the nonexchangeable pool by dissolving away the calcium and phosphate deposits of bone. During this process, the collagen of bone may also be broken down. Because collagen is the only protein of the body containing the amino acid hydroxyproline, any increase either in its concentration in blood or in its excretion into urine is indicative of dissolution of the protein matrix of bone.

Other osteocytes (osteoblasts) form bone from the calcium and phosphate in plasma. These cells appear to be influenced by a rising blood level of calcitonin. Thus, in contrast to what one might expect, bone is a dynamic tissue. It is constantly being broken down and reformed, a process called remodeling.

The typical, mature bone mineral is microcrystalline calcium hydroxyapatite, $Ca_{10}(PO_4)_6(OH)_2$. The formation of apatite crystals during calcification is a complicated process. The mineral is amorphous after precipitation and matures into microcrystalline apatite later. The compositions of the initial precipitate and of the fluid at the site of mineral deposition are not known with certainty.

As with the steroid hormones studied in earlier chapters, the ionized calcium of plasma is in equilibrium with the protein-bound calcium. The equilibrium is influenced by changes in the pH of blood. A small rise in plasma pH can reduce the concentration of ionized calcium and increase the calcium bound to protein. Thus, it can be demonstrated in many humans that an increase in respiratory rate and depth sufficient to result in an excess loss of carbon dioxide from blood can induce a rise in the pH of blood. This may be accompanied by a decrease in ionized calcium concentration in blood, followed by increased neuromuscular excitability and twitching.

An additional equilibrium exists between calcium and phosphate ions in plasma and calcium phosphate. If calcium concentration of plasma is elevated to a sufficient level, the equilibrium reaction will be shifted toward calcium phosphate. This may then precipitate in soft tissues of the body. A rule of thumb is that when the product of the calcium and phosphate concentrations exceeds 55 mg/100 ml, deposition of calcium phosphate is likely to occur. The normal value is 10×3, or 30 mg/100 ml.

3. *The Kidneys as a Source of Calcium.* Calcium can be lost from plasma into perspiration (about 50 mg/day) and feces and urine (250–300 mg/day). (*Q. 10-5*) *Would you expect free or bound calcium to be filtered at the glomeruli of the kidneys?* Calcium enters blood from the intestines, from reabsorption in the renal tubules, and from dissolution of bone. Less than 0.5% of the calcium in the skeleton can exchange with plasma. (*Q. 10-6*) *What is this fraction of the total skeletal calcium called?* Of these three sources the quantity of calcium reabsorbed by the renal tubules of the normal human each day (about 11,000 mg) is far greater than that absorbed from the gastrointestinal tract (about 400 mg) or as a result of resorption of bone (about 600 mg). About 99% of all calcium filtered at the glomeruli of the kidneys is reabsorbed by the renal tubules. About 60% of the renal tubular reabsorption of calcium occurs in the proximal tubule. The remainder occurs in the ascending limb of the loop of Henle and in the distal tubule. Reabsorption in the distal tubule appears to occur under the influence of PTH.

The excreted calcium generally is complexed either with citrate or phosphate. The urinary excretion of calcium may be either increased or decreased depending on the amount filtered at the level of the glomeruli. The renal handling of calcium and sodium appears to be similar and interdependent. For example, changes in dietary intake of sodium are accompanied by parallel changes in urinary excretions of sodium and calcium. The two processes can be separated experimentally by administration of mineralocorticoid hormones that induce reabsorption of sodium by renal tubules without affecting the reabsorption of calcium. (*Q. 10-7*) *Do you recall the name of the potent mineralocorticoid hormone secreted by the adrenal gland?*

B. PHOSPHATE HOMEOSTASIS

Most of the inorganic phosphate in the body (80–90%, 500–800 g) is in the skeleton in association with calcium as hydroxyapatite. The remainder (approximately 100 g) is found in soft tissues, largely in the form of organic phosphorus compounds. These are important in cellular energetics (e.g., ATP), as intracellular messengers (e.g., cAMP), in enzymes, and so on.

The concentration of phosphate in plasma is more variable than that of calcium and is 3 to 4.5 mg/100 ml in adults (4.0–7.0 mg/100 ml in children). Variations in plasma concentration of phosphate may represent shifts between extra- and intracellular compartments. About 45% of phosphate in plasma is in ionized form. The majority of the remainder is present in plasma as soluble complexes.

Since ionized phosphate and ionized calcium are in equilibrium with calcium phosphate in plasma, any increases in ionized calcium, such as may occur in certain chronic renal diseases, may result in precipitation of calcium phosphate in soft tissues.

About 800 to 1500 mg of phosphate is ingested daily with dairy products, cereals, and meats by adult Americans. It is absorbed efficiently, primarily in the jejunum of the intestine. At very low levels of intake, as much as 90% of the ingested phosphate may be reabsorbed. Absorption of phosphate occurs in all portions of the small intestine, but the rate of absorption is highest in the duodenum. (*Q. 10-8*) *In which portion of the intestine is the rate of absorption of calcium highest?* As is the case with calcium, phosphate is absorbed by a dual process: an active transport mechanism and passive diffusion. About 60 to 65% of the ingested phosphate is absorbed, as opposed to approximately 20% of ingested calcium. In general, factors increasing intestinal absorption of calcium also increase intestinal absorption of phosphate; thus vitamin D increases the absorption of both calcium and phosphate. The active transport processes for calcium and phosphate are separate; and the interaction of vitamin D with these processes is not well understood.

Phosphate is excreted primarily by the kidney (500–1500 mg/day) although some phosphate is excreted in feces. The normal reabsorption of phosphate by renal tubules amounts to about 80% of the filtered load but may be modified by increases and decreases in intake. The proximal tubules of the kidneys actively reabsorb most of the phosphate contained in the glomerular filtrate. Reabsorption of phosphate also occurs in the distal convoluted tubule, but to a much lesser extent. Reabsorption in both proximal and distal tubules is inhibited by PTH through an increase in the formation of cAMP. A persistent elevation in the concentration of PTH in blood can result in an increased urinary excretion of phosphate accompanied by a decreased concentration of phosphate in plasma.

SECTION 10-2: POST-TEST QUESTIONS

1. Name three organs contributing to the maintenance of a relatively constant concentration of calcium in plasma.
   a.
   b.
   c.
2. Acidification is important in the absorption of calcium from the _____.
3. Calcium is the most abundant cation in the body. (True/False)
4. About 99% of the body's calcium is located in the skeleton. (True/False)

5. Name the three depots containing the remaining 1% of the body's calcium.
   a.
   b.
   c.
6. The total concentration of calcium in plasma is a. _____ mg/100 ml. Of this, b. _____ mg/100 ml is bound to protein and another c. _____ mg/100 ml is complexed to citrate, lactate, and other ions, and d. _____ mg/100 ml is ionized. Of these, it is the e. _____ calcium that is important physiologically.
7. A portion of the calcium in bone is in equilibrium with the calcium in plasma. This is the a. _____ pool of calcium. It constitutes about b. _____% of the total calcium in bone. The remainder of the bone calcium is called the c. _____ pool. It is this pool of calcium that is affected by d. _____ hormone.
8. Of the three organs concerned with the maintenance of a constant concentration of calcium in plasma, the _____ handle the greatest amount of calcium daily.
9. The majority of phosphate in the body is located in the _____.
10. The concentration of phosphate in plasma is less variable than the concentration of calcium. (True/False)
11. A major dietary source of both calcium and phosphate is dairy products. (True/False)
12. An acute increase in parathyroid hormone concentration in blood is accompanied by a decrease in urinary excretion of calcium and an increase in urinary excretion of phosphate. (True/False)
13. Increases in the concentration of hydroxyproline in blood or urine are indicative of what pathologic situation?

SECTION 10-2: POST-TEST ANSWERS

1. a. Intestines
   b. Skeleton
   c. Kidneys
2. intestines (duodenum)
3. True
4. True
5. a. Plasma
   b. Extracellular fluid
   c. Soft tissues
6. a. 10
   b. 3
   c. 1 or 2
   d. 5 to 6
   e. ionized
7. a. exchangeable
   b. 1
   c. nonexchangeable
   d. parathyroid
8. kidneys

9. skeleton
10. False
11. True
12. True
13. Dissolution of the protein matrix (i.e., collagen) of bone.

SECTION 10-3: SYNTHESIS AND PHYSIOLOGICAL ACTIONS OF VITAMIN D

OBJECTIVES:

The student should be able to:
1. Name the metabolite of vitamin D_3 that is believed to be the biologically active form.
2. Discuss the sequence in which the biologically active form of vitamin D_3 is synthesized physiologically, including the organs important in the synthetic process and their contribution.
3. State a role for vitamin D in the intestinal absorption of calcium.
4. State a role for vitamin D in the resorption of calcium and phosphate from bone.

A. SYNTHESIS OF 1,25-DIHYDROXY VITAMIN D_3

It was pointed out in Section 10-2 that vitamin D is important for the movement of calcium across the wall of the small intestine. A deficiency of vitamin D in children has long been associated with a disease called rickets and with osteomalacia in adults. Both of these conditions result from failure to absorb a sufficient amount of calcium from the small intestine to calcify bones properly. The bones of a vitamin D-deficient child are soft and as a result, they become deformed.

Vitamin D_3 is produced in skin by ultraviolet irradiation from the sun. An unstable, previtamin D_3 is an intermediate in this process. The source of vitamin D_3 is 7-dehydrocholesterol, which is present in abundance in skin (see Figure 10-2). Vitamin D_3, made either in the skin or absorbed from ingested food, becomes attached to a carrier protein (α_2-globulin) in plasma and is transported to the liver. Here the compound undergoes hydroxylation at position 25 on the molecule as a result of action by enzymes located in hepatic microsomes (see Figure 10-2). This transformation makes the compound several-fold more potent than vitamin D_3 (cholecalciferol). The newly hydroxylated compound is again attached to a carrier protein in plasma and transported to the kidneys, where it is hydroxylated at position 1 by enzymes located in the mitochondria of renal cells. This compound, 1,25-dihydroxycholecalciferol, is 5 to 10 times more potent than 25-hydroxycholecalciferol. It is also the most rapidly acting metabolite of vitamin D_3. It appears at present that 1,25-dihydroxycholecalciferol [1,25(OH)$_2$D$_3$] is the biologically active form of vitamin D.

The production of vitamin D_3 (cholecalciferol) appears to be controlled only by the amount of sunlight to which the skin is exposed. In addition, the 25-hydroxylation of vitamin D_3 by the liver appears to be limited only by the availability of the substrate. There is, however, some evidence of a local product inhibition of the 25-hydroxylation process in the liver. By contrast, the production of 1,25(OH)$_2$D$_3$ by the kidneys is influenced by the concentration of PTH in plasma. Rising levels of PTH are associated with a stimulation of the renal enzymes concerned with 1-α-hydroxylation of 25(OH)D$_3$.

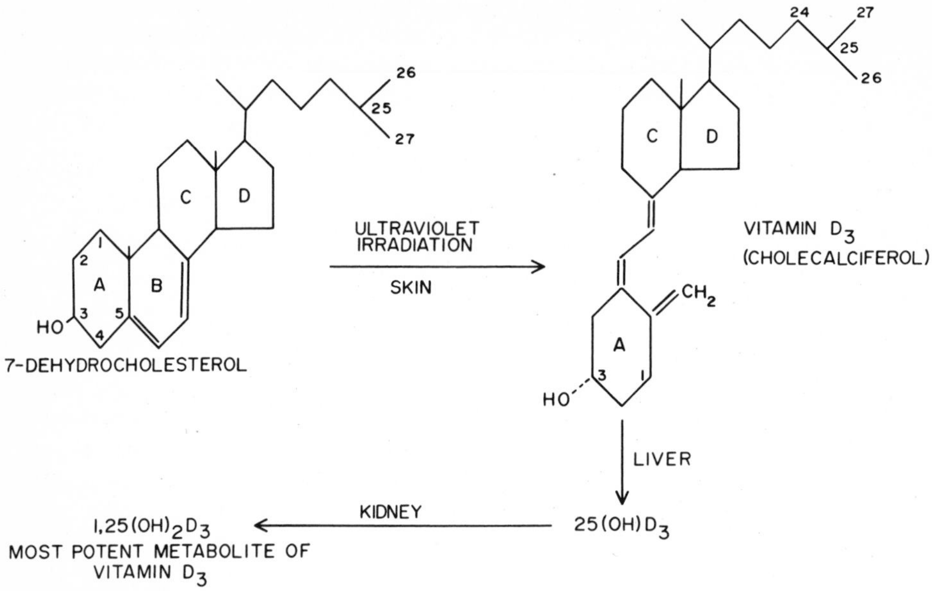

FIGURE 10-2: The biosynthetic pathway for the formation of the most potent metabolite of vitamin D$_3$, 1,25-dihydoxycholecalciferol [1,25(OH)$_2$D$_3$].

Recent studies suggest that the activity of this enzyme actually is increased by both the reduction in intracellular concentration and the increase in urinary excretion of phosphate brought about by an increase in the concentration of PTH in plasma. Thus, it has been shown that parathyroidectomized rats, maintained on a low-phosphorus, high-calcium diet, can synthesize 1,25(OH)$_2$D$_3$. Present evidence therefore suggests that PTH is not absolutely necessary for the induction of this renal hydroxylase enzyme and that a reduction in the concentration of phosphate in plasma can also increase its activity. Although the effect of PTH on the 1α-hydroxylation of 25(OH)D$_3$ may be indirect, any situation increasing the secretion of PTH will result in a consequent increase in 1-α-hydroxylation of 25(OH)D$_3$ as long as this substrate is available. (*Q. 10-9*) *Can you name two situations that should produce an increase in the 1α-hydroxylation of 25(OH)D$_3$ as a result of an increase in the secretion of PTH?* The interrelation between the effect of increasing concentrations of PTH and decreasing concentrations of phosphate on renal 1α-hydroxylation of 25(OH)D$_3$ is discussed in Section 10-3-D.

Although it would be pleasing theoretically if calcitonin had an inhibitory effect on the renal enzyme 25-OH-D-1 α-hydroxylase, careful studies in rats infused continuously with calcitonin have failed to demonstrate such an effect. (*Q. 10-10*) *Why would this be a pleasing possibility?*

A source of vitamin D that has been exploited commercially is ergocalciferol or vitamin D$_2$, which is produced by ultraviolet irradiation of the ergosterol produced naturally by plants and yeasts. Vitamin D$_2$ undergoes essentially the same hydroxylation reactions in vivo as vitamin D$_3$. In man, vitamins D$_2$ and D$_3$ are equipotent. Vitamin D$_2$ is used commercially as a vitamin supplement in milk.

Researchers active in this field have also been helpful in synthesizing the vitamin D compound, 1α(OH)D$_3$. (*Q. 10-11*) *In what clinical situations would you expect the use of this compound to be important therapeutically?*

As was the case with steroid hormones, vitamin D_3, $25(OH)D_3$, and $1,25(OH)_2D_3$ are secreted into bile by the liver and are reabsorbed in the intestines. This enterohepatic circulation of vitamin D is important in the conservation of this compound. However, it also means that any situation that induces excessive fecal loss of fats and bile acids can induce a deficiency of vitamin D.

B. PHYSIOLOGIC EFFECTS OF VITAMIN D ON THE INTESTINE

Vitamin D was cited earlier for its role in increasing the transport of both calcium and phosphate from the lumen of the gastrointestinal tract into the extracellular fluid. The primary events that are important for the transport of calcium are initiated by vitamin D in the cells of the intestinal mucosa. The first event is the binding of $1,25(OH)_2D_3$ to a specific receptor in the cytoplasm of the cell, similar to the receptors for steroid hormones discussed in earlier chapters (see Figure 1-3). The vitamin D-receptor complex undergoes an activational step that increases the likelihood of its association with chromatin acceptors within the nucleus. This interaction leads to the de novo synthesis of mRNA and proteins. At least four separate proteins are believed to be synthesized, one of which is designated as calcium binding protein. It is the calcium binding protein that may be essential for maintenance of the transport process for calcium in the intestine. This may then constitute the mechanism by which vitamin D affects calcium transport from the intestine to blood. The functions of the remaining three proteins that are also synthesized under the influence of vitamin D are unknown. (Q. 10-12) Why would you expect vitamin D to act by way of a mobile receptor rather than a fixed receptor?

Vitamin D is also important for the active transport of phosphate from the intestine to the extracellular fluid. Thus, vitamin D is involved in two separate transport processes in the intestine, one for calcium and one for phosphate.

The relative potencies of vitamin D_3, $25(OH)D_3$, and $1,25(OH)_2D_3$ in stimulating the absorption of calcium are expressed by the ratio $1:4:13$. When a vitamin D_3 deficiency occurs, or when there is a failure to produce the most active metabolite of vitamin D_3, $1,25(OH)_2D_3$, the absorption of calcium from the gastrointestinal tract falls to subnormal levels. Calcium absorption may be returned toward normal by ingestion of a diet very high in calcium. Syndromes similar to a deficiency of vitamin D_3 are produced by abnormalities of metabolism of vitamin D_3. (Q. 10-13) What problems with vitamin D would you expect to find in patients with advanced renal disease? It is worth pointing out here that vitamin D-dependent rickets is believed by a number of investigators to be related to an inability of the kidney to produce sufficient quantities of $1,25(OH)_2D_3$.

C. PHYSIOLOGIC EFFECTS OF VITAMIN D ON BONE

Vitamin D acts in concert with PTH to increase the mobilization of calcium and phosphate from bone to blood. Bone mineral and matrix are resorbed simultaneously with the release of calcium, phosphate, and hydroxyproline into extracellular fluid. The cells of bone have receptors for PTH. Activation of the receptors in turn activates the cAMP system.

It has recently been shown that a specific receptor is also available to $1,25(OH)_2D_3$ in bone and that this compound can stimulate the production of a calcium binding protein in the bone of rachitic chicks, just as it does in the intestine. However, the two calcium binding proteins appear to be different biochemically. Although a calcium binding protein has now been identified in bone, its role in the mobilization of calcium and phosphate induced by PTH is unclear. This may be because the mechanism of action of

PTH on bone is also unclear. Although it is well recognized for its role in mobilization of calcium and phosphate from bone, it may also play a role in the *formation* of bone. Thus, small amounts of PTH administered to parathyroidectomized rats *increase* bone mass. Furthermore, studies of the kinetics of calcium exchange in patients with hyperparathyroidism show high rates not only of bone resorption but also of bone formation. However, the rate of resorption is usually greater than the rate of formation.

Present knowledge suggests that the primary action of PTH is on bone resorption and that its effect on bone formation may be secondary. It would appear that the role of PTH is to maintain the concentration of calcium in blood, which assures normal neuromuscular activity, cellular metabolism, and so on. The maintenance of the metabolism of bone may be its secondary role. Thus, at present the mechanism by which the calcium binding protein of bone (whose production is stimulated by the action of vitamin D) and the cAMP system of bone (which is stimulated to activity by PTH) interact to release calcium and phosphate from bone into blood is unknown.

Hypoparathyroidism can be treated by administration of vitamins D_2 or D_3, or a synthetic analogue of vitamin D called dihydrotachysterol, which is about five times more potent than vitamin D_3. As a result, the 3β-hydroxyl group occupies a position comparable to that occupied by the 1α-hydroxyl group of $1,25(OH)_2D_3$. Since dihydrotachysterol has biologic activity in nephrectomized rats, it would appear that it only needs to be hydroxylated at the 25 position by the liver to exert its full biologic effect. Compared to $1,25(OH)_2D_3$, however, 500 to 1000 times more dihydrotachysterol is required to produce similar effects in nephrectomized animals.

Hypoparathyroidism is often treated with pharmacologic doses of vitamin D_3 (1 million or more units per day). This is about 2500 times the daily dose required by normal adults. Such large doses of vitamin D_3 appear to act both directly on bone to stimulate resorption and on the intestines to induce absorption of calcium. Both of these actions effectively raise the concentration of calcium in plasma to normal. In man, a delay of about 10 hours occurs between administration of either dihydrotachysterol or vitamin D_3 and the observation of a biologic effect. In contrast, administration of $1,25(OH)_2D_3$ may produce a biologic effect within 2 to 3 hours. (*Q. 10-14*) *What do you think accounts for the long latent period for a response to vitamin D_3?*

Vitamin D is absorbed from the upper duodenum and the distal ileum of the gastrointestinal tract. After absorption, it appears to be associated with cylomicra before it becomes attached to its α_2-globulin binding protein in plasma. Vitamin D is stored in virtually every tissue of the body. Major amounts are stored in adipose tissue and skeletal muscle. This probably accounts for the very small amounts excreted into urine (1–2% of an injected dose per day) and feces (2–6% of an injected dose in 2 days).

D. VITAMIN D AS A HORMONE

$1,25(OH)_2D_3$ is considered by some investigators to be a hormone because the sole site of its production is the kidney. It is also the physiologically important form of vitamin D and acts on intestine and bone as target tissues. The concentration of calcium in plasma could function as a feedback signal to help control the synthesis $1,25(OH)_2D_3$. When the concentration decreases, the secretion of PTH is increased and the activity of the renal hydroxylating enzyme is also increased. This results in the production of increased amounts of $1,25(OH)_2D_3$, which increases the transport of calcium from the intestine and acts with PTH to increase resorption of calcium and phosphate from bone. When the concentration of calcium in plasma increases, the production of $1,25(OH)_2D_3$ is greatly depressed in favor of the relatively inactive metabolite $24,25(OH)_2D_3$ (see Figure 10-3). (*Q. 10-15*) *How is this reminiscent of the peripheral metabolism of thyroxine?*

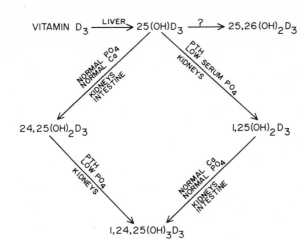

FIGURE 10-3: The metabolites of vitamin D_3 and the conditions that are known to be conducive to the formation of the various metabolites, showing the organ or organs in which the metabolite is formed. (*Adapted from:* Deluca, 1976.)

It was mentioned in Section 10-3-A that a reduction in the concentration of phosphate in plasma also stimulates 1α-hydroxylation of $25(OH)D_3$, even in parathyroidectomized rats. Since a reduction in the concentration of phosphate in plasma suppresses the secretion of PTH in intact animals, the resulting stimulation of secretion of $1,25(OH)_2D_3$ increases intestinal absorption of phosphate and its concentration in plasma. Although transport of calcium is also increased under these conditions, its concentration in plasma changes very little. Since the secretion of PTH is suppressed under these conditions, bone resorption does not occur.

E. PHYSIOLOGIC EFFECTS OF VITAMIN D ON THE KIDNEY

A number of studies suggests that the various metabolites of vitamin D inhibit the excretion of calcium and phosphate by the kidney of parathyroidectomized animals. Too little is currently known about these effects to suggest a mechanism by which vitamin D and its metabolites may act.

SECTION 10-3: POST-TEST QUESTIONS

1. Vitamin D_3 undergoes metabolic activation. What is the name of the biologically active metabolite of vitamin D_3? _____

2. The precursor of vitamin D_3, 7-dehydrocholesterol, is ingested in large amounts with food. (True/False)

3. Vitamin D_3 is produced from 7-dehydrocholesterol in the a. _____ as a result of b. _____.

4. The liver is important in the process of forming the biologically active form of vitamin D because a. _____. The kidney also contributes by b. _____. Which of these is influenced by PTH?
   c. _____
   _____.

5. Vitamin D is hydrophobic and relatively insoluble in plasma. Why isn't this a significant problem physiologically?

6. Why is the presence or absence of an enterohepatic circulation for vitamin D important in man?

7. What is the name of the metabolite of vitamin D_3 that is formed when plasma concentration of calcium is elevated? a. _____ How does this metabolite play a role in the maintenance of calcium homeostasis? b.

8. A metabolite of thyroxine with minimal biologic activity is also produced peripherally in circumstances when an increased metabolic activity is undesirable. What is the name of this metabolite?

9. Vitamin D appears to act in intestinal mucosal cells by way of a. _____ receptors. After transport to the nuclei, the cells are stimulated to produce b. _____. In this process, a c. _____ _____ is produced that is important in the transport of calcium from the lumen of the gut to the blood. How does PTH appear to be involved in this process? d.

10. Vitamin D acts in concert with _____ to increase the mobilization of calcium and phosphate from bone to blood.
11. The mechanism by which this interaction stimulates the mobilization of these ions is well understood. (True/False)
12. Parathyroid hormone acts on bone by way of the cAMP system. (True/False)
13. Vitamin D may act on bone by a mechanism similar to its action on intestinal mucosal cells to stimulate the release of calcium and phosphate from bone into blood. Essential to this mechanism is the production of _____
_____.
14. Vitamin D_3 can induce the mobilization of calcium and phosphate from bone in the absence of PTH but only if the doses are _____.
15. A deficiency of the precursors of biologically active vitamin D in food during childhood can result in a disease called a. _____. What characterizes it? b.

How can this disease still occur when there is an adequate intake of the precursors of biologically active vitamin D?
c.

SECTION 10-3: POST-TEST ANSWERS

1. 1,25-Dihydroxycholecalciferol [1,25(OH)$_2$D$_3$]
2. False
3. a. skin
   b. ultraviolet irradiation by the sun
4. a. It hydroxylates vitamin D$_3$ at position 25.
   b. Hydroxylating 25-hydroxy vitamin D$_3$ at position 1.
   c. The hydroxylation of 25(OH)D$_3$ in the kidney may be influenced by PTH.
5. Vitamin D is carried in blood bound to an α_2-globulin.
6. The presence of the enterohepatic circulation for vitamin D is important in man for the conservation and recycling of vitamin D.
7. a. 24,25-Dihydroxy vitamin D$_3$.
   b. 24,25(OH)$_2$D$_3$ is much less potent biologically than 1,25(OH)$_2$D$_3$, and its preferential synthesis under these conditions reduces the formation of the biologically active derivative, hence the absorption of calcium from the gastrointestinal tract.
8. Reverse triiodothyronine (rT$_3$)
9. a. mobile
   b. at least four proteins
   c. specific calcium binding protein.
   d. Indirectly. PTH exerts an important influence on the kidney in its hydroxylation of 25(OH)D$_3$ at position 1 on the molecule. It is the 1,25(OH)$_2$D$_3$ that acts on intestinal mucosa to increase the transport of calcium across it.
10. parathyroid hormone
11. False
12. True
13. a specific calcium binding protein
14. clearly above the physiologic level
15. a. rickets
    b. Failure to absorb calcium from the gastrointestinal tract with resultant softness of the bones. In children, this results in distortion of the bones.
    c. Rickets could still be produced if the kidney failed to hydroxylate 25(OH)D$_3$ at position 1 on the molecule.

SECTION 10-4: MECHANISMS CONTROLLING THE CONCENTRATION OF CALCIUM IN PLASMA

OBJECTIVES:

The student should be able to:
1. Describe the consequence of both a rise and a fall in the concentration of parathyroid hormone on the concentration of calcium in plasma.
2. Describe the role of vitamin D in the maintenance of the concentration of calcium in plasma.
3. Describe the role of calcitonin in the maintenance of the concentration of calcium in plasma.

There are three major overlapping negative feedback loops that are important in the maintenance of calcium homeostasis. These are the control loops associated with absorption of calcium from the intestine, resorption of calcium from bone, and reabsorption of calcium from the urine by renal tubules.

A model for control of the concentration of calcium in serum is shown in Figure 10-4. This "butterfly" model has three overlapping loops that interlock and relate to one another through the concentration of ionic calcium, parathyroid hormone, and calcitonin. The two sets of loops on the left (A) and right (B) represent feedback mechanisms that increase and decrease serum calcium concentration, respectively. Limb 1 is the feedback limb representing the relation between bone and the concentration of calcium in serum; whereas limb 2 represents the relation between intestinal absorption of calcium and concentration of calcium in serum. Limb 3 represents the relation between renal excretion of calcium and concentration of calcium in serum.

If the concentration of calcium in serum decreases, the secretion of PTH increases while that of calcitonin is turned off. The increased concentration of PTH in serum acts a) via pathway 1A to increase bone resorption of calcium in conjunction with $1,25(OH)_2D_3$, b) via pathway 2A to stimulate production of $1,25(OH)_2D_3$ by the kidney and thereby increase the reabsorption of calcium by the intestine, and c) via pathway 3A to decrease the renal excretion of calcium. All these pathways serve to return to normal the reduced concentration of calcium in serum that initiated the increased rate of secretion of PTH. If the concentration of calcium in serum increases, the secretion of calcitonin increases while that of PTH decreases. The combination of events proceeds as follows:

1. It acts via pathway 1B to decrease bone resorption of calcium. This occurs in part because the rate of secretion of PTH is reduced and in part because the resultant increased concentration of phosphate in serum depresses the production of $1,25(OH)_2D_3$ by the kidney.
2. The depressed production of $1,25(OH)_2D_3$ also results in a reduction in the absorption of calcium from the intestine via pathway 2B.
3. The reduction in secretion of PTH results in an increase in the renal excretion of calcium via pathway 2C.

The combination of these events serves to reduce the concentration of calcium in serum. The "butterfly" loops thus provide a convenient method for coordinating the various

FIGURE 10-4: The "butterfly" model for visualizing the mechanisms involved in the control of the concentration of calcium in serum; see text for details of operation: PTH = parathyroid hormone, CT = calcitonin, SCa^{++} = serum calcium, SPi = serum phosphate, UP_1 = urine phosphate. (*Source:* Arnaud, 1978.)

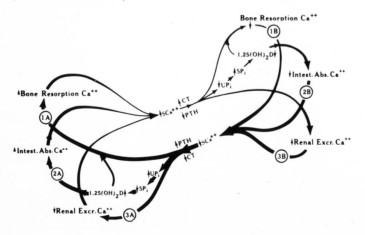

events that occur when the concentration of calcium in serum either increases or decreases.

A shortcoming of the butterfly model is its failure to provide information about the time constants or the limitations of the responses of the various elements of the model. This difficulty cannot be overcome because this information, for the most part, has not been obtained. Hence, this system cannot, at present, be defined in more precise terms.

The butterfly model is also useful in illustrating the effects of hyperparathyroidism on the control system. In primary hyperparathyroidism a large increase in the synthesis and secretion of PTH occurs as a consequence of a parathyroid tumor. The net effect is to stimulate activity in all three limbs on the left side of the model (Figure 10-4). Thus, there is increased bone resorption (limb 1A), decreased concentration of phosphate in serum, increased production of $1,25(OH)_2D_3$, increased absorption of calcium from the intestine (limb 2A), and, in the early stages of the disease, increased reabsorption of calcium by the kidney (limb 3A). All these actions are a consequence of an increased rate of secretion of PTH, and they all contribute to the increased concentration of calcium in serum. This is the hallmark of primary hyperparathyroidism.

One might expect the increase in the concentration of calcium in serum to initiate counterregulatory responses, as would happen under normal circumstances. This does not occur under the conditions just outlined because the parathyroid tumor is unresponsive to the elevated concentration of calcium in serum. On the other hand, the capacity of calcitonin to influence the concentration of calcium in serum in the presence of overwhelming amounts of PTH is very limited. As a result, all feedback loops on the right side of Figure 10-4 are virtually nonfunctional. As the disease progresses and serum calcium rises to high levels, renal excretion of calcium occurs in spite of the increased rate of secretion of PTH. (Q. 10-16) *With what other hormone does a similar renal response to continuing hormone stimulation occur?* The calcium escape is important because it provides protection against a potential life-threatening hypercalcemia. The unfortunate aspect of this response is that it contributes to the development of renal stones, a common problem in primary hyperparathyroidism.

The usual treatment of primary hyperparathyroidism is the surgical removal of the tumor. When this has been accomplished, a readjustment of the activities of the loops occurs until the concentration of calcium in the serum is returned to normal.

In unusual cases of primary hyperparathyroidism, it is sometimes necessary to treat the patient with oral doses of phosphate. (Q. 10-17) *What effect would you expect an elevation in the concentration of phosphate in serum to have on the concentration of calcium in the serum of such patients?*

The butterfly model can be very helpful in understanding many of the mechanisms controlling the concentration of calcium in serum. The student should not, however, consider it to be complete or final; but rather, it should serve as a point of reference to which new discoveries in this field can be related.

SECTION 10-4: POST-TEST QUESTIONS

1. What is the regulated variable in the butterfly model?

2. Name the three organs which are affected by an increase in the concentration of PTH in serum.
   a.
   b.
   c.

3. Describe the way each of these organs contributes to increase the concentration of calcium in serum.

   a.

   b.

   c.

4. An increase in the concentration of calcitonin in serum is accompanied by three principal responses. Describe these responses.

   a.

   b.

   c.

5. Accidental removal of the parathyroid glands during thyroidectomy would be expected to result in what effect on the concentrations of calcium and phosphate in serum?

   a.

   Could you treat such a patient chronically with parathyroid hormone?

   b.

   What other therapy could be used?

   c.

   How does it act?

   d.

SECTION 10-4: POST-TEST ANSWERS

1. Serum concentration of calcium
2. a. Bone
   b. Intestine
   c. Kidneys
3. a. Increase in dissolution of bone increases the release of calcium in blood.
   b. Increase in the absorption of calcium from the intestine contributes to the increase in concentration of calcium in serum.
   c. Increase in reabsorption of calcium from the urine contributes to the increase in concentration of calcium in serum.
4. a. A decreased dissolution of bone as a result of the accompanying decrease in the concentration of PTH in serum.
   b. A decreased absorption of calcium from the intestine as a result of a decrease in $1,25(OH)_2D_3$ resulting from an elevation in the concentration of phosphate in serum.
   c. An increased renal excretion of calcium resulting mainly from a decrease in the concentration of PTH in serum.
5. a. A reduction in the concentration of calcium and an increase in the concentration of phosphate in serum would occur.
   b. Yes, but synthetic PTH is available commercially only as PTH_{1-34}, and it is expensive. Second, it would need to be injected frequently each day, since its half-life is about 15 minutes (see Section 10-1).
   c. Vitamin D_3 could be used in very high doses. It can be taken orally and is relatively inexpensive.
   d. Vitamin D_3, after conversion to $1,25(OH)_2D_3$, acts on both the bones and the intestines to increase the concentration of calcium in serum.

SELECTED REFERENCES

Arnaud, C. D., 1978, Calcium homeostasis: regulatory elements and their integration, *Federation Proceedings* 37: 2557.

Austin, L. A. and Heath, H., III, 1981, Calcitonin—physiology and pathophysiology, *New England Journal Of Medicine* 304: 269.

Cohn, D. V. and MacGregor, R. R., 1981, The biosynthesis, intracellular processing, and secretion of parathormone, *Endocrine Reviews* 2: 1.

De Luca, H. F., 1976, Vitamin D endocrinology, *Annals Of Internal Medicine* 85: 367.

Kumar, R., 1980, The metabolism of 1,25-dihydroxyvitamin D_3, *Endocrine Reviews* 1: 258.

ANSWERS TO TEXT QUESTIONS

CHAPTER 1: ANSWERS TO TEXT QUESTIONS

Q.1. The surface area of the plasma membrane would continue to increase with each episode of exocytosis.

Q.2. Positively charged calcium ions may neutralize the negative charges in the plasma membrane of the secretory granule, thus facilitating the fusion of the granular and cellular membranes. Since calcium ions are well known for their ability to initiate contraction of myofibrillar elements (e.g., in striated muscle), they may interact in exocytosis by initiating similar events in the plasma membrane of the secretory granule.

Q.3. This would be expected to occur in the gonads (testis and ovary).

Q.4. If the binding affinity for the hormone is low, it will dissociate more readily from its carrier than if the binding affinity is high.

Q.5. Given the following equilibrium for T_4 and TBG in blood:

$$T_4 + TBG \underset{k_2}{\overset{k_1}{\rightleftharpoons}} T_4 \cdot TBG$$

These findings may be the result of either a decrease in the rate of association (i.e., k_1) between the hormone (T_4) and the protein (TBG) or an increase in the rate of dissociation (i.e., k_2) of the hormone-protein complex ($T_4 \cdot TBG$). Although the former possibility seems unlikely, since PBI has been shown to increase under these conditions, the latter possibility remains a viable alternative. A third possibility arises from the fact that estrogens are known to increase the production of TBG, as well as other carrier proteins such as transcortin (see Chapter 5) and testosterone binding globulin (see Chapter 6), this would be expected to decrease the concentration of free T_4 (and T_3) transiently. Thus the feedback mechanisms would come into play to return the concentration of the free hormones to normal. One might expect this to lead to an increase in the rate of production of T_4 and T_3; however, experimental evidence suggests that this is not the case.

Q.6. One would expect protein-type hormones that cannot penetrate cellular membranes readily to be bound to this type of receptor.

Q.7. One would expect steroid-type hormones that readily penetrate cellular membranes to be bound to this type of receptor.

Q.8. A receptor with a K_d of 10^{-8} mole/liter has a lower affinity for its ligand than a receptor with a K_d of 10^{-10} mole/liter.

Q.9. These substances can inhibit the production of proteins throughout the body. This fact obscures the possibility of determining an effect on a specific enzyme system. Such studies can be done only in vitro.

Q.10. The specificity of the chemical determination may be such that the metabolites of the hormone may be included in the measurement of the hormone itself. The bioassay measures only the biologically active forms of the hormones.

Q.11 In circumstances of abnormal secretion by an endocrine organ producing a protein-type hormone, excessive quantities of the prohormone may be produced and appear in the circulation in higher than normal amounts. In a radioimmunoassay the prohormone may not be distinguished from the hormone, although the biologic activity of the prohormone may be significantly less than that of the hormone.

CHAPTER 2: ANSWERS TO TEXT QUESTIONS

Q.1. Pituitary tumors most often grow dorsally out of the sella and thus pose a potential threat to damage neural tissue. The optic chiasm is in the greatest jeopardy, and visual field deficits can be used in the diagnosis of one of these tumors.

Q.2. The neurohypophysis receives extensive innervation from the supraoptic and paraventricular nuclei of the hypothalamus. The adenohypophysis receives no innervation from the brain that is known to influence its secretory activity.

Q.3. No. Most veins have valves that prevent blood from flowing in a retrograde direction.

Q.4. Yes. The capillaries of the median eminence (and other circumventricular organs of the brain) do not exhibit the so-called blood-brain barrier. This barrier normally prevents the passage of large molecules through the fenestrations of the endothelial cells lining most other capillaries. Capillaries in most brain regions have tight junctions between the endothelial cells and layer of glial "end feet" (terminal processes of protoplasmic astrocytes). Capillaries in the median eminence appear to lack these specializations.

Q.5. A hormone reaching the base of the brain via either the internal carotid or the basilar artery will enter the posterior communicating artery. Branches from this artery supply the ventromedial nucleus of the hypothalamus.

Q.6. A hormone can leave the internal carotid or the posterior communicating artery and enter the superior hypophyseal artery. A hormone can also leave the internal carotid artery and enter the middle or inferior hypophyseal artery. In the former situation the hormone can pass through the external and internal plexuses of the hypothalamus and enter the capillaries that supply (and receive) blood to (and from) the adenohypophysis. In the latter situation the hormone can pass into the capillary plexus in the neurohypophysis and eventually enter the adenohypophysis via the dense capillary network that interconnects the neuro- and adenohypophyses. Once in the adenohypophysis the hormone can leave the capillaries by diffusing through the fenestrations between the endothelial cells and then diffusing to their target cells.

Q.7. Adenohypophyseal hormones can diffuse into the capillaries that interconnect the adeno- and neurohypophyses. Once in the neurohypopohysis the adenohypophyseal hormone can be transported via the so-called portal capillaries directly to the external plexus of capillaries lining the base of the hypothalamus.

Q.8. ADH (vasopressin) has been shown to possess CRH-like activity in both clinical and laboratory studies. In laboratory animals the concentration of ADH in portal blood has been shown to be much greater than in the general circulation. In rodents subjected to adrenalectomy, the immunoreactive histochemical staining of ADH-containing neurons that project to capillary loops in the median eminence have been shown to undergo a marked increase. However, other evidence has shown that ADH is not the only biochemical with CRH-like activity. In rats with a genetic absence of ADH, ACTH and glucocorticoid concentrations are essentially normal, suggesting either that the mutant rats have adapted to their unusual situation or that ADH plays a minimal role (at best) in the physiologic regulation of ACTH secretion.

Q.9. ADH has some oxytocinlike activity and oxytocin has some ADH-like activity.

Q.10. The neurophysins are contained in the same dense cored vesicle as the neurohypophyseal hormone. Both these biochemicals are believed to be produced by posttranslational cleavage of the same protein prohormone. When the vesicle fuses with the plasma membrane of the axon terminal in the neurohypophysis, the entire contents of the vesicle have the potential of being released—this includes the neurophysin as well as the neurohypophyseal hormone.

Q.11. No. The hormone released in response to an acute stimulus is undoubtedly already present in the axon terminals of the neurohypophysis. Experiments suggest that this hormone is stored in a so-called readily releasable pool.

Q.12. Thirty minutes.

Q.13. Nicotine-stimulated neurophysin (NSN).

Q.14. One interpretation of these data is that the osmotic and blood volume stimuli activate different populations of magnocellular ADH neurons. It is possible, however, that a differential regulation of interneurons could also explain these data.

CHAPTER 3: ANSWERS TO TEXT QUESTIONS

Q.1. Organs such as the salivary glands and stomach can trap iodide ions. Since they lack the thyroglobulin molecule and the necessary peroxidase enzymes, these organs cannot synthesize thyroid hormone.

Q.2. In the early stages of the disease the patient will have an increase in the concentration of free thyroid hormone in serum. This results in an increased urinary loss of free T_4 and an increase in the rate of hepatic metabolism. The net effect is an increase in the turnover of thyroid hormones.

Q.3. The acute stimulation of the secretion of TSH in response to the administration of TRH does not require the de novo synthesis of proteins. These findings do not preclude the possibility that de novo synthesis of proteins is required for the increased synthesis of TSH that results from the administration of TRH.

Q.4. To test for dysfunction at the level of the thyroid gland (i.e., insensitivity to TSH), the patient can be given TSH and the production of thyroid hormone can be monitored. To test for dysfunction at the level of the pituitary gland (i.e., insensitivity to TRH and/or insensitivity or supersensitivity to the negative feedback actions of thyroid hormones), the patient can be given TRH with and without pretreatment with various doses of thyroid hormones.

Q.5. If the patient is hypothyroid due to hypofunction at any level, thyroid hormone replacement therapy can be prescribed. If the patient is hyperthyroid (due to hyperfunction at either the thyroid or pituitary gland), the condition is generally treated with antithyroid drugs such as propylthiouracil. Alternatively, surgical or radiation ablation of the thyroid gland combined with thyroid hormone replacement therapy may be prescribed.

Q.6. Hyperthyroid patients would be expected to present with elevated metabolic rates, heat production, and body temperature. Thus, when these individuals are challenged with an increase in the ambient temperature, they are more susceptible than euthyroid individuals to the potentially destructive effects of further elevations in body temperature. In hypothyroid patients the opposite situation would be expected.

Q.7. If the rate of absorption of hexose and pentose sugars across the gut wall is decreased, the rate of increase in the concentration of blood glucose and the release of insulin in response to that increase would also be reduced. Thus, in hypothyroid individuals, the glucose tolerance test should yield a more sluggish or protracted and, possibly, blunted response.

Q.8. The following list summarizes some of the possible ways in which hypothyroidism could be produced. Some of the examples are purely hypothetical and probably rarely if ever occur in nature. Examples of possible ways in which hyperthyroidism could be produced are left to the student's imagination.

a. Decrease in the dietary intake of iodide ions.

b. Decrease in the metabolically driven, active transport of iodide ions into the follicular cells of the thyroid gland.

c. Increase in the excretion of iodide ions by the kidney.

d. Decrease in the synthesis, availability, and/or activity of the peroxidase enzyme found in follicular cells. This enyzme is required for the oxidation of iodide ions to iodine and for the iodination of the tyrosyl residues contained in the thyroglobulin molecule. A genetically induced deficiency of catabolism of this enzyme could also result in hypothyroidism.

e. Decrease in the synthesis, availability (e.g., it could be bound to an antibody), and/or activity (e.g., exposure of the appropriate tyrosyl residues to the peroxidase enzyme) of thyroglobulin. An increase in its rate of catabolism could also result in hypothyroidism.

f. Decrease in the ability of the follicular cells to store (and/or retrieve from storage) the iodinated thyroglobulin.

g. Decrease in the synthesis (or increase in the catabolism), availability, activity, and/or specificity (e.g., cleavage of the iodinated thyroglobulin molecule at inappropriate locations) of the protease enzymes found in the follicular cells. These enzymes are essential for the release of the iodinated thyroglobulin from the pinocytotic vesicles (i.e., colloid droplets) and for the degradation of this protein to form T_4, T_3, MIT, and DIT.

h. Increase in the release of thyroglobulin from the follicular cells into blood. This could result in an increased formation of antibodies to this essential protein.

i. Increase in the synthesis (or decrease in the catabolism) and/or binding capacity and avidity of thyroid binding globulin in blood.

j. Decrease in the rate of peripheral deiodination of T_4 to T_3 or an increase in the production of rT_3, T_2, and/or T_1.

k. Increase in the ability of the liver to conjugate thyroid hormones, by induction of hepatic enzymes.

l. Decrease in the synthesis (or increase in the catabolism), availability, and/or activity of the enzyme β-glucuronidase in the small intestine. This enzyme is essential for the removal of the glucuronide moiety from the conjugated thyroid hormones, thus permitting the reabsorption of these hormones into the blood.

m. Decrease in the synthesis (e.g., due to a brain lesion), release, and/or action (e.g., decrease in the number and/or activity of membrane-associated receptors for TRH on the thyrotropes) of TRH.

n. Decrease in the synthesis (e.g., nonresponsiveness to TRH), release, and/or action (e.g., decrease in the number and/or activity of membrane-associated receptors for TSH on the follicular cells of the thyroid gland) of TSH.

Q.9. The thyroid gland and the kidneys compete for iodide ions. When more of an injected dose of radioactive iodide is excreted by way of the kidneys, less is available for uptake by the thyroid gland. This therefore decreases the 24-hour uptake by the thyroid gland.

Q.10. Yes. The excretion of iodide ions by the kidney is increased by natriuretic agents leading to a reduction in the availability of iodide ions to the thyroid gland.

Q.11. TSH acts on the thyroid gland to stimulate the synthesis and secretion of thyroid hormones, which in turn feed back to suppress the synthesis and secretion of TSH (i.e., via negative feedback at the level of the pituitary gland). Since an increase in the synthesis of thyroid hormones requires an increase in the uptake of iodide, the administration of TSH would be expected to increase iodide ion accumulation by the thyroid gland, whereas the administration of T_4 or T_3 should suppress the uptake of iodide ion by the thyroid gland.

Q.12. Thyroperoxidase.

Q.13. The dose of T_4 that inhibits completely the release of radioactivity from the thyroid gland is a direct reflection of the amount of T_4 necessary to suppress the secretion of TSH (i.e., negative feedback). Thus, although the secretion of thyroid hormones requires the actions of TSH, this assay provides only indirect evidence on the rate of thyroid hormone section.

Q.14. The specific activity of ^{131}I-labeled thyroid binding globulin should be higher in the hypothyroid patient than in the euthyroid or hyperthyroid individual because of an increase in the availability of unoccupied receptor sites on the TBG.

Q.15. The exogenous T_4 and T_3 would suppress the secretion of TSH (i.e., negative feedback), thus reducing the tropic stimulation of thyroid hormone synthesis and iodide ion (radiolabeled and nonradiolabeled) uptake by the thyroid gland.

Q.16. No. The exogenous T_4 or T_3 would be expected to bind to the plasma proteins in the same manner as the endogenous thyroid hormones. Thus even though the secretion of endogenous thyroid hormones would be expected to be suppressed with this therapy, the exogenous thyroid hormones should be able to maintain the PBI at normal or above normal values.

Q.17. It is a direct measure of pituitary function and is not confounded by the possibility of a dysfunction at the level of the thyroid gland. The direct measurement of TSH before and after the administration of either T_4 or T_3 provides direct information concerning both the basal rate of TSH secretion (which of course is a reflection of numerous factors including the secretion of TRH and the responsiveness of the thryotrope to that TRH) and the ability of thyroid hormones to suppress the secretion of TSH.

Q.18. Initiation of thyroxine replacement therapy.

Q.19. Initiation of thyroxine replacement therapy.

Q.20. There is no compelling reason to use TSH or TRH replacement therapy, since thyroxine replacement therapy can resolve the problem at comparatively low cost and little inconvenience to the patient. Both TSH and TRH have a relatively short half-life and as such the maintenance of an adequate thyroid hormone concentration in blood could be difficult. Furthermore, an inexpensive source of pure human TSH has not been found.

Q.21. A high rate of oxygen consumption is typical for hyperthyroid individuals.

Q.22. Since rT_3 has less than 2% of the metabolic activity of T_3, it has a much reduced capacity to stimulate an increase in the calorigenic and other actions attributable normally to T_3. Any increase in the production of rT_3 at the expense of the production of T_3 would therefore be expected to result in a reduction in metabolic rate (i.e., oxygen consumption).

CHAPTER 4: ANSWERS TO TEXT QUESTIONS

Q.1. The adrenal medulla can be regarded as a terminal ganglion within the sympathetic nervous system.

Q.2. One of the characteristics of the parasympathetic nervous system consists of its comparatively specific (i.e., anatomically restricted) responses to stimulation.

Q.3. The anatomic arrangements are similar. The preganglionic parasympathetic axons of the pelvic nerve distribute to the terminal ganglia within the organs they eventually innervate as a plexus of axons associated with the blood vessels to those organs. The postganglionic sympathetic axons emerging from the lateral and collateral ganglia also distribute to their target organs as a plexus of axons associated with the blood vessels to these same organs. There are exceptions to both these generalizations.

Q.4. By inhibiting the enzyme responsible for catabolizing the neurotransmitter, it would be logical to predict that the response to stimulation of the parasympathetic nerves would be magnified due to an increase in the half-life of the pre- and postganglionic neurotransmitter.

Q.5. Thyroxine (tetraiodothyronine, T_4) and triiodothyronine (T_3).

Q.6. Negative.

Q.7. They originate from neural crest tissue.

Q.8. The fusion of the membrane of the granule with the plasma membrane permits the entire contents of the granule to be released into the extracellular space. Thus the dopamine-β-hydroxylase is released during exocytosis in much the same manner as the neurophysins are released during the release of the neurohypophyseal hormones (see Section 2-3).

Q.9. A greater proportion of the norepinephrine would be subject to catabolism by catechol-O-methyltransferase, and as such it should be detected as an increase in the concentration of free and conjugated forms of normetanephrine (NMN) in urine.

CHAPTER 5: ANSWERS TO TEXT QUESTIONS

Q.1. 11-Deoxycortisol and 11-deoxycorticosterone.

Q.2. Steroid hormones possess little, if any, intrinsic antigenicity. They are comparatively small molecules whose structural features have been conserved apparently over a wide range of animal species (and evolutionary development). Therefore, to develop antibodies to steroids they often must first be linked chemically to a protein that is recognized as "foreign" to the immune system of the animal used to generate the antibodies. This protein-steroid complex may stimulate the production of numerous different antibodies, only a few of which may be able to recognize the special features of the steroid hormone.

Q.3. Cortisol and cortisone.

Q.4. Less. With serious congestion of the liver, the rate of catabolism of cortisol would be expected to be reduced (i.e., the half-life would be increased). Therefore, a given dose of cortisol would be expected to exert a greater and/or more prolonged effect than the same dose given to someone with normal liver function.

Q.5. This suggests that the zona glomerulosa is not controlled primarily by the anterior pituitary gland and the secretion of ACTH.

Q.6. Since the process of synthesis and secretion of glucocorticoid hormones requires the tropic actions of ACTH, a suppression in the concentration of ACTH in blood due to the negative feedback actions of the exogenous glucocorticoids would be expected to lead to a depression in the production of endogenous glucocorticoids. A reduction in the synthesis of these hormones is associated with a reduction in the size of the zonae fasciculata and reticularis of the adrenal cortex.

Q.7. Shortly after removal of one adrenal gland the concentration of cortisol in blood would be expected to be reduced, but this reduction would probably be only temporary, since the secretion of ACTH would be expected to increase because of the reduction in the magnitude of the negative feedback signal. After the remaining adrenal gland has restored the concentration of cortisol in blood to near normal, the increased secretion of ACTH would also be expected to return to near normal.

Q.8. No. The pattern of secretion of cortisol and ACTH during the light and dark periods of the day appears to be shifted approximately 8 hours later than that displayed by aldosterone and renin. For example, the concentration of cortisol in blood reaches a maximum during the early morning hours (8 A.M. in Figure 5-14), whereas the concentration of aldosterone in blood reaches a maximum during the late evening hours (12 P.M. in Figure 5-20).

Q.9. The concentration of ACTH in plasma would be expected to be elevated because of the loss of the negative feedback actions of the endogenous glucocorticoids.

Q.10. If the patients cannot display an increase in the production of glucocorticoids in response to the administration of ACTH, it would be unwise to test them with metyrapone, since the assay for an increase in ACTH secretion (due to the reduction in cortisol production following the inhibition of 11β-hydroxylase) is an increase in the production of glucocorticoid hormone precursors by the possibly defective adrenal gland.

Q.11. No. Since the test itself involves measurement of the concentration of cortisol in blood, administration of this hormone exogenously would obscure the measurement.

Q.12. The patients should have a low concentration of potassium in the blood, since the aldosterone secreted by the tumor would be expected to stimulate the excretion of potassium. The high rates of sodium reabsorption that normally accompany the excretion of potassium are blocked in these patients by the actions of "third factor." The alkalosis is a by-product of the continued excretion of potassium. Bicarbonate ions are reabsorbed to balance the chloride ions that are excreted along with the potassium ions. The net result is an increase in the pH of the plasma.

Q.13. The secretion of renin would be expected to be reduced because of the negative feedback actions of aldosterone exerted by way of the long feedback loop (see Figure 5-18).

Q.14. The reduced ability of the adrenal gland to secrete cortisol in response to exogenous ACTH in an individual with secondary adrenal hypofunction is probably the result of an atrophy of the zonae fasciculata and reticularis. The zona glomerulosa (i.e., the source of the aldosterone) should not have atrophied, and thus it should be able to display a marked increase in the synthesis and secretion of aldosterone in response to the administration of exogenous ACTH.

Q.15. In secondary adrenocortical insufficiency the zonae fasciculata and reticularis (and to a much lesser extent, the zona glomerulosa) of the adrenal gland are commonly in an atrophic state due to the absence of trophic stimulation by endogenous ACTH. Therefore, exogenous ACTH should be administered for at least 3 days to allow sufficient time for the steroidogenic capacity of the atrophic cell layers to be restored to a level where a measurable increase in the production of glucocorticoids is readily apparent. In primary adrenocortical insufficiency the atropic adrenal gland continues to remain unresponsive to stimulation by ACTH even after 3 days of successive exposure to the tropic hormone.

Q.16. These females would be expected to be virilized, but not hypertensive. They should have an increased rate of adrenal androgen synthesis and secretion (due to the increase in the secretion of ACTH and the decrease in the conversion of 17α-OH-progesterone to nonandrogenic products) and a decreased rate of glucocorticoid and mineralocorticoid synthesis and secretion (both of which are due to the reduction in 21-hydroxylase activity). The increase in the secretion of ACTH is due to the reduction in the negative feedback signal, which results from the reduction in the secretion of cortisol.

Q.17. The sulfated conjugates of etiocholanolone and androsterone.

CHAPTER 6: ANSWERS TO TEXT QUESTIONS

Q.1. The testes contain a number of temperature-sensitive enzymes essential for the continued viability of the sperm.

Q.2. Vasectomy should not have any detrimental effects on the production and secretion of testosterone, since the steroid is secreted into the testicular veins and not into the ductus deferens.

Q.3. The interstitial cells of Leydig appear to lack the microsomal enzyme 21-hydroxylase, which is essential for the conversion of progesterone and 17α-OH-progesterone and 11-deoxycorticosterone and 11-deoxycortisol, respectively.

Q.4. The cells of the zona glomerulosa are specialized for the synthesis and secretion of the mineralocorticoid aldosterone; those in the zona fasciculata produce the glucocorticoid cortisol, and androstenedione. The cells of the zona reticularis produce the bulk of the adrenal androgens, although these cells also have the capacity to synthesize and secrete cortisol.

Q.5. Because TeBG has such a high affinity for testosterone, an increase in the concentration of TeBG in blood has a dramatic effect on the concentration of free testosterone. Once testosterone is bound to TeBG, it is not dissociated easily.

Q.6. The virilizing potency of circulating androgens should be increased as a direct result of the reduction in the total binding capacity of TeBG and the consequent increase in the concentration of free androgens in blood.

Q.7. Since the effects of TeBG and total testosterone production are in the same direction in both cases, it is possible that there would be little if any effect on the concentration of free testosterone in blood.

Q.8. Steroids are lipids and as such should have little difficulty penetrating the lipid portions of the plasma membrane.

Q.9. Humans and animals with the Tfm mutation usually respond in an essentially normal fashion to estrogens, since the receptors for these steroids should be unaffected by this mutation.

Q.10. Except for an abnormally formed penis, these men have a virilized appearance.

Q.11. The problem of cross-reactivity is increased greatly with these hormones because of the identity of the α-chains and the marked similarity of the β-chains.

Q.12. No. α-LH/β-FSH should exhibit similar physiologic responses to native FSH (i.e., α-FSH/β-FSH); α-LH/β-LH is native LH.

Q.13. α-FSH/β-LH should behave similar to native LH, α-FSH/β-TSH should behave similar to native TSH, and α-TSH/β-FSH should behave similar to native FSH.

Q.14. The decrease in the MCR and the consequent increase in the biopotency of gonadotropins following gonadectomy (or reduced secretion of gonadal steroids) should increase the efficacy of these hormones in negative feedback regulation of testicular steroidogenesis.

Q.15. Since inhibition of the phosphodiesterase enzyme should lead to an increase in the half-life, hence concentration of cAMP, theophylline and caffeine should increase the potency of LH in stimulating steroid biosynthesis in the Leydig cells.

Q.16. Since the standard genomic mechanism of steroid action requires the de novo synthesis of mRNA and proteins, hence a diploid chromosome number, it is not clear what the function of these receptors would be in a haploid cell. Since the genetic locus for the androgen receptor (i.e., the Tfm locus) is found on the short arm of the X chromosome, haploid germ cells that contain the Y chromosome would not carry the genetic information essential for the synthesis of the androgen receptor. In Tfm/Y mice there are no testosterone receptors and spermatogenesis is arrested at the first meiotic division, but in Tfm/Y—+/Y chimeric phenotypic males spermatogenesis appears to be normal (i.e., they are fertile). Since Tfm/Y—+/Y chimeric males can produce Tfm/X female siblings when mated with a X/X normal female, some of the Tfm sperm must have been viable. This viability is undoubtedly the result of the essential supportive actions of +/Y Sertoli (and epididymal) cells, which will, of course, have normal receptors for testosterone.

Q.17. If Gn-RH analogues can be shown to inhibit the actions of native Gn-RH, it should be possible to use these agents to block the secretion of LH (and FSH), hence to inhibit gametogenesis in both sexes. Unfortunately, this therapy would also produce a functional castration and the consequent onset of impotence.

Q.18. No. Given the episodic and pulsatile nature of the secretion of testosterone and LH, respectively, it is imperative that multiple sampling over time be performed to gain an appreciation of the range of hormone concentration that may be possible at any given time of day.

Q.19. Many pituitary and hypothalamic hormones exhibit a pulsatile pattern of secretion. For example, oxytocin is released in a pulsatile fashion.

Q.20. The increase in the concentration of Gn-RH is further increased with hypophysectomy because the negative influence of the short feedback loop is lost. This effect is exaggerated in the castrated individual, in whom the concentration of gonadotropins would be expected to be elevated because of the loss of the negative feedback actions of the testicular androgens.

Q.21. Testosterone secretion should be depressed following the administration of pharmacologic doses of exogenous estrogen.

Q.22. Estrogen can inhibit the secretion of testosterone by acting directly on the biosynthetic enzymes of the testes and by acting in the brain and pituitary to inhibit the secretion of LH.

Q.23. Androgen binding protein.

CHAPTER 7: ANSWERS TO TEXT QUESTIONS

Q.1. The adrenal gland is also divided into cortical and medullary regions.

Q.2. No. The first wave of spermatogenesis occurs during puberty.

Q.3. The effects of radiation damage on gametogenesis should be more lasting in women than in men because at birth women have all the primary oocytes that they will ever produce, whereas men continue to produce new primary spermatocytes throughout most of adulthood.

Q.4. Whenever nonidentical twins are produced there must have been at least two follicles that reached the final stages of maturation. Identical twins are produced from the same ovum; hence only one Graafian follicle would have been required.

Q.5. Whereas the time required for the completion of oogenesis is approximately 14 days, the time required for the completion of spermatogenesis has been estimated to be at least 64 days.

Q.6. Four.

Q.7. The follicular and luteal phases are each approximately 14 days long.

Q.8. The interstitial cells of Leydig are responsible for the production of testosterone; whereas the Sertoli cells convert this androgen into estradiol.

Q.9. Transcortin (corticosteroid binding globulin).

Q.10. Testosterone binding globulin.

Q.11. Albumin.

Q.12. glucuronide; sulfate

Q.13. The activation of a steroid receptor increases the affinity of the steroid-receptor complex for its nuclear acceptors.

Q.14. This fibrinolysin helps to prevent the clotting of the blood released during the menstrual discharge.

Q.15. Fourteen days, although there is considerable variability even at these ages.

Q.16. Ten to fourteen days.

Q.17. Menarche can be defined as the age at which periodic menstruation and ovarian cyclicity begins (i.e., at puberty). Menopause can be defined as the age at which periodic menstruation and ovarian cyclicity ceases (i.e., during late middle age).

Q.18. The contractions of the uterine myometrium during menstruation should assist in the expulsion of the necrotic endometrial tissue.

Q.19. A high percentage of cornified cells should be present in the Pap smears taken from these patients.

Q.20. Three to five days.

Q.21. Two. One α-chain and one β-chain.

Q.22. The α-chains have the same amino acid sequence for LH, FSH, and TSH. The β-chains also show a surprising degree of similarity across these three hormones.

Q.23. The metabolic clearance rate of FSH (and to a lesser extent, LH) is reduced following gonadectomy. This effect is attributed to the pleomorphism produced by changes in the number of sialic acid residues attached to the glycoprotein hormone.

Q.24. No. Ovulation is the result of a combination of three major factors: the thinning of the follicular wall, the enzymatic weakening of the intercellular adhesions of the follicular wall, and the contraction of the theca externa cells found in the follicular wall.

Q.25. Estradiol.

Q.26. The actions of estradiol and progesterone in the uterine endometrium during the luteal phase are characterized by a continuation in cellular hypertrophy, increased mucus production, increased length of the spiral arteries, and increased edema.

Q.27. Corpus albicans.

Q.28. Fallopian tube.

Q.29. Six days after ovulation.

Q.30. Somatostatin, vasoactive intestinal protein (vasotocin), angiotensin, etc.

Q.31. LH.

Q.32. The placenta acts as a barrier to many compounds in the mother's blood supply. Thus, hPL is not transferred easily to the growing fetus.

Q.33. They should undergo contraction in response to the increased availability of oxytocin.

Q.34. The concentration of ACTH would be expected to decrease in the face of increasing concentration of cortisol because of the negative feedback actions of this steroid.

Q.35. The myometrium should undergo contractions in response to the increased availability of oxytocin, which is released in response to suckling.

Q.36. The Gn-RH is synthesized on ribosomes, packaged into vesicles by the Golgi apparatus, transported from the soma of the parvicellular neuron to its axon terminal by an energy-dependent mechanism (i.e., neuroplasmic or axoplasmic flow), and released from the axon terminal by a stimulus-secretion-coupling-dependent exocytotic mechanism into either the perivascular space near the capillary loops of the internal and external plexus or the periventricular space near the third ventricle. In the former situation the Gn-RH may diffuse directly into the fenestrated capillaries of the hypothalamohypophyseal blood system (i.e., portal blood supply); in the latter situation it may diffuse through the third ventricle to the floor of the infundibular recess, where it may be taken up by the tanycytes and transported to the capillary loops of the internal plexus. The hormone is transported within the hypothalamohypophyseal capillaries to the adenohypophysis, wherein it diffuses through the fenestrated endothelial lining of the capillaries to make contact with the plasma membranes of the gonadotropes.

Q.37. No. Gn-RH is synthesized and released in several other regions of the brain (e.g., preoptic area and ventral tegmental area). The action of Gn-RH in these other brain regions is not clear in humans, but animal studies suggest that it may serve a role in modulating reproductive behavior.

Q.38. This operation would interrupt the hypothalamohypophyseal blood system and thus prevent the transport of PIH from the hypothalamus to the adenohypophysis at which inhibition of secretion normally occurs.

Q.39. Lactotropes. Since prolactin is the only adenohypophyseal hormone to primarily be under negative regulation, it is not surprising that increased secretion of this hormone is associated commonly with adenohypophyseal tumors.

Q.40. The release of adenohypophyseal hormones such as LH and FSH is believed to be activated by the actions of cAMP produced in response to the actions of their HHHs with receptors located on the plasma membrane.

Q.41. It is directly related, since L-DOPA is the immediate precursor for dopamine.

Q.42. One mechanism could invoke the concomitant release of somatostatin, which would block the release of TSH induced by the actions of TRH.

Q.43. There is no single correct answer to this question. Use your imagination to come up with some novel approaches.

Q.44. The growing follicles provide the principal source of estradiol during the follicular (i.e., proliferative) phase; the corpus luteum provides the principal source of this hormone during the luteal (i.e., secretory) phase.

Q.45. The cells in the external layer of the granulosa cell mass that begin to undergo luteinization before ovulation.

Q.46. The secretion of Prl is highly susceptible to stress and as such it is difficult to obtain stable measurements even under laboratory conditions.

Q.47. As long as the lighting cycle is not shifted, the pattern of secretion of ACTH and cortisol should remain the same even if the sleep cycle is shifted.

Q.48. If the normal pattern and magnitude of ovarian hormone secretion is recreated with exogenous hormones, there should be a greater probability of a large increase in the secretion of LH and FSH similar to that observed in normal women before ovulation. There is no guarantee, however, that this increased availability of gonadotropins will lead to a greater probability of ovulation, since there may be more pathologic alteration in the ovaries of these women than simply a reduced capacity to synthesize and secrete estradiol and progesterone.

Q.49. Normally women do not ovulate during pregnancy. The high concentrations of progesterone in the blood of these women should prevent the release of Gn-RH from the hypothalamus in much the same manner as it does during the luteal phase of the menstrual cycle.

Q.50. No. Neurons containing Gn-RH have been reported to exist in numerous other brain regions including the amygdala, the ventral tegmental area, and the preoptic area.

Q.51. The secretion of Prl should be increased following these lesions because of the loss of the neurons producing PIH or the loss of the tissue through which this hormone is transported to the pituitary.

Q.52. Gn-RH, like many other hormones, is secreted normally in a pulsatile fashion. Tonic exposure of membrane-bound receptors to their appropriate hormone ligand often leads to a desensitization and eventual down-regulation (i.e., internalization) of the receptors.

Q.53. Desensitization and/or down-regulation of membrane-bound receptors for Gn-RH and processing of the nuclear estrogen-receptor-acceptor complex are definite possibilities; however, the self-termination may simply be a reflection of the fact that the rate of secretion has exceeded the rate at which the release pool of LH can be replenished.

Q.54. In the last few days of the luteal phase the ability of LH to stimulate the synthesis and secretion of progesterone and estradiol by the cells of the corpus luteum is known to be diminished markedly. This self-terminating response in the face of relatively invariant levels of the tropic hormone is due apparently to the desensitization and eventual down-regulation (i.e., internalization) of the receptors for LH found on the plasma membranes of these cells.

Q.55. There is no single correct answer to this question. Use your imagination. Do you think that the steroid might affect the relative distribution of the gonadotropin in the various intracellular pools?

Q.56. Inhibin is synthesized by the Sertoli cells of the testes.

Q.57. Transection of the infundibular stalk should lead to an increase in the tonic rate of secretion of Prl (due to the loss of PIH) and a decrease in the tonic rate of secretion of LH (due to the loss of Gn-RH).

Q.58. TRH can be catabolized rapidly by blood-borne peptidases.

Q.59. The competitive inhibition of COMT activity by the catechol estrogens would be expected to increase the local concentrations of endogenous catecholamines such as dopamine. This effect could contribute to the effectiveness of the catechol estrone in inhibiting the secretion of Prl.

Q.60. No. A lesion in that region of the hypothalamus would be expected to destroy neurons that synthesize and secrete PIH (i.e., dopamine). This, of course, should lead to an increase not a decrease in the secretion of Prl.

Q.61. There is no single correct answer to this question. Use your imagination.

Q.62. These results might be interpreted as suggesting that L-DOPA has a greater effect (in an acute situation) on the secretion of Prl and LH than it does on the synthesis of these hormones. That is, synthesis may continue while secretion is inhibited. Thus, following the cessation of the inhibition of secretion, a greater than normal rate of secretion may result from the greater than normal magnitude of the release pool of Prl and LH.

CHAPTER 8: ANSWERS TO TEXT QUESTIONS

Q.1. The close similarity between the chemical structures of growth hormone, prolactin, and placental lactogen would be expected to increase the probability of producing antibodies that display significant cross-reactivity for all three hormones.

Q.2. There are many examples of hormones that undergo metabolic activation in vivo including testosterone, thyroxine, angiotensin I, vitamin D, and estrone.

Q.3. Prolactin.

Q.4. Prolactin is chemically very similar to growth hormone, with 161 of its amino acids in the same sequence as in growth hormone.

Q.5. Serotonin is thought to be involved in increasing the secretion of prolactin.

Q.6. The secretion of LH and prolactin are inhibited by the administration of L-DOPA.

Q.7. Prolactin.

Q.8. Caffeine and theophylline. They increase the concentration of cAMP by inhibiting the catabolism of this cyclic nucleotide by the phosphodiesterase enzyme.

Q.9. The observation suggests that either the target cells and receptors for growth hormone are distributed in many regions of the body or else they are more localized to a limited number of regions, one of which is responsible for the production of another factor or hormone that is responsible for stimulating growth. The second factor may have receptors in many regions of the body. Obvious candidates for this factor are the somatomedins produced in the liver.

Q.10. Yes. Since growth hormone stimulates an increase both in the uptake of amino acids and in their incorporation into proteins, the availability of amino acids for the urea cycle would be expected to be diminished.

Q.11. 5 to 10 mg. Thus, the 8-mg dose used in the experiment outlined in Table 8-2 represents an equivalent of approximately one whole pituitary gland.

Q.12. Yes. The metabolic acidosis seen in diabetes mellitus is also characterized by an increased mobilization of fats, an increased production of acetoacetic acid and β-hydroxybutyrate by the liver, and the appearance of a rapid and deep pattern of breathing that lowers the concentration of bicarbonate in blood.

Q.13. The half-life of somatomedins in blood is reduced in hypophysectomized animals. This reduction is thought to be the result of a diminution in the production of a carrier protein for the somatomedins that is synthesized normally in the liver by the actions of growth hormone.

Q.14. It is a small peptide composed of a single chain of 14 amino acids linked by a single disulfide bond.

Q.15. These findings might be interpreted as suggesting that the receptors for somatostatin in the membranes of the A- and B-cells of the pancreas recognize slightly different aspects to the somatostatin molecule.

Q.16. Growth hormone and thyroid stimulating hormone.

Q.17. The observation that blood samples taken from Laron dwarfs are characterized by high concentrations of growth hormone and low concentrations of somatomedins could be interpreted as support for the possibility that somatomedins feed back in a negative manner to regulate the secretion of growth hormone.

Q.18. Since the concentration of growth hormone and somatomedins in the blood of the African pigmy is not reduced greatly compared to a "normal" individual, it has been speculated that the unusually short stature of these people is the result of an insensitivity of their tissues to somatomedins. The possibility that such an insensitivity may be the result of a reduction in the number and/or activity of receptors for somatomedins has not been resolved completely.

CHAPTER 9: ANSWERS TO TEXT QUESTIONS

Q.1 No. One of the few definitions of an endocrine gland that all endocrinologists would agree to is that a hormone is not transported from the gland by a system of ducts.

Q.2. It acts to inhibit the secretion of at least nine other hormones, including insulin, pancreatic and gut glucagon, motilin, gastrin, vasoactive intestinal peptide, gastric inhibitory polypeptide, and the two adenohypophyseal hormones, growth hormone and thyroid stimulating hormone.

Q.3. A hormone secreted by one islet cell into the extracellular fluid could be taken into another cell by endocytosis. The hormone could also be secreted into blood and returned by this route to another islet cell.

Q.4. The surface area of the plasma membrane of the B-cells in the islets of Langerhans would have to increase slightly with each episode of secretion of insulin. This, of course, does not occur, thus adding to the support for the theory that the vesicular membranes are retrieved by endocytosis.

Q.5. The thyroid gland stores a comparatively large quantity of thyroid hormones (in the form of iodinated thyroglobulin) in the lumen of its follicles.

Q.6. The antibodies would reduce the biologic effectiveness of the exogenous insulin by binding to the antigenic sites of the "foreign" insulin molecule and thus render it inactive.

Q.7. If there are 4 units of insulin per gram of pancrease and 24 units per milligram of insulin, there are 166 μg of insulin per gram of pancreas.

Q.8. Assuming that the patient still has some functional B-cells in his islets of Langerhans, this operation should have an effect equivalent to increasing the secretion of insulin by 40–50%, thus reducing the need for exogenous insulin.

Q.9. If the receptor were a phospholipid, the phospholipase would be expected to reduce, not increase, the binding of insulin.

Q.10. Most peptide and protein hormones appear to initiate their molecular effects through the so-called second messenger, cAMP. Examples of protein and peptide hormones that appear to utilize this mechanism of action are ACTH, LH, FSH, and glucagon.

Q.11. Guanylate cyclase.

Q.12. There are many possible interpretations of these findings. For example, insulin, and/or its fragments that still retain the antigenic recognition sites (but possibly not the biologic activity) of the parent protein, may be taken up by certain cells (by carrier-mediated transport, active uptake, or some other mechanism) and transported by diffusion to the lysosomes, which (further) cleave the insulin molecule into fragments (some of which may retain the antigenic, but not the biologic potency of the parent chemical). After being released from the lysosome and taken up by the nucleus of the cell, these fragments may bind within the nucleus to the chromatin in a biologically relevant manner, leading to the de novo synthesis of specific messenger RNAs and proteins. Alternatively, the binding to the nuclear material may be nonspecific and serve no relevant biologic function.

Q.13. Again there are several possible interpretations of these observations. For example, it may turn out that the receptors in insulin-insensitive tissues are in fact different in some fashion from those found in insulin-sensitive cells and that this difference is responsible for the failure or success of insulin to stimulate glucose uptake by the cell. It may turn out that there really are no differences in the receptor molecule in the two types of cell but there is a difference in the coupling of that receptor to an effector system, which must be activated to stimulate the normal physiologic response to insulin.

Q.14. The rapid catabolism of insulin (endogenous and exogenous) makes it difficult to maintain appropriate (and not excessive) concentrations of insulin in blood. As a result of this problem, the normal treatment of diabetics with systemic injections of insulin does not maintain the concentration of glucose in blood within the same range as that achieved by endogenous insulin (and other hormones) in the nondiabetic individual.

Q.15. Somatostatin inhibits the secretion of these hormones as well as that of growth hormone, thyroid stimulating hormone, pancreatic glucagon, motilin, and gastrin.

Q.16. Growth hormone and the somatomedins also appear to increase the uptake of amino acids and the incorporation of those amino acids into tissue proteins.

Q.17. When the concentration of glucose in blood is low (i.e., during fasting), the rates of secretion of glucagon and epinephrine increase, leading to an increase in glycogenolysis and lipolysis. The latter process results in an increase in the concentration of free fatty acids in blood. These lipids are required as substrates for the generation of metabolic energy in the liver during gluconeogenesis. The free fatty acids are catabolized in the liver through the β-oxidation cycle to form the so-called ketones acetoacetate and β-hydroxybutyrate. During conditions of an increased concentration of glucose in blood, the secretion of insulin increases, leading to a decrease in lipolysis and a consequent reduction in the production of ketones by the liver.

Q.18. Several hormones exhibit this pattern of secretion (e.g., FSH and LH).

Q.19. Dopamine (i.e., PIH). The inhibition of the secretion of prolactin secretion from the lactotropes of the adenohypophysis by dopamine is thought to involve the inhibition of calcium influx.

Q.20. A given dose of somatostatin inhibits the secretions of both insulin and glucagon to the same extent (see Section 8-5).

Q.21. The shorter lasting insulin could be administered before ingestion of meals, whereas the longer lasting insulin could be used as a maintenance dose.

Q.22. Epinephrine, growth hormone, and glucagon (see Figure 9-7).

Q.23. Carbon dioxide (acid) is blown off by way of the lungs.

Q.24. One may speculate that there is a resetting of the set point for control of glucocorticoid concentration of the blood.

Q.25. Reduce the dosage of insulin administered.

CHAPTER 10: ANSWERS TO TEXT QUESTIONS

Q.1. Exocytosis.

Q.2. Under normal circumstances, no pro-PTH or fragments of PTH are released from the parathyroid gland.

Q.3. Stored thyroid hormone may last several months; whereas there is essentially no storage for steroid hormones.

Q.4. It is the free, rather than the bound, hormone that is important physiologically.

Q.5. Free calcium.

Q.6. Exchangeable stores.

Q.7. Aldosterone.

Q.8. Duodenum.

Q.9. A low-calcium diet and reduced absorption of calcium from the intestines, as well as a parathyroid tumor, would be expected to increase the secretion of PTH and consequently the hydroxylation of 25(OH)D$_3$.

Q.10. Since calcitonin opposes the action of PTH on bone, it would be of some interest if it also were found to counteract the effect of PTH to induce the renal enzyme that converts $25(OH)D_3$ to $1,25(OH)_2D_3$.

Q.11. This compound would be useful in patients with renal disease who are unable to hydroxylate $25(OH)D_3$.

Q.12. Vitamin D is a lipid-soluble compound that has little difficulty traversing the cellular membrane.

Q.13. Patients with advanced renal disease generally are unable to hydroxylate $25(OH)D_3$.

Q.14. Vitamin D_3 must be hydroxylated successively by enzymes in the liver and kidneys. This undoubtedly accounts for a portion of the delay.

Q.15. In the case of thyroxine, peripheral conversion to reverse triiodothyronine rather than triiodothyronine greatly diminishes its physiologic effects.

Q.16. Aldosterone.

Q.17. It would be expected to reduce the concentration of calcium in serum because an elevation in the concentration of phosphate inhibits the hydroxylation of $25(OH)D_3$.

COMPREHENSIVE POST-TEST

A. MULTIPLE CHOICE QUESTIONS (ONE CORRECT ANSWER PER QUESTION)

1. Experimental proof that a hormone is produced as a result of protein synthesis can be obtained by the use of certain compounds such as:
   a. Theophylline (a xanthine compound)
   b. Metyrapone
   c. Propylthiouracil
   d. Actinomycin D
   e. Oubain

2. Which of the following hormones does *not produce* a response in its target tissue by activation of protein kinase enzymes?
   a. TSH
   b. Parathyroid hormone
   c. FSH
   d. ACTH
   e. Insulin

3. Which of the following hormones exhibits a *decrease* in its biologic half-life under the conditions listed?
   a. FSH following castration
   b. Somatomedin following hypophysectomy
   c. Thyroxine following treatment with estrogens
   d. a, b, and c
   e. None of the above

4. Hypophysectomy results in all the following *except:*
   a. Atrophy of the thyroid gland
   b. Growth retardation if performed before puberty
   c. Deficiency of aldosterone
   d. Cessation of the menstrual cycle
   e. Impaired testosterone secretion

5. Which of the statements *accurately* describes an example of the physiologic regulation of a *proteolytic enzyme?*
   a. The synthesis of fibrinolysin *increases* in the uterine endometrium following cessation of exposure to estrogens.
   b. The concentration of plasmin *increases* in the Graafian follicle following exposure to FSH.

    c. The secretion of renin from the juxtaglomerular cells *increases* following exposure to angiotensin II.

    d. The proteolytic destruction of PTH in the parathyroid gland *decreases* during prolonged hypercalcemia.

    e. All the above

6. Stimulus-secretion coupling is a mechanism for hormone release that includes:

    a. Calcium entry into the cell storing the hormone

    b. Exocytosis of vesicles following their incorporation into the plasma membrane

    c. Increase in cyclic nucleotide production in the cell producing the hormone

    d. a and b only

    e. a, b, and c

7. Which of the following statements about parathyroid hormone is correct?

    a. It is transported in blood bound to a carrier protein.

    b. Its secretion decreases in response to an increasing concentration of free calcium in plasma.

    c. It inhibits loss of phosphate from bone.

    d. It is secreted by the parafollicular or C cells.

    e. None of the above.

8. Promotion of gluconeogenesis, maintenance of the rate of glomerular filtration by the kidneys, and suppression of the secretion of a hypothalamic releasing factor are all thought to be physiologically important effects of:

    a. Glucagon

    b. Somatomedins

    c. Aldosterone

    d. Cortisol

    e. Triiodothyronine

9. If the pituitary gland is transplanted successfully from the sella turcica to the kidney capsule:

    a. The concentration of glucose in blood increases.

    b. The thyroid gland becomes hypertrophied.

    c. The concentration of sodium in plasma decreases.

    d. The concentration of calcium in plasma decreases.

    e. None of the above

10. Which of the following hormones exhibits a sleep-associated pattern of secretion?

    a. Cortisol

    b. Aldosterone

    c. ACTH

    d. Growth hormone

    e. None of the above

11. Which of the following statements about human chorionic gonadotropic hormone (hCG) is correct?

    a. It is secreted by the cytotrophoblast of the placenta.

    b. It is regulated by the negative and positive feedback actions of estrogen.

    c. It stimulates FSH receptors in the ovary.

    d. It's secretion parallels that of human placental lactogen (hPL).

    e. It's secretion is stimulated by placental LH-RH.

12. Which of the following statements is *incorrect*? The midcycle surge of FSH:

    a. induces the mucification (i.e., an expansion of the hyaluronic acid matrix) of the granulosa cell cumulus surrounding the egg.

    b. increases the plasmin activity in the follicular fluid.

    c. stimulates the contraction of the Graafian follicle.

    d. requires a small preovulatory surge of progesterone.

    e. all the above.

13. Which of the following statements about growth hormone is correct?
    a. Its content in the pituitary increases with age.
    b. Like insulin and thyroid hormones, it can be obtained from slaughterhouse animals for human use.
    c. It is important in facilitating the closure of the epiphyses of the long bones.
    d. It stimulates the secretion of somatomedin from the kidney.
    e. It requires cortisol for its effect on growth.

14. The observed effects of administered glucagon would include:
    a. Hyperglycemia
    b. Glycogenolysis
    c. Lipolysis
    d. Insulin secretion
    e. All the above

15. A hypersecreting tumor of the zona glomerulosa of the adrenal cortex would most logically be associated with:
    a. Decreased secretion of ACTH
    b. Hypokalemia
    c. Marked muscle wasting
    d. Moon facies
    e. An increase in plasma renin activity

16. Hypophysectomy is known to ameliorate the effects of experimentally induced diabetes mellitus by:
    a. Inhibiting the metabolism of insulin
    b. Decreasing secretion of epinephrine
    c. Decreasing secretion of antidiuretic hormone
    d. Decreasing secretion of glucocorticoids
    e. Decreasing secretion of T_4 and T_3

17. Which of the following hormones have *metabolites that do not* have biologic activity equal to, or greater than, the parent compound?
    a. Angiotensin II
    b. Testosterone
    c. Tetraiodothyronine
    d. Aldosterone

18. Glucocorticoids are important physiologically in:
    a. Regulation of the concentration of sugar in blood by counteracting the effects of insulin
    b. The deposition of liver glycogen
    c. The release of amino acids from muscle proteins
    d. Suppressing antiinflammatory and immune responses
    e. All the above

19. Estrogen administration to adult males should be expected to lead to:
    a. Inhibition of spermatogenesis
    b. A decrease in plasma renin activity
    c. Stimulation of breast development
    d. Stimulation of prolactin secretion
    e. Increased production of thyroxine binding globulin

20. Which of the following hormones is usually *not* bound tightly to a carrier protein when circulating in situ?
    a. Aldosterone
    b. Cortisol
    c. Testosterone
    d. Thyroxine
    e. None of the above

B. TRUE-FALSE QUESTIONS

1. A significant proportion of the daily secretion of thyroid hormones is excreted into urine as thyroxine and triiodothyronine. (True/False)
2. Enterohepatic circulation refers to the blood flow to the liver, as affected by thyroid hormones. (True/False)
3. Activation of cellular processes by glucagon is mediated by the cAMP system. (True/False)
4. Thyroxine plays a role in the maintenance of the concentration of glucose in blood by facilitating the absorption of glucose from the gastrointestinal tract. (True/False)
5. Pituitary reserve for ACTH may be tested by administration of a pharmacologic inhibitor of the adrenal 11β-hydroxylase enzyme. (True/False)
6. A deficiency of parathyroid hormone is characterized by hyperphosphatemia (high concentration of phosphorus in the blood). (True/False)
7. The onset of menstruation occurs as a consequence of an acute fall in plasma gonadotropin concentration. (True/False)
8. Secretion of aldosterone can be stimulated by an increase in the concentration of potassium in blood. (True/False)
9. Hypophysectomy (removal of pituitary gland) is known to reduce the elevated concentration of sugar in blood of animals with diabetes mellitus. (True/False)
10. Bilateral adrenalectomy is accompanied by hyperkalemia (increased concentration of potassium in blood). (True/False)
11. Aldosterone controls sodium and potassium concentrations in secretions of salivary glands, sweat glands, colon, and kidneys. (True/False)
12. Cushing's syndrome (hyperadrenocorticism) can occur with a perfectly normal level of cortisol in plasma determined at 9 A.M. (True/False)
13. Failure of a patient to respond to an infusion of ACTH with an increase either in the concentration of cortisol in blood or in excretion of 17-hydroxysteroids into urine indicates primary adrenocortical insufficiency. (True/False)
14. Synthetic steroid hormones frequently are more effective orally than their natural counterparts because the synthetic analogues have a longer half-life. (True/False)
15. The first and rate-limiting enzymatic step in the metabolism of cortisol is A-ring reduction. (True/False)
16. Following removal of the pituitary gland, the responsiveness to a fixed dose of insulin is reduced. (True/False)
17. Hypophysectomized animals are unable to maintain a normal sodium balance when given a diet deficient in sodium (True/False)
18. Oral contraceptives are known to increase the renin substrate concentration in blood. (True/False)
19. Epinephrine increases blood sugar primarily through increased liver glycogenolysis. (True/False)
20. Hypersecretion of growth hormone in prepubertal humans results in gigantism with disproportionately long legs and short trunk. (True/False)
21. The basal level of heat production can be correlated directly with serum concentrations of thyroid hormones. (True/False)
22. Severe chronic vitamin D deficiency results in an inability to absorb calcium from the small intestine. (True/False)
23. Diabetic ketoacidosis can be compared to the starvation state because the pivotal disturbance is the reduced availability of glucose to cells. (True/False)
24. The number of β-adrenergic receptors for epinephrine (i.e., maximal binding capacity) in cardiac tissue decreases in response to exposure to triiodothyronine. (True/False)

25. A marked increase in skin pigmentation could logically be associated with an elevation in the concentration of ACTH in plasma. (True/False)
26. Insulin is degraded in the liver to C-peptides and proinsulin. (True/False)
27. The hyperthyroidism of Graves' disease is accompanied by an elevated concentration of thyroid stimulating hormone in plasma. (True/False)
28. Growth hormone acts directly on the long bones of prepubertal humans to close the epiphyses. (True/False)
29. In the female, the excretion of 17-ketosteroids into urine is a very good measure of adrenal androgen production. (True/False)
30. Secretion of growth hormone can be stimulated by an infusion of the amino acid arginine. (True/False)
31. Vitamin D_3, enhances bone resorption at *physiologic* doses. (True/False)
32. The deiodinating enzyme in thyroid follicular cells is important in the release of T_4 and T_3 into blood. (True/False)
33. β-Glucuronidase is an enzyme found in liver that is important in glycogenolysis. (True/False)
34. Present knowledge indicates that renin is secreted by the juxtaglomerular apparatus of the kidneys. (True/False)
35. The concentration of angiotensin II in blood is regulated by the concentration of aldosterone in blood. (True/False)
36. In the absence of a functional thyroid gland, the growth and mental development of an infant will be retarded. (True/False)
37. A patient in severe diabetic ketoacidosis will breathe at a reduced frequency. (True/False)
38. The adrenogenital syndrome is accompanied by elevated levels of cortisol in blood. (True/False)
39. Reverse T_3 is an abnormal form of thyroid hormone produced by the diseased thyroid gland. (True/False)
40. Newly released insulin from the pancreatic gland goes directly to the liver, where 50% of it is destroyed. (True/False)
41. The neurohypophysis receives a direct arterial input from the superior hypophyseal artery; whereas the adenohypophysis receives its direct arterial input from the middle and inferior hypophyseal arteries. (True/False)
42. Follicular atresia is thought to be due to the actions of androgens produced in the ovary in response to the stimulatory actions of FSH. (True/False)
43. cAMP appears to play an integral role in *both* FSH- and testosterone-stimulated androgen binding protein biosynthesis in the Sertoli cells. (True/False)
44. The number of cytoplasmic receptors for progesterone (i.e., maximal binding capacity) in the endometrium is estrogen dependent. (True/False)
45. The suckling-induced increase in the secretion of oxytocin from the neurohypophysis is preceded by an increase in the firing rate (i.e., action potential frequency) of magnocellular neurons found in the paraventricular nucleus of the hypothalamus. (True/False)
46. Mutations at the Tfm locus on the X chromosome typically produce an individual who fails to respond to androgens because the enzyme necessary for the conversion of testosterone to dihydrotestosterone is either absent or defective. (True/False)
47. Sleep is a primary physiologic stimulus for secretion of growth hormone in man. (True/False)
48. Whereas stress stimulates the release of corticotrophin releasing hormone, it typically inhibits the release of oxytocin. (True/False)
49. The oxytocin released during an acute stimulus (e.g., suckling) is not the oxytocin synthesized in response to that stimulus. (True/False)

50. Following the exocytotic release of ADH, the vesicular membrane is endocytosed back into the axon terminal, wherein it is reutilized for the packaging of more hormone. (True/False)

51. Secretion of progesterone from the corpus luteum is not required in the later stages of pregnancy because progestins are produced by the fetal adrenal. (True/False)

52. Chondrocyte hyperplasia is stimulated in vivo (i.e., in the whole animal), but not in vitro (i.e., in an isolated preparation removed from the animal and bathed in an artificial plasma), by growth hormone. (True/False)

53. Increases in both blood plasma osmotic pressure and blood volume can be expected to produce an additive increase in the release of vasopressin. (True/False)

54. The glucuronide conjugates of testosterone serve as a storage pool of this important androgen. (True/False)

55. The 5α-reduction of testosterone to dihydrotestosterone appears to be very important in testosterone-stimulated growth of the seminal vesicles and prostate. (True/False)

56. The efficacy of the negative feedback actions of testosterone on secretion of LH in human males is increased dramatically following long-term castration. (True/False)

57. De novo biosynthesis of C-18 estrogens from C-21 progestins requires the intermediate formation of C-19 androgens. (True/False)

58. Less than half the insulin activity in blood determined biologically exhibits insulinlike immunologic activity when determined by a radioimmunoassay. (True/False)

59. The insulin response to a glucose challenge in obese individuals is blunted relative to that observed in nonobese individuals. (True/False)

60. Administration of insulin to a nondiabetic individual at a dose sufficient to result in a large fall in the concentration of glucose in blood will stimulate an increase in the secretion of glucagon and epinephrine. (True/False)

C. NATIONAL BOARD FORMAT QUESTIONS

$$a = 1, 2, 3 \quad b = 1, 3 \quad c = 2, 4 \quad d = 4 \text{ only} \quad e = \text{all}$$

1. Which of the following statements *accurately characterize* one of the basic principles of radioimmunoassays?
   1. In general it is easier to develop antibodies against steroid hormones than against peptide hormones.
   2. In principle it should be possible to develop a radioimmunoassay to virtually any hormone that can be purified.
   3. One of the major advantages of radioimmunoassay over the bioassays is their general lack of cross-reactivity with biochemically similar hormones.
   4. Since it is possible to measure biologically inactive hormone with a radioimmunoassay, these assays may have limited usefulness in some pathologic situations.

2. Which of the following statements *accurately characterize* one of the basic principles of steroid catabolism?
   1. Ring A reduction usually is the rate-limiting step in the catabolism of estrogens.
   2. The 16α-hydroxylation pathway from estrone to estriol is now thought to be the major metabolic route for the catabolism of conjugated estrogens.

3. The methylating enzyme catechol-O-methyltransferase performs the rate-limiting step in the conversion of estrogens to catechol estrogens in the liver.
4. Glucoronic acid conjugation is not considered to be an important step in the catabolism of adrenal androgens.

3. Which of the following statements *accurately characterize* one of the basic principles of the genomic mechanism of steroid actions in mammalian tissues?
   1. The activation of a steroid-receptor complex usually is required before its interaction with its intranuclear acceptor molecules.
   2. Although we generally think of receptors as being specific for a given steroid, a given cell may have receptors for more than one steroid.
   3. Steroid-receptor interactions usually are not irreversible.
   4. The dissociation of the steroid from its receptor usually is required before translocation across the nuclear membrane.

4. Which of the following situations *should lead* to a *suppression* in the secretion of ACTH?
   1. Insulin-induced hypoglycemia
   2. Final exam stress
   3. Administration of metyrapone
   4. Administration of cortisol

5. Which of the indicated pharmacologic agents *could be used* to treat the hyperthyroidism associated with Graves' disease?
   1. Antagonists of receptors for TRH
   2. Inhibitors of the synthesis of T_4 and T_3
   3. Inhibitors of the secretion of TSH
   4. Inhibitors of the peripheral deiodination of T_4 and T_3

6. Which of the indicated biochemicals and/or physiologic conditions *is thought* to be involved in the regulation of the synthesis of thyroxine?
   1. TSH
   2. Availability of iodide ion
   3. Negative feedback of circulating T_4 and T_3 at the level of the adenohypophysis
   4. ACTH

7. Which of the following responses *is induced* by epinephrine?
   1. Increases in the concentration of glucose in blood
   2. Increases in the conversion of inactive to active phosphorylase in the liver
   3. Increases in the concentration of free fatty acids in plasma
   4. Increases in heart rate

8. Which of the following responses *is induced* by glucagon?
   1. Hyperglycemia
   2. Glycogenolysis
   3. Lipolysis
   4. Reduction in the secretion of insulin

9. Which of the following conditions *is characteristic* for a female patient with inadequate adrenal 11β-hydroxylase activity?
   1. Hypotensive and nonvirilized
   2. Hypertensive and nonvirilized
   3. Hypotensive and virilized
   4. Hypertensive and virilized

10. Which of the following statements *accurately describe* some facet of spermatogenesis in the *adult* human?
    1. The elevation of scrotal temperature to normal internal body temperature levels results in a reduction in spermatogenesis due to the inhibition of certain temperature-sensitive metabolic processes (e.g., protein synthesis).

a = 1, 2, 3   b = 1, 3   c = 2, 4   d = 4 only   e = all

2. Testosterone-receptor-acceptor interactions within the spermatid are required for the completion of the final stages of sperm maturation.
3. Contrary to many standard texts, FSH is facilitatory, but not absolutely required for the completion of spermatogenesis in the adult human male.
4. FSH exerts its facilitatory actions on the process of spermatogenesis through an increase in the production of *both* ABP and estradiol in the testis.

11. Which of the following statements *accurately describe* some facet of the endometrial cycle in the adult women?
    1. The amount of desquamation in a given region of the uterus during menstruation is roughly proportional to the extent of estrogen-progestin-induced elongation of the spiral arteries in that region.
    2. Although the rapid proliferation of the endometrial epithelium requires the actions of estrogen, the rapid increase in the production of mucus during the secretory phase of the cycle does not require the actions of estrogen.
    3. The reepithelization of the denuded endometrial mucosa actually begins before the completion of the previous menstrual discharge.
    4. The myometrium is *never* damaged during menstruation because it is protected by the presence of the basal layer of the endometrium, which of course contains the epithelial cells specialized for the regeneration of the functional layer of the endometrium.

12. Which of the following statements *accurately characterize* the biosynthesis of the principal adrenal, testicular, and ovarian steroid hormones?
    1. The tropic hormone (e.g., LH) acts at the step in the biosynthetic path at which pregnenolone is converted to progesterone.
    2. The tropic hormone (e.g., ACTH) facilitates the uptake of cholesterol by the synthetic cell (e.g., a zona fasciculata cell).
    3. A mutation in the gene controlling the production of the steroid metabolizing enzyme 3β-hydroxydehydrogenase would likely cause a serious medical problem, but it should not be fatal.
    4. The synthesis of cortisol requires the sequential activity of both mitochondrial and microsomal (i.e., smooth endoplasmic reticulum) enzymes.

13. Which of the following is a *correct example* of up- or down-regulation of receptors?
    1. FSH receptors on granulosa cells in response to LH during the follicular phase of the ovarian-menstrual cycle.
    2. Estradiol receptors in endometrial epithelial cells in response to progesterone during the luteal phase of the ovarian-menstrual cycle.
    3. LH receptors on corpus luteum cells in response to the continued exposure to LH during the luteal phase of the ovarian-menstrual cycle.
    4. ACTH receptors on zona reticularis cells of the fetal adrenal gland in response to prolactin from the fetal pituitary during the last days of gestation.

14. Which of the following hormones *does not* initiate its principal biologic action in the indicated target tissue or cell through *stimulating an increase* in the activity of the enzyme, adenylate cyclase?
    1. Insulin in striated muscle
    2. $1,25(OH)_2D_3$ in the small intestine
    3. Triiodothyronine in the thyrotropes of the adenohypophysis
    4. Aldosterone in the distal tubule of the kidney

15. Which of the following hormones *undergoes* metabolic *activation* in the indicated tissue or cell?
    1. Testosterone in the prostate

2. Estrone in the uterine endometrium
3. Vitamin D_3 in the liver
4. TRH in the thyrotropes of the adenohypophysis
16. Which of the following hormones *does not undergo* metabolic *activation* in the indicated tissue or cell?
    1. Tetraiodothyronine in the liver
    2. Testosterone in striated muscle
    3. Angiotensin I in lung tissue
    4. ACTH in the adrenal cortex
17. The concentration of which of the following hormones *increases* following an acute unexpected hemorrhage?
    1. Aldosterone
    2. Antidiuretic hormone
    3. Angiotensin II
    4. Prolactin
18. According to present knowledge, which of the following hormones is synthesized as a result of *posttranslational* modification of a precursor or prohormone?
    1. Insulin
    2. Prolactin
    3. Parathyroid hormone (PTH)
    4. ACTH
19. Which of the following hormones *is not* secreted via *exocytosis* following its synthesis?
    1. Angiotensin II
    2. Gn-RH
    3. Cortisol
    4. Growth hormone
20. Which of the following statements is *true* regarding the multihormonal regulation of the concentration of *glucose* in blood of the *nondiabetic* human?
    1. The administration of cortisol extends the duration of the increase in the concentration of glucose in blood following the administration of glucagon and epinephrine.
    2. The administration of a glucose load, as in a glucose tolerance test, increases the secretion of insulin, whereas an increase in the seretion of glucagon, epinephrine, and growth hormone often requires the development of frank hypoglycemia.
    3. The administration of cortisol leads to an increase in the *de novo* synthesis of certain transaminase enzymes in liver, which facilitate the conversion of amino acids to gluconeogenic substrates.
    4. The administration of somatostatin can temporarily reduce the "basal" concentrations of insulin, glucagon, and growth hormone.
21. The synthesis of estradiol and/or estrone is *increased* in which of the indicated tissues or cells after the administration of the following exogenous agents?
    1. Theca interna cells of the ovary after administration of LH
    2. Sertoli cells of the testis after administration of FSH
    3. Granulosa cells of the ovary after administration of dihydrotestosterone
    4. Placenta after the administration of prostaglandin $F_{2\alpha}$
22. When a pituitary gland is transplanted successfully from the sella turcica to the kidney capsule, which of the following endocrine conditions *is likely* to result *for the reasons indicated?*
    1. A marked increase in the secretion of growth hormone due to the loss of the tonic inhibition produced normally by somatostatin.

a = 1, 2, 3   b = 1, 3   c = 2, 4   d = 4 only   e = all

2. A marked reduction in spermatogenesis in an adult male due to the loss of the tropic actions of FSH on the Sertoli cells.

3. A marked increase in the secretion of prolactin due to the increased secretion of catechol estrone by the hypothalamus (and/or liver).

4. A marked increase in urination (polyuria) due to the decreased secretion of antidiuretic hormone.

23. Which of the following statements *accurately* describes an endocrine consequence of hypophysectomy *for the reasons indicated?*

1. Inability to maintain proper sodium balance due to the loss of appropriate stimulation for secretion of aldosterone.

2. A chronic suppression of the immune system due to the loss of appropriate stimulation for secretion of cortisol.

3. Inability to maintain proper concentrations of glucose in blood due to the loss of appropriate stimulation for secretion of insulin.

4. A chronic reduction in collagen biosynthesis in the epiphysial growth plates due to the loss of appropriate stimulation for secretion and action of somatomedin.

24. The synthesis of progesterone (as an intermediate and/or as a final secretory product) is *increased* in which of the situations listed below?

1. Zona reticularis of the adrenal cortex after administration of ACTH.

2. External layer of granulosa cells in the Graafian follicle after administration of LH.

3. Zona glomerulosa of the adrenal cortex after administration of angiotensin III.

4. Sertoli cells of the testis after administration of FSH.

25. Which of the following statements *accurately describes* some facet of the process of ovulation?

1. The rupture of the Graafian follicle requires the combination of several effects including the thinning of the follicular wall, the reduction in the strength of the intercellular adhesions in the follicular wall, and the contraction of the theca externa cells, which make up the external layer of the follicular wall.

2. The increase in intrafollicular pressure that precedes ovulation is due to the increased production of intrafollicular fluids (stimulated by the actions of estradiol on the theca interna cells) and to the increased production of the intercellular matrix separating the cumulus cells (stimulated by the increased production of LH immediately before ovulation).

3. An increase in the synthesis of progesterone and a decrease in the synthesis of estradiol usually occurs within the Graafian follicle before ovulation.

4. When the oocyte leaves the follicle (i.e., during ovulation) it already has completed the second division of meiosis and is now ready for fertilization by the haploid spermatozoa within the Fallopian tube.

26. A surprising number of hormones once thought to be synthesized exclusively in either nonneural or neural tissues are now thought to be produced by both these general classes of cell types. Which of the following statements *accurately describe* one of these examples?

1. Somatostatin is synthesized both in the hypothalamus and in the pancreas.

2. The decapeptide commonly known as Gn-RH or LH-RH is now known to be synthesized both in the hypothalamus and in the cytotrophoblast.

3. The biogenic amine hormone epinephrine is now known to be synthesized both in the brain and in the adrenal medulla.

4. The potent vasoconstrictor angiotensin II is now thought to be synthesized both in the brain and in the lung.

27. Which of the following statements *accurately describe* some feature of the hypo-thalamopituitary blood supply?
    1. The adenohypophysis receives direct arterial input from at least three arteries.
    2. The hypothalamohypophyseal vessels (*which are described accurately as veins*) can be used to transport hormones to the pituitary from the hyothalamus, and vice versa.
    3. There is little or no mixing of blood between the adenohypophysis and the neurohypophysis.
    4. The capillaries that supply the median eminence of the hypothalamus are somewhat unusual in that they apparently are not protected by the so-called blood-brain barrier, which of course is advantageous in the transport of peptide HHHs from the hypothalamic neurons to the adenohypophysis.
28. Which of the following generalities is *valid* for humans?
    1. Both sexes have the potential to display both negative and positive feedback regulation of the secretion of LH, when challenged under the appropriate endo-crine situation.
    2. Follicle stimulating hormone is essential for the completion of gametogenesis in both sexes during adulthood.
    3. An injection of TRH usually results in a larger increase in the secretion of prolactin in a woman than it does in a man.
    4. A mutation at the Tfm locus in the genome results in a loss of the 5α-reductase enzyme in the male only, because this gene is segregated to the Y chromosome.
29. Which of the following statements is *valid* regarding the synthesis and secretion of insulin in the human?
    1. Synthesis and secretion are increased during conditions of acute hyperglycemia.
    2. Synthesis occurs in the B-cells of the pancreas.
    3. Secretion may be inhibited by somatostatin and facilitated by growth hormone.
    4. The cleavage of proinsulin to insulin is thought to occur primarily in the liver.
30. Which of the following statements is *valid* regarding the synthesis, secretion, and/or catabolism of the catecholamines produced in the adrenal medulla?
    1. The synthesis of dopamine occurs primarily in the dense cored vesicles, whereas the synthesis of norepinephrine and epinephrine occurs primarily in the cytoplasm.
    2. The human adrenal secretes more epinephrine than norepinephrine.
    3. The secretion of adrenal medullary catecholamines is thought to be stimulated by the release of norepinephrine from the sympathetic preganglionic axons terminal.
    4. Along with norepinephrine and epinephrine, the adrenal medulla also releases the enzyme dopamine β-hydroxylase, as a direct consequence of the process of vesicular exocytosis.

ANSWERS TO COMPREHENSIVE POST-TEST

A. MULTIPLE CHOICE QUESTIONS

1. d	6. d	11. e	16. d
2. e	7. b	12. c	17. d
3. b	8. d	13. c	18. e
4. c	9. e	14. e	19. b
5. b	10. d	15. b	20. a

B. TRUE-FALSE QUESTIONS

1. False	16. False	31. False	46. False
2. False	17. False	32. False	47. True
3. True	18. True	33. False	48. True
4. True	19. True	34. False	49. True
5. True	20. False	35. False	50. False
6. True	21. True	36. True	51. False
7. False	22. True	37. False	52. True
8. True	23. True	38. False	53. False
9. True	24. False	39. False	54. False
10. True	25. True	40. True	55. True
11. True	26. False	41. False	56. False
12. True	27. False	42. False	57. True
13. True	28. False	43. False	58. False
14. True	29. True	44. True	59. False
15. True	30. True	45. True	60. True

C. NATIONAL BOARD FORMAT QUESTIONS

1. Correct answer = c (2, 4)
   1. Incorrect becasue it usually is easier to develop antibodies against peptides than it is against steroids.
   2. Correct.
   3. One of the major disadvantages of radioimmunoassays is the problem of cross-reactivity.
   4. Correct.

2. Correct answer = d (4 only)
   1. Incorrect because A-ring reduction generally is not involved in the catabolism of estrogens.
   2. Incorrect because the catechol estrogens are now considered to be part of the major route of estrogen catabolism in the liver (i.e., 2- and 4-hydroxylation pathways).
   3. Incorrect because COMT is a catabolic enzyme that methylates both catecholamines and the catechol estrogens.
   4. Correct because the sulfates are the principal conjugated forms of adrenal androgen catabolites (i.e., from androsterone and etiocholanolone).
3. Correct answer = a (1, 2, 3)
   1. Correct. Activation may involve a conformation change and/or an aggregation of the steroid-receptor complex with other macro- and small molecules.
   2. Correct (e.g., epithelial cells of the uterine endometrium).
   3. Correct, although the binding may have a very high affinity constant.
   4. Incorrect because the steroid-receptor complex diffuses through the nuclear pores without dissociating. The steroid-plasma protein carrier must dissociate before diffusion of the steroid across the plasma membrane of the cell.
4. Correct answer = d (4 only)
   1. Incorrect. The insulin-induced hypoglycemia may in fact lead to an increase in the secretion of ACTH because this condition may be stressful to the individual.
   2. Incorrect because stress (both physical and mental) can easily produce an increase in the secretion of ACTH.
   3. Incorrect because metyropone is an 11β-hydroxylase inhibitor. The consequent reduction in the synthesis of cortisol will lead to a reduction in the negative feedback suppression of the secretion of ACTH.
   4. Correct. The secretion of ACTH will be reduced by the negative feedback actions of cortisol in the adenohypophysis and hypothalamus.
5. Correct answer = c (2, 4)
   1. Incorrect because the problem in Graves' disease is an antibody that mimics the action of TSH in the thyroid. Thus an inhibtion of the actions of TRH will have no beneficial effect on the course of the disease.
   2. Correct because direct inhibition of the synthesis of thyroid hormones will of course block the actions of the TSH-like antibody.
   3. Incorrect for the same reasons as outlined in (1).
   4. Correct because in most cases T_3 appears to be the active form of thyroid hormone.
6. Correct answer = a (1, 2, 3)
   1. Correct. TSH stimulates the synthesis and release of thyroid hormones.
   2. Correct. Iodide deficiency can lead to a reduction in the synthesis of thyroid hormones, which in turn leads to a reduction in the negative feedback suppression of TSH. The resulting hypersecretion of TSH leads to an enlargement of the thyroid gland.
   3. Correct. It is now thought that one of the mechanisms whereby T_4 and T_3 suppress the secretion of TSH involves a reduction in the number of membrane-associated receptors for TRH (i.e., heterologous down-regulation) on the thyrotropes.
   4. Incorrect. ACTH is involved in the production of adrenocortical hormones.
7. Correct answer = e (all)
   1. Correct. Epinephrine produces an increase in glucogenolysis.
   2. Correct.
   3. Correct. Epinephrine produces an increase in lipolysis.
   4. Correct. β-adrenergic actions.

8. Correct answer = a (1, 2, 3)
   1. Correct. Glucagon increases glycogenolysis.
   2. Correct.
   3. Correct.
   4. Incorrect. The increase in the concentration of sugar in blood leads to an increase in the secretion of insulin.

9. Correct answer = d (4 only)
   1. Incorrect
   2. Incorrect.
   3. Incorrect.
   4. Correct. The reduction in 11β-hydroxylase activity (due to genetics, drugs, or other causes) leads to a decrease in the secretion of cortisol. This in turn produces an increase in the secretion of ACTH (due to the reduction in the negative feedback actions of cortisol) followed by increases in the production of adrenal androgens (thus virilization) and 11-deoxycorticosterone (11-DOC), which has considerable mineralocorticoid activity (thus hypertension).

10. Correct answer = b (1, 3)
    1. Correct.
    2. Incorrect. The haploid spermatid does not appear to possess the high-affinity mobile receptors for androgens necessary for the elicitation of the genomic mechanism of steroid action. Recall the experiments with the Tfm/+ X/+ chimeras (see Answer to Text Question 6-16).
    3. Correct. FSH is now thought to be obligatory in spermatogenesis only during the first wave of sperm production at puberty. Both testosterone and FSH can stimulate the production of ABP in adulthood, and only testosterone is required absolutely for the completion of spermatogenesis.
    4. Incorrect. Although FSH does stimulate an increase in the production of both ABP and estrogen in the Sertoli cells of the testis, the estrogen clearly is not facilitatory to spermatogenesis, since it can diffuse to the adjacent Leydig cells in which it can reduce the synthesis of testosterone.

11. Correct answer = b (1, 3)
    1. Correct
    2. Incorrect. Although the production of mucus is ascribed commonly to the actions of progesterone, estrogen is required for that action through its stimulation of the production of the intracellular receptors for progesterone.
    3. Correct. The reepithelization appears to begin within 36 hours after the onset of menstrual hemorrhaging and it is completed usually within 140 hours.
    4. Incorrect. The myometrium is involved occasionally in the desquamation, necrosis, and hemorrhaging of menstruation. This may only be in a few regions of the uterus, but it can happen. As described in Section 7-3, there is no such thing as a basal layer that contains endometrial epithelial cells specialized for the regeneration of the denuded endometrium. All the endometrial epithelial cells have the potential for hyperplasia and consequent regeneration of the mucosa.

12. Correct answer = d (4 only)
    1. Incorrect. LH acts at the step at which cholesterol is converted to pregnenolone.
    2. Incorrect. ACTH facilitates the release of cholesterol esters and the uptake of cholesterol by the mitochondria, but it does not facilitate the uptake of cholesterol by the zona fasciculata cells.
    3. Incorrect. This is a fatal mutation due to the loss of virtually all steroids.
    4. Correct.

13. Correct answer = b (1, 3)
    1. Correct. FSH stimulates an increase in the number and/or activity of LH receptors; whereas LH stimulates a decrease in the number and/or activity of FSH receptors.
    2. Incorrect. Estradiol stimulates an increase in the *de novo* synthesis of receptors for progesterone; whereas progesterone does not appear to have a facilitatory or inhibitory influence on the synthesis of receptors for estrogen.
    3. Correct. Normal desensitization of the corpus luteum to the actions of LH. This is thought to lead to a down-regulation of the receptors for LH unless the synthesis of hCG is stimulated following implantation of the fertilized blastocyst.
    4. Incorrect. Prolactin is thought to produce an increase in the number and/or activity of the receptors for ACTH in the fetal adrenal cortex.
14. Correct answer = e (all)
    1. Correct, although the mechanism of insulin action is still unclear.
    2. Correct. $1,25(OH)_2D_3$ exerts its actions via a genomic mechanism similar to that utilized for the adrenal and gonadal steroid hormones.
    3. Correct. T_3 interacts with intranuclear receptors to stimulate a genomic response.
    4. Correct. Aldosterone actions are believed to be mediated by the standard genomic mechanisms typical of most steroid hormone actions.
15. Correct answer = a (1, 2, 3)
    1. Correct. Testosterone is converted to dihydrotestosterone.
    2. Correct. Estrone is converted to estradiol.
    3. Correct. Vitamin D_3 is converted to $1,25(OH)_2D_3$.
    4. Incorrect. TRH may in fact be catabolized by membrane-associated peptidases.
16. Correct answer = c (2, 4)
    1. Incorrect. T_4 is converted to T_3.
    2. Correct. Testosterone, rather than dihydrotestosterone, is believed to be the active androgen in striated muscle.
    3. Incorrect. Angiotensin I is converted to angiotensin II.
    4. Correct. There is no evidence for the metabolic activation of ACTH in the adrenal.
17. Correct answer = e (all)
    1. Correct. Secretion of aldosterone should be increased as a result of the stimulatory actions of both angiotensin II (and III) and ACTH (secreted in response to the stress).
    2. Correct. Concentrations in blood of both ADH and nicotine-stimulated neurophysin are increased following hemorrhage. ADH (vasopressin) has vasoconstrictor activity in addition to its actions on the distal tubule of the kidney.
    3. Correct. The concentration of angiotensin II in blood increases because of the increase in secretion of renin from the JGA. Renin is of course required for the conversion of renin substrate to angiotensin I.
    4. Correct. The secretion of Prl is very susceptible to stress.
18. Correct answer = e (all)
    1. Correct. Proinsulin is converted into insulin.
    2. Correct. Preprolactin is converted into prolactin.
    3. Correct. Proparathyroid hormone is converted into parathyroid hormone.
    4. Correct. Opiocorticotropin is converted into ACTH and other peptides including the endorphins.
19. Correct answer = b (1, 3)
    1. Correct. Angiotensin II is synthesized in the blood from angiotensin I.

    2. Incorrect. Gn-RH is secreted via exocytosis from the parvicellular neurons of the hypothalamus.

    3. Correct. Cortisol is a steroid, hence it is not synthesized or stored in vesicles.

    4. Incorrect. Growth hormone is secreted via exocytosis from the somatotropes.

20. Correct answer = e (all)

    1. Correct. Cortisol appears to prevent the down-regulation of both glucagon and epinephrine.

    2. Correct.

    3. Correct.

    4. Correct.

21. Correct answer = c (2, 4)

    1. Incorrect. LH stimulates an increase in the synthesis of androgen by the theca interna cells, but the synthesis of estrogen occurs in the granulosa cells.

    2. Correct. FSH stimulates the aromatization of testosterones to estradiol in the Sertoli cells.

    3. Incorrect. Dihydrotestosterone acts to inhibit FSH-stimulated aromatization.

    4. Correct. The action of prostaglandin $F_{2\alpha}$ in the placenta shortly before parturition leads to a reduction in the secretion of progesteron and an increase in the secretion of estradiol.

22. Correct answer = d (4 only)

    1. Incorrect. The secretion of growth hormone would be reduced dramatically, but not because of the loss of the effects of somatostatin.

    2. Incorrect. Spermatogenesis would be reduced dramatically, but because of the loss of LH-stimulated testosterone production, not FSH-stimulated ABP production, which can also be maintained by testosterone.

    3. Incorrect. The secretion of prolactin would be increased dramatically, but not because of the increased actions of catechol estrone, which acts to suppress the secretion of prolactin.

    4. Correct.

23. Correct answer = d (4 only)

    1. Incorrect. The secretion of aldosterone is not reduced to any major extent by the loss of ACTH from the adenohypophysis.

    2. Incorrect. Glucocorticoids act to suppress the immune system; thus a reduction in their synthesis and secretion following the loss of ACTH would not be expected to produce a chronic suppression of the immune system.

    3. Incorrect. The secretion of insulin is thought to be stimulated by the actions of glucose directly in the pancreas.

    4. Correct. Growth hormone would of course be lost; hence the secretion of the somatomedins should be depressed severely.

24. Correct answer = a (1, 2, 3)

    1. Correct. The synthesis of progesterone is increased as a consequence of the increased synthesis of cortisol (i.e., progesterone is an intermediate in the biosynthesis of cortisol).

    2. Correct. The secretion of progesterone is stimulated directly by the actions of LH.

    3. Correct. Angiotensin III stimulates an increase in the synthesis of aldosterone, which of course leads to an increase in the production of its intermediate, progesterone.

    4. Incorrect. FSH stimulates an increase in the aromatization of preexisting testosterone in the Sertoli cells.

25. Correct answer = b (1, 3)

1. Correct.
2. Incorrect. There is no increase in intrafollicular pressure. FSH, not LH, stimulates the production of the intercellular matrix between the cumulous (granulosa) cells.
3. Correct.
4. Incorrect. Fertilization is required for the completion of the second meiotic division, and this in turn requires the estrogen-stimulated maturation of the ovum through the direct actions of this steroid in the attached cumulous cells.

26. Correct answer = e (all)
    1. Correct.
    2. Correct.
    3. Correct.
    4. Correct.

27. Correct answer = d (4 only)
    1. Incorrect. The arterial supply to the adenohypophysis is always indirect. The superior, middle, and inferior hypophyseal arteries supply blood to the adenohypophysis, but only after the blood has passed through a capillary network.
    2. Incorrect. The portal vessels are not veins, they are capillaries.
    3. Incorrect.
    4. Correct.

28. Correct answer = b (1, 3)
    1. Correct. In gonadectomized male and female humans it is possible to produce a midcycle-like increase in the secretion of LH if the appropriate estrogen treatment is administered.
    2. Incorrect. FSH is essential for spermatogenesis only during the first wave of sperm production during puberty.
    3. Correct. Presumably because of the increased production of Prl in the lactotrope due to the presence of estrogens.
    4. Incorrect. The Tfm locus is responsible for the production of the androgen receptor and not the 5α-reductase enzyme. Furthermore, the Tfm locus is found in the X chromosome and not in the Y chromosome.

29. Correct answer = a (1, 2, 3)
    1. Correct.
    2. Correct.
    3. Correct.
    4. Incorrect. Proinsulin cleavage to form insulin occurs primarily in the pancreas.

30. Correct answer = c (2, 4)
    1. Incorrect. The synthesis of DA occurs primarily in the cytoplasm, whereas the synthesis of NE occurs in the vesicles, and the synthesis of E occurs in the cytoplasm.
    2. Correct.
    3. Incorrect. Acetylcholine is the transmitter utilized by the preganglionic neurons.
    4. Correct.

INDEX

ILLUSTRATION AND TABLE CREDITS

We would like to thank the authors and publishers listed below for granting permission to reproduce previously published illustrations and tables. These acknowledgments are listed by chapter.

CHAPTER 1

Martin, J. B., Reichlin, S., and Brown, G. M., 1977, *Clinical Neuroendocrinology*, Philadelphia: F. A. Davis Co., p. 30, Fig. 13.

CHAPTER 2

Bergland, R. M., and Page, R. B., 1979, "Pituitary-Brain Vascular Relations: A New Paradigm," in *Science* 204: 18–24, Figs. 1, 2, 11, 12, and 13.

Clattenburg, R. E., 1974, *Can. J. Neurol. Sci.* 1:41, Fig. 1.

Cross, B. A., Dyball, R. E. J., Dyer, R. G., Jones, D. W., Lincoln, J. F., Morris, J. F., and Pickering, B. T., 1975, *Recent Progr. Horm. Res.* 31: 243, Figs. 9 and 18.

Douglas, W. W., 1974, *Handbook of Physiology*, Sect. 7: Endocrinology, 4: 1, R. O. Greep, and W. H. Sawyer (Eds.), Baltimore: Williams and Wilkins, p. 211, Fig. 30.

Ezrin, C. et al., 1979, *Systematic Endocrinology*, 2nd ed., New York: Harper and Row, p. 46.

Junqueira, L. C., and Carneiro, J., 1980, *Basic Histology*, 3rd ed., Los Altos: Lange Medical Publications, p. 416, Fig. 21–7.

Kendall, J. W., Jacobs, J. J., and Kramer, R. M., 1972, *Brain-Endocrine Interactions*, K. M. Knigge, D. E. Scott, and A. Weindl (Eds.), New York: S. Karger, p. 343, Fig. 1.

Rasmussen, Andrew T., 1973, *The Principal Nervous Pathways*, 3rd ed. (Copyright 1945, MacMillan Publishing Co., Inc., renewed 1973, Theodore B. Rasmussen and Charlotte Roberts).

Turner, C. Donnell, and Bagnara, Joseph T., 1976, *General Endocrinology*, 6th ed. (Copyright 1976 by W. B. Saunders Company. Copyright 1948, 1955, 1960, 1966, and 1971 by W. B. Saunders Company. Reprinted by permission of Holt, Rinehart and Winston).

Villee, Claude A., Walker, Warren F., Jr., and Barnes, Robert D., 1978, *General Zoology*, 5th ed. (Copyright 1978 by W. B. Saunders Company. Copyright 1958, 1963, 1968, and 1973 by W. B. Saunders Company. Reprinted by permission of Holt, Rinehart and Winston).

Zimmerman, E. A., and Antunes, J. A., 1976, *J. Histochem. and Cytochem.* 24: 807, Fig. 1.

CHAPTER 3

Edelman, I. S., 1974, *New Engl. J. Med.* 290: 1303.

CHAPTER 4

Koelle G. B., 1970, *Pharmacological Basis of Therapeutics*, L. S. Goodman (Ed.), New York: MacMillan, p. 427, Fig. 21.7.

CHAPTER 5

Bethune, J. E., 1975, *The Adrenal Cortex*, The Upjohn Co., p. 23, Fig. 30; p. 24, Fig. 31; p. 25, Fig. 32; p. 36, Fig. 42.

Catt, K. J., 1970, *The Lancet* 1: 1275.

Davis, J. O., 1971, *Circ. Res.* 28: 301, Fig. 1. (Reprinted by permission of the American Heart Association.)

Ham, A. W., and Cormack, D. H., 1979, *Histology*, 8th ed., Philadelphia: J. B. Lippincott Co., p. 814, Fig. 25–29.

Laragh, J. H., Baer, L., Brunner, H. R., Buhler, F. R., Sealey, J. E., and Vaughan, E. D., Jr., *Hypertension Manual*, J. H. Laragh (Ed.), New York: Yorke Medical Books, Technical Publishing, a Division of Dun-Donnelley Publishing Corporation, a Company of Dun & Bradstreet Corporation, p. 320, Fig. 2.

Liddle, G. W., 1965, *Physiol. Physicians* 3: 7.

Sambhi, M. P., 1973, *Ann. Inter. Med.* 79: 411, Figs. 13 and 14.

CHAPTER 6

Barry, J., 1977, *Cell Tissue Res.* 181: 1, Fig. 10.

Bloom, W., and Fawcett, D. W., 1975, *A Textbook of Histology*, 10th ed., Philadelphia: W. B. Saunders, Co., p. 839, Fig. 32–37.

Cooke, B. A., van der Molen, H. J., and Setchell, B. P., 1973, *Res. Reprod.* 5: 6, The International Planned Parenthood Federation, Fig. 5.

Farquhar, M. G., 1971, *Mem. Soc. Endocrinol.* 19: 79, Fig. 16.

Ham, A. W., and Cormack, D. H., 1979, *Histology*, 8th ed., Philadelphia: J. B. Lippincott Co., p. 875, Fig. 27-1.

Junqueira, L. C., and Carneiro, J., 1980, *Basic Histology*, 3rd ed., Los Altos: Lange Medical Publications, p. 446, Fig. 23-3.

Luttge, W. G., Hall, N. R., and Wallis, C. J., 1975, in *Sexual Behavior—Pharmacology and Biochemistry*, M. Sandler and G. L. Gessa (Eds.), New York: Raven Press, pp. 341–363.

Means, A. R., Fakunding, J. L. Huckins, C., Tindall, D. J., and Vitale, R., 1976, *Recent Progr. Horm. Res.* 32: 477: Fig. 23.

Plant, T. M., Hess, D. L., Hotchkiss, J., and Knovil, E., 1978, *Endocrinology* 103: 535, Figs. 2, 6, and 7.

Setchell, B. P., Davies, R. V., and Main, S. J., 1977, in *The Testis*, Vol. 4, A. D. Johnson, and W. R. Gomes (Eds.), New York: Academic Press, p. 93, Fig. 1.

Waites, G. N. H., 1970, in *The Testis*, Vol. 4, A. D. Johnson, and W. R. Gomes (Eds.), New York: Academic Press, p. 191, Fig. 1.

Weitzman, E., Boyer, R., Kapen, S., and Hellman, L., 1975, *Recent Progr. Horm. Res.* 31: 399, Fig. 19.

CHAPTER 7

Dickinson, R. L., 1933, *Human Sex Anatomy*, Baltimore: Williams and Wilkins, p. 43.

Ferin, M., 1979, *J. Steroid Biochem.* 11: 1015, Fig. 3.

Gorbman, A., and Bern, H. A., 1962, *A Textbook of Comparative Endocrinology*, New York: John Wiley & Sons, Inc., p. 253.

Groom, G. V., 1977, *J. Reprod. Fert.* 51: 273, Fig. 3.

Ham, A. W., and Cormack, D. H., 1979, *Histology*, 8th ed., Philadelphia: J. B. Lippincott Co., p. 846, Fig. 26-12 and p. 856, Fig. 26-33.

Hoff, J. D., Lasley, B. K., Wang, C. F., and Yen, S. S. C., 1977, *J. Clin. Endocrinol. Metab.* 44: 302, Figs. 3 and 4.

Hwang, P., Guyda, H., and Friesen, H., 1971, *Proc. Nat. Acad. Sci. (U.S.A.)* 68: 1902, Fig. 3.

Jacobs, L. S., Snyder, P. J., Utiger, R. D., and Daughaday, W. H., 1973, *J. Clin. Endocrinol. Metab.* 36: 1069, Fig. 4.

Jensen, D., 1980, *The Principles of Physiology*, 2nd ed., New York: Appleton-Century-Crofts; p. 974, Fig. 67-3 and p. 978, Fig. 67-6.

Knobil, E., 1974, *Recent Progr. Hor. Res.* 30: 1, Fig. 12.

Laborde, N., Carril, M., Cheviakoff, S., Croxatto, H. D., Pedroza, E., and Rosner, J. M., 1976, *J. Clin. Endocrinol. Metab.* 43: 1157, Fig. 3.

Lachelin, G. C. L., Leblanc, H., and Yen, S. S. C., 1977, *J. Clin. Endocrinol. Metab.* 44: 728, Fig. 1.

Liggins, G. C., Fairclough, R. J., Grieves, S. A., Kendall, J. Z., and Knox, B. S., 1973, *Recent Progr. Horm. Res.* 29: 111, Fig. 19.

Luttge, W. G., 1979, in *Endocrine Control of Sexual Behavior,* C. Beyer (Ed.), New York: Raven Press, pp. 341–363.

Miyake, A., Kawamura, Y., Aono, T., and Kurachi, K., 1980, *Acta Endocrinologica* 93: 257, Fig. 5.

Nakai, Y., Plant, T. M., Hess, D. L., Keogh, E. J., and Knobil, E., 1978, *Endocrinology,* 102: 1008, Fig. 5.

Noel, G. L., Suh, H. N., and Frantz, A. G., 1974, *J. Clin. Endocrinol. Metab.* 36: 1255, Fig. 1; and 38: 413, Fig. 1.

Sassin, J. F., 1972, "Human Prolactin: 24-Hour Pattern with Increases Release during Sleep," in *Science* 177: 1205–1207, Fig. 2.

Warwick, R., and Williams, P. L., 1973, *Gray's Anatomy,* 35th British Edition, Edinburgh: Churchill Livingstone, p. 1351, Fig. 8.176 and p. 1365, Fig. 8.191.

Weitzman, E., Boyer, R., Kapen, S., and Hellman, L., 1975, *Recent Progr. Horm. Res.* 31: 399, Fig. 18.

Yen, S. S. C., 1977, *J. Reprod. Fert.* 51: 181, Fig. 1.

CHAPTER 8

Cochinov, R. H., and Daughaday, W. H., 1976, *Diabetes* 25: 994, Fig. 2.

Friesen, H. G., 1977, *Clinical Endocrinology: A Survey of Current Practice,* C. Ezrin, J. O. Godden, and P. G. Walfish (Eds.), New York: Appleton-Century-Crofts, p. 60.

Gerich, J. E., 1976, *Metabolism* 25: 1505, Fig. 1.

Luft, R., Efendic, S., and Hokfelt, T., 1978, *Diabetologia* 14:1, Figs. 6 and 7.

Merimee, T. J., and Rabin, D., 1973, *Metabolism* 22: 1235, Fig. 1.

Takahashi, Y., Kipnis, D. M., and Daughaday, W. H., 1968, *J. Clin. Investigation* 47: 2079, Fig. 2.

Tannenbaum, G. S., and Martin, J. B., 1976, *Endocrinology* 98: 562, Fig. 2.

Van Wyk, J. J., and Underwood, L. E., 1978, *Hospital Practice* 13 (8): 57, 64, and 66.

Zhand, G. R., Steinke, J., and Renold, A. E., 1960, *Proc. Soc. Exp. Biol. Med.* 105: 455–459.

CHAPTER 9

Cahill, G. F., Jr., 1977, in *Clinical Endocrinology: A Survey of Current Practice,* C. Ezrin, J. O. Godden, and P. G. Walfish (Eds.), New York: Appleton-Century-Crofts: p. 18, Fig. 4 and p. 19, Fig. 2.

Perley, M., and Kipnis, D. M., 1966, *Diabetes* 15: 867, Fig. 2.

Unger, R. H., 1974, in *Endocrine Physiology,* Vol. 5, S. M. McCann (Ed.), Baltimore: University Park Press, p. 197, Fig. 6.20.

Woods, S. C., and Porte, D., Jr., 1978, *Advan. Metab. Disord.* 9: 289, Fig. 1.

CHAPTER 10

Arnaud, C. D., 1978, *Fed. Proc.* 37: 2557, Fig. 1.

De Luca, H. F., 1976, *Ann. Inter. Med.* 5: 367, Fig. 2.